Material-Tissue Interfacial Phenomena

Related titles

Pre-prosthetic and Maxillofacial Surgery

(ISBN 978-1-84569-589-7)

Bioactive Glasses

(ISBN 978-1-84569-768-6)

Bone Substitute Biomaterials

(ISBN 978-0-85709-497-1)

Cellular Response to Biomaterials
(ISBN 978-1-84569-547-7)

Woodhead Publishing Series in Biomaterials:
Number 124

Material-Tissue Interfacial Phenomena

Contributions from Dental and Craniofacial Reconstructions

Edited by

Paulette Spencer

and

Anil Misra

ELSEVIER

AMSTERDAM • BOSTON • CAMBRIDGE • HEIDELBERG
LONDON • NEW YORK • OXFORD • PARIS • SAN DIEGO
SAN FRANCISCO • SINGAPORE • SYDNEY • TOKYO
Woodhead Publishing is an imprint of Elsevier

WP
WOODHEAD
PUBLISHING

Woodhead Publishing is an imprint of Elsevier
The Officers' Mess Business Centre, Royston Road, Duxford, CB22 4QH, United Kingdom
50 Hampshire Street, 5th Floor, Cambridge, MA 02139, United States
The Boulevard, Langford Lane, Kidlington, OX5 1GB, United Kingdom

Notices
Knowledge and best practice in this field are constantly changing. As new research and experience broaden our understanding, changes in research methods, professional practices, or medical treatment may become necessary.

Practitioners and researchers must always rely on their own experience and knowledge in evaluating and using any information, methods, compounds, or experiments described herein. In using such information or methods they should be mindful of their own safety and the safety of others, including parties for whom they have a professional responsibility.

To the fullest extent of the law, neither the Publisher nor the authors, contributors, or editors, assume any liability for any injury and/or damage to persons or property as a matter of products liability, negligence or otherwise, or from any use or operation of any methods, products, instructions, or ideas contained in the material herein.

Library of Congress Cataloging-in-Publication Data
A catalog record for this book is available from the Library of Congress

British Library Cataloguing-in-Publication Data
A catalogue record for this book is available from the British Library

ISBN: 978-0-08-100330-5 (print)
ISBN: 978-0-08-100341-1 (online)

Publisher: Matthew Deans
Acquisition Editor: Laura Overend
Editorial Project Manager: Lucy Beg
Production Project Manager: Poulouse Joseph
Designer: Greg Harris

Typeset by TNQ Books and Journals

Contents

List of contributors

B.S. Bohaty University of Missouri-Kansas City, Kansas City, MO, United States

E. Bresciani São Paulo State University, São José dos Campos, São Paulo, Brazil

H. Chai Tel Aviv University, Tel Aviv, Israel

L. Cheng University of Maryland, Baltimore, MD, United States; Sichuan University, Chengdu, China

A. Chughtai New York University College of Dentistry, New York, NY, United States

J.L. Ferracane Oregon Health & Science University, Portland, OR, United States

F. Garcia-Godoy University of Tennessee Health Science Center, Memphis, TN, United States

S.E.P. Gonçalves São Paulo State University, São José dos Campos, São Paulo, Brazil

G.T.-J. Huang University of Tennessee Health Science Center, Memphis, TN, United States

C.Y. Koga Ito Universidade Estadual Paulista (UNESP), São Paulo, Brazil

F. Li Fourth Military Medical University, Xian, China; University of Maryland, Baltimore, MD, United States

G.M.G. Lima Universidade Estadual Paulista (UNESP), São Paulo, Brazil

U. Lohbauer Universitätsklinikum Erlangen, Friedrich-Alexander Universität Erlangen-Nürnberg, Erlangen, Germany

O. Marangos Cyprus University of Technology, Limassol, Cyprus

A. Misra University of Kansas, Lawrence, KS, United States

W.M. Palin University of Birmingham, Birmingham, United Kingdom

R. Parthasarathy Tennessee State University, Nashville, TN, United States

J.H. Purk University of Missouri-Kansas City, Kansas City, MO, United States

F. Sene State University of Londrina, Londrina, Brazil

V. Singh University of Kansas, Lawrence, KS, United States

P. Spencer University of Kansas, Lawrence, KS, United States

C. Tamerler University of Kansas, Lawrence, KS, United States

M.H. Tanaka Universidade Estadual Paulista (UNESP), São Paulo, Brazil

R. Trushkowsky New York University College of Dentistry, New York, NY, United States

F.S. Utku Yeditepe University, Istanbul, Turkey

M.D. Weir University of Maryland, Baltimore, MD, United States

M.S. Wolff New York University College of Dentistry, New York, NY, United States

H.H.K. Xu University of Maryland, Baltimore, MD, United States

Q. Ye University of Kansas, Lawrence, KS, United States

E. Yuca University of Kansas, Lawrence, KS, United States; Yildiz Technical University, Istanbul, Turkey

K. Zhang University of Maryland, Baltimore, MD, United States; Capital Medical University, Beijing, China

L. Zhang Fourth Military Medical University, Xian, China; University of Maryland, Baltimore, MD, United States

Y. Zhang New York University College of Dentistry, New York, NY, United States

Woodhead Publishing Series in Biomaterials

1 **Sterilisation of tissues using ionising radiations**
Edited by J. F. Kennedy, G. O. Phillips and P. A. Williams
2 **Surfaces and interfaces for biomaterials**
Edited by P. Vadgama
3 **Molecular interfacial phenomena of polymers and biopolymers**
Edited by C. Chen
4 **Biomaterials, artificial organs and tissue engineering**
Edited by L. Hench and J. Jones
5 **Medical modelling**
R. Bibb
6 **Artificial cells, cell engineering and therapy**
Edited by S. Prakash
7 **Biomedical polymers**
Edited by M. Jenkins
8 **Tissue engineering using ceramics and polymers**
Edited by A. R. Boccaccini and J. Gough
9 **Bioceramics and their clinical applications**
Edited by T. Kokubo
10 **Dental biomaterials**
Edited by R. V. Curtis and T. F. Watson
11 **Joint replacement technology**
Edited by P. A. Revell
12 **Natural-based polymers for biomedical applications**
Edited by R. L. Reiss et al
13 **Degradation rate of bioresorbable materials**
Edited by F. J. Buchanan
14 **Orthopaedic bone cements**
Edited by S. Deb
15 **Shape memory alloys for biomedical applications**
Edited by T. Yoneyama and S. Miyazaki
16 **Cellular response to biomaterials**
Edited by L. Di Silvio
17 **Biomaterials for treating skin loss**
Edited by D. P. Orgill and C. Blanco
18 **Biomaterials and tissue engineering in urology**
Edited by J. Denstedt and A. Atala

19 **Materials science for dentistry**
B. W. Darvell
20 **Bone repair biomaterials**
Edited by J. A. Planell, S. M. Best, D. Lacroix and A. Merolli
21 **Biomedical composites**
Edited by L. Ambrosio
22 **Drug–device combination products**
Edited by A. Lewis
23 **Biomaterials and regenerative medicine in ophthalmology**
Edited by T. V. Chirila
24 **Regenerative medicine and biomaterials for the repair of connective tissues**
Edited by C. Archer and J. Ralphs
25 **Metals for biomedical devices**
Edited by M. Niinomi
26 **Biointegration of medical implant materials: Science and design**
Edited by C. P. Sharma
27 **Biomaterials and devices for the circulatory system**
Edited by T. Gourlay and R. Black
28 **Surface modification of biomaterials: Methods analysis and applications**
Edited by R. Williams
29 **Biomaterials for artificial organs**
Edited by M. Lysaght and T. Webster
30 **Injectable biomaterials: Science and applications**
Edited by B. Vernon
31 **Biomedical hydrogels: Biochemistry, manufacture and medical applications**
Edited by S. Rimmer
32 **Preprosthetic and maxillofacial surgery: Biomaterials, bone grafting and tissue engineering**
Edited by J. Ferri and E. Hunziker
33 **Bioactive materials in medicine: Design and applications**
Edited by X. Zhao, J. M. Courtney and H. Qian
34 **Advanced wound repair therapies**
Edited by D. Farrar
35 **Electrospinning for tissue regeneration**
Edited by L. Bosworth and S. Downes
36 **Bioactive glasses: Materials, properties and applications**
Edited by H. O. Ylänen
37 **Coatings for biomedical applications**
Edited by M. Driver
38 **Progenitor and stem cell technologies and therapies**
Edited by A. Atala
39 **Biomaterials for spinal surgery**
Edited by L. Ambrosio and E. Tanner
40 **Minimized cardiopulmonary bypass techniques and technologies**
Edited by T. Gourlay and S. Gunaydin
41 **Wear of orthopaedic implants and artificial joints**
Edited by S. Affatato
42 **Biomaterials in plastic surgery: Breast implants**
Edited by W. Peters, H. Brandon, K. L. Jerina, C. Wolf and V. L. Young

43 **MEMS for biomedical applications**
Edited by S. Bhansali and A. Vasudev
44 **Durability and reliability of medical polymers**
Edited by M. Jenkins and A. Stamboulis
45 **Biosensors for medical applications**
Edited by S. Higson
46 **Sterilisation of biomaterials and medical devices**
Edited by S. Lerouge and A. Simmons
47 **The hip resurfacing handbook: A practical guide to the use and management of modern hip resurfacings**
Edited by K. De Smet, P. Campbell and C. Van Der Straeten
48 **Developments in tissue engineered and regenerative medicine products**
J. Basu and J. W. Ludlow
49 **Nanomedicine: Technologies and applications**
Edited by T. J. Webster
50 **Biocompatibility and performance of medical devices**
Edited by J.-P. Boutrand
51 **Medical robotics: Minimally invasive surgery**
Edited by P. Gomes
52 **Implantable sensor systems for medical applications**
Edited by A. Inmann and D. Hodgins
53 **Non-metallic biomaterials for tooth repair and replacement**
Edited by P. Vallittu
54 **Joining and assembly of medical materials and devices**
Edited by Y. (Norman) Zhou and M. D. Breyen
55 **Diamond-based materials for biomedical applications**
Edited by R. Narayan
56 **Nanomaterials in tissue engineering: Fabrication and applications**
Edited by A. K. Gaharwar, S. Sant, M. J. Hancock and S. A. Hacking
57 **Biomimetic biomaterials: Structure and applications**
Edited by A. J. Ruys
58 **Standardisation in cell and tissue engineering: Methods and protocols**
Edited by V. Salih
59 **Inhaler devices: Fundamentals, design and drug delivery**
Edited by P. Prokopovich
60 **Bio-tribocorrosion in biomaterials and medical implants**
Edited by Y. Yan
61 **Microfluidic devices for biomedical applications**
Edited by X.-J. James Li and Y. Zhou
62 **Decontamination in hospitals and healthcare**
Edited by J. T. Walker
63 **Biomedical imaging: Applications and advances**
Edited by P. Morris
64 **Characterization of biomaterials**
Edited by M. Jaffe, W. Hammond, P. Tolias and T. Arinzeh
65 **Biomaterials and medical tribology**
Edited by J. Paolo Davim
66 **Biomaterials for cancer therapeutics: Diagnosis, prevention and therapy**
Edited by K. Park

67 **New functional biomaterials for medicine and healthcare**
E. P. Ivanova, K. Bazaka and R. J. Crawford
68 **Porous silicon for biomedical applications**
Edited by H. A. Santos
69 **A practical approach to spinal trauma**
Edited by H. N. Bajaj and S. Katoch
70 **Rapid prototyping of biomaterials: Principles and applications**
Edited by R. Narayan
71 **Cardiac regeneration and repair Volume 1: Pathology and therapies**
Edited by R.-K. Li and R. D. Weisel
72 **Cardiac regeneration and repair Volume 2: Biomaterials and tissue engineering**
Edited by R.-K. Li and R. D. Weisel
73 **Semiconducting silicon nanowires for biomedical applications**
Edited by J. L. Coffer
74 **Silk biomaterials for tissue engineering and regenerative medicine**
Edited by S. Kundu
75 **Biomaterials for bone regeneration: Novel techniques and applications**
Edited by P. Dubruel and S. Van Vlierberghe
76 **Biomedical foams for tissue engineering applications**
Edited by P. Netti
77 **Precious metals for biomedical applications**
Edited by N. Baltzer and T. Copponnex
78 **Bone substitute biomaterials**
Edited by K. Mallick
79 **Regulatory affairs for biomaterials and medical devices**
Edited by S. F. Amato and R. Ezzell
80 **Joint replacement technology Second edition**
Edited by P. A. Revell
81 **Computational modelling of biomechanics and biotribology in the musculoskeletal system: Biomaterials and tissues**
Edited by Z. Jin
82 **Biophotonics for medical applications**
Edited by I. Meglinski
83 **Modelling degradation of bioresorbable polymeric medical devices**
Edited by J. Pan
84 **Perspectives in total hip arthroplasty: Advances in biomaterials and their tribological interactions**
S. Affatato
85 **Tissue engineering using ceramics and polymers Second edition**
Edited by A. R. Boccaccini and P. X. Ma
86 **Biomaterials and medical-device associated infections**
Edited by L. Barnes and I. R. Cooper
87 **Surgical techniques in total knee arthroplasty (TKA) and alternative procedures**
Edited by S. Affatato
88 **Lanthanide oxide nanoparticles for molecular imaging and therapeutics**
G. H. Lee
89 **Surface modification of magnesium and its alloys for biomedical applications Volume 1: Biological interactions, mechanical properties and testing**
Edited by T. S. N. Sankara Narayanan, I. S. Park and M. H. Lee

90 **Surface modification of magnesium and its alloys for biomedical applications Volume 2: Modification and coating techniques**
Edited by T. S. N. Sankara Narayanan, I. S. Park and M. H. Lee
91 **Medical modelling: The application of advanced design and rapid prototyping techniques in medicine Second Edition**
Edited by R. Bibb, D. Eggbeer and A. Paterson
92 **Switchable and responsive surfaces and materials for biomedical applications**
Edited by Z. Zhang
93 **Biomedical textiles for orthopaedic and surgical applications: Fundamentals, applications and tissue engineering**
Edited by T. Blair
94 **Surface coating and modification of metallic biomaterials**
Edited by C. Wen
95 **Hydroxyapatite (HAP) for biomedical applications**
Edited by M. Mucalo
96 **Implantable neuroprostheses for restoring function**
Edited by K. Kilgore
97 **Shape memory polymers for biomedical applications**
Edited by L. Yahia
98 **Regenerative engineering of musculoskeletal tissues and interfaces**
Edited by S. P. Nukavarapu, J. W. Freeman and C. T. Laurencin
99 **Advanced cardiac imaging**
Edited by K. Nieman, O. Gaemperli, P. Lancellotti and S. Plein
100 **Functional marine biomaterials: Properties and applications**
Edited by S. K. Kim
101 **Shoulder and elbow trauma and its complications: Volume 1: The shoulder**
Edited by R. M. Greiwe
102 **Nanotechnology-enhanced orthopedic materials: Fabrications, applications and future trends**
Edited by L. Yang
103 **Medical devices: Regulations, standards and practices**
Edited by S. Ramakrishna, L. Tian, C. Wang, S. L. and T. Wee Eong
104 **Biomineralisation and biomaterials: Fundamentals and applications**
Edited by C. Aparicio and M. Ginebra
105 **Shoulder and elbow trauma and its complications: Volume 2: The elbow**
Edited by R. M. Greiwe
106 **Characterisation and design of tissue scaffolds**
Edited by P. Tomlins
107 **Biosynthetic polymers for medical applications**
Edited by L. Poole-Warren, P. Martens and R. Green
108 **Advances in polyurethane biomaterials**
Edited by S. L. Cooper
109 **Nanocomposites for musculoskeletal tissue regeneration**
Edited by H. Liu
110 **Thin film coatings for biomaterials and biomedical applications**
Edited by H. J. Griesser
111 **Laser surface modification of biomaterials**
Edited by R. Vilar
112 **Biomaterials and regenerative medicine in ophthalmology Second edition**
Edited by T. V. Chirila and D. Harkin

113 **Extracellular matrix-derived medical implants in clinical medicine**
Edited by D. Mooradian
114 **Wound healing biomaterials: Volume 1: Therapies and regeneration**
Edited by M. S. Ågren
115 **Wound healing biomaterials: Volume 2: Functional biomaterials**
Edited by M. S. Ågren
116 **Materials for the direct restoration of teeth**
J. Nicholson and B. Czarnecka
117 **Science and principles of biodegradable and bioresorbable medical polymers**
Edited by X. Zhang
118 **Medical biosensors for point of care (POC) applications**
Edited by R. Narayan
119 **Biocompatibility of dental biomaterials**
Edited by R. Shelton
120 **Bioresorbable polymers for biomedical applications: From fundamentals to translational medicine**
Edited by G. Perale
121 **Bioinspired materials for medical applications**
Edited by L. Rodrigues and M. Mota
122 **Chitosan based biomaterials Volume 1: Fundamentals**
Edited by J. A. Jennings and J. D. Bumgardner
123 **Chitosan based biomaterials Volume 2: Tissue engineering and therapeutics**
Edited by J. A. Jennings and J. D. Bumgardner
124 **Material-tissue interfacial phenomena: Contributions from dental and craniofacial reconstructions**
Edited by P. Spencer and A. Misra
125 **Mechanical testing of orthopaedic implants**
Edited by E. Friis
126 **Management of periprosthetic joint infections (PJIs)**
Edited by A. J. Arts and J. A. P. Guerts
127 **Bone response to dental implant materials**
Edited by A. Piattelli
128 **Orthodontic applications of biomaterials: A clinical guide**
Edited by T. Eliades & W. A. Brantley
129 **Biofilms and implantable medical devices: Infection and control**
Edited by Y. Deng & W. Lv

Preface

During the past two to three decades, there has been a surge in the design, development, and use of new materials for the repair and reconstruction of dental and craniofacial tissues. In spite of the intense focus and the clear need, few, if any, of the synthetic materials achieve the complexity or robust behavior of native biological materials/systems. The differences between synthetic and biological systems are particularly evident when dissimilar materials of widely varying properties are combined. In these synthetic material systems, the interfacial regions are invariably defective and typically, the location where failure initiates.

This book represents a practice-inspired approach to understanding both the material/tissue interfacial phenomena, and the threat that damage, discrepancies, and deficiencies at the interface pose to the repair and reconstruction of dental and craniofacial tissues. The book is intended to engage a diverse audience of scientists, engineers, and clinical investigators. The early chapters represent the clinical need and problems in restoring form, function, and esthetics to dental and craniofacial tissues. The fundamental properties and multiscale characterization of materials, tissues, and material/tissue interfacial structures, relevant to dental and craniofacial repair, are discussed in subsequent chapters. The behavior of materials, tissues, and material/tissue interfacial structures is complicated by a variety of physical, chemical, and mechanical factors. Factors such as nonlinearity and rate and time dependence confound the interpretation and comparison of data measured at different scales and with various testing modalities. Measurement techniques at spatial scales ranging from nano- to micrometers are imperfect. In view of these challenges, later chapters are devoted to the multiscale mathematical and computational models that are required for realistic data interpretation. The final chapters highlight emerging techniques for addressing interfacial failures relevant to dental and craniofacial reconstruction. Peptide, protein, and cellular engineering are particularly promising approaches for the rational design of integrated material/tissue interfaces.

We thank all of the authors for their insightful contributions. We are grateful to Laura Overend, Lucy Beg, Poulouse Joseph, and the team at Woodhead Publishing for their enthusiasm, support, and patience throughout this project. We express our appreciation to the patients who inspired us to write this book. We thank our teachers, students, and colleagues for their encouragement. We are forever grateful to our families. This book would not have been possible without the unwavering support of our families.

Paulette Spencer and Anil Misra
Lawrence, KS, USA, 2016

Part One

Dental and craniofacial reconstructions using biomaterials

Clinical presentation: reconstruction using composite materials

1

B.S. Bohaty[1], *F. Sene*[2]
[1]University of Missouri-Kansas City, Kansas City, MO, United States; [2]State University of Londrina, Londrina, Brazil

1.1 Historical overview of composite resins and resin components in dentistry

The use of resin composite for repair and reconstruction can be traced to the pioneering work of Drs Buonocore and Bowen more than 50 years ago. Michael Buonocore has been credited with the development of the technique to "condition" enamel with acid for producing a roughened surface that could be infiltrated by acrylic filling materials. Through this work, Buonocore was able to demonstrate the micromechanical bonding capabilities of an etching and infiltration system (Buonocore, 1955). The widespread application of this technique to dental restorative materials was not recognized, however, until a hybrid monomer, (2,2-bis[4-(2-hydroxy-3-methacryloxypropoxy) phenyl]-propane) "Bis-GMA" was synthesized with properties that were conducive for use in the oral cavity (Bowen, 1963).

The first reports of using etched enamel as a means to attach and retain direct filling materials to tooth structure appeared in the literature in the 1970s (Laswell et al., 1971). By this time, etching enamel, prior to restoring with resin-based materials or prior to placing orthodontic brackets, was gaining popularity and was being increasingly utilized (Bowen, 1984).

The early composite resin restorative materials were plagued by clinical failures due to polymerization shrinkage, marginal leakage, and color mismatch. These products were usually chemically cured and lacked handling properties, which allowed direct placement into tooth preparations (Puckett et al., 2007). The evolution of composite resins continued, and new formulations were designed to improve the esthetics and decrease the challenges in establishing and maintaining marginal integrity.

Differences in composite resin formulations are linked to the various clinical applications for this material. However, in general, composites are composed of (1) some type of matrix, usually a dimethacrylate; (2) filler particles; (3) a coupling agent; and (4) various chemicals designed to mediate the polymerization reaction and process (Ferracane, 2011).

Most dental resin composites use the organic matrix, Bis-GMA, as the base monomer. Since Bis-GMA is extremely viscous, it is often combined with other monomers such as triethyleneglycol dimethacrylate, urethane dimethacrylate, or others to achieve the level of viscosity needed for use in dental composites (Ferracane, 1995).

Material-Tissue Interfacial Phenomena. http://dx.doi.org/10.1016/B978-0-08-100330-5.00001-7

In an effort to mitigate the problems associated with polymerization shrinkage and the accompanying contraction stresses, manufacturers turned their attention and effort toward the development of epoxy-based silorane systems as a replacement for traditional dimethacrylate systems. Although some of the initial studies regarding mechanical properties with this system indicated less shrinkage and good mechanical properties (Ilie and Hickel, 2006), at least one clinical trial has indicated that marginal adaptation of silorane-based composites was inferior to the traditional nanocomposite system (Schmidt et al., 2011). The development of various monomer systems that will offer improved properties and clinical durability is a challenge for manufacturers and researchers.

Filler particles are used to increase strength, decrease polymerization shrinkage, and decrease water sorption. These particles are usually delineated by size and have been modified extensively by manufacturers to improve the strength and polishability. The newest generation of composite resins is characterized by higher filler particle density, approximately 78 wt% (Chen et al., 2010), and smaller filler particle size, eg, 5–100 nm (Ilie and Hickel, 2006).

The coupling agents used in dental composites have not changed dramatically over time. A typical coupling agent is 3-methacryloxypropyltrimethoxysilane. This coupling agent is bifunctional, ie, it has chemical groups that react with the organic matrix and other groups that react with the inorganic filler particles. The use of a coupler in the composite formulation enhances the bonding between the inorganic and organic components of the dental composite (Ferracane, 2011).

The basic composition of resin composites used in dentistry has thus remained relatively constant over several decades. In contrast, the use of composite materials by practicing dentists has increased dramatically over the past few decades. This increase is traced primarily to patient preferences for esthetic restorations and to the concerns about mercury in the environment (Sensi et al., 2007).

1.2 Bonding substrates: enamel and dentin

Human enamel is one of the most mineralized tissues in the human body. The composition of enamel is 96 wt% inorganic materials, 4 wt% organic materials, and water. The inorganic material is predominantly composed of calcium phosphate related to the hexagonal hydroxyapatite, whose chemical formula is $Ca_{10}(PO_4)_6 \cdot (OH)_2$ (Gwinett, and Matsui, 1967; Carvalho et al., 2000). Bonding resin materials to this structure has been for the most part successful by using an acid to render the surface microporous (Fig. 1.1). The prepared surface can then be penetrated by low-viscosity resins (Gwinett and Matsui, 1967). Although the technique has been slightly modified and new products developed and introduced over time, the general tenet of using acid in concentrations of 35–40% to etch enamel and provide micromechanical retention for resin composites has endured. Bonding to enamel has been proved to be successful and reliable over decades of clinical use (Kugel and Ferrari, 2000). The composition of human enamel is relatively well understood, and its chemical components demonstrate a fairly consistent response to acid conditioning and resin infiltration.

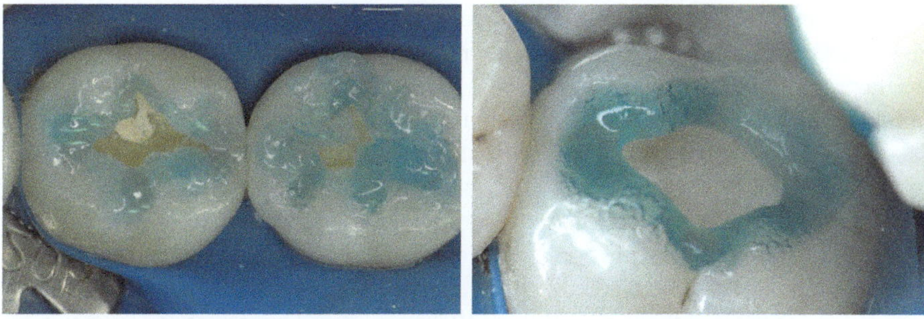

Figure 1.1 Acid etch process to prepare enamel.

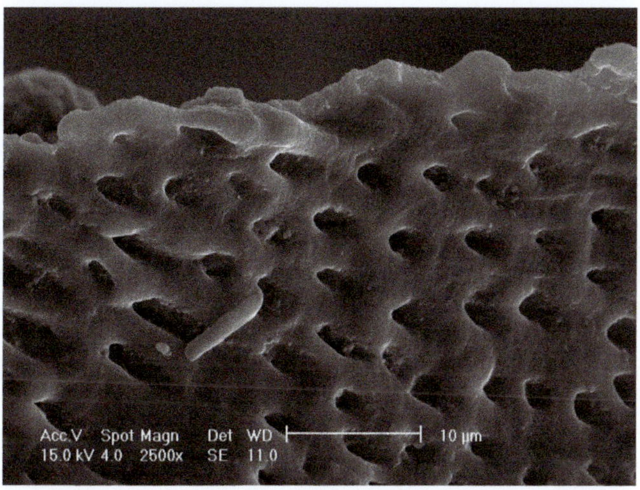

Figure 1.2 Scanning electron microscope photomicrograph of dentinal tubules.

Dentin is a complex, biologic substrate. The structural components of dentin consist of approximately 50 vol% mineral, 30 vol% organic matrix (primarily Type I collagen) and 20 vol% water (Ten Cate, 1994). The composition of this hydrated organic complex is not static, ie, the composition is influenced by the relative position of the dentin within the tooth, the age of the dentin, and the presence or absence of disease (Marshall et al., 1997). One of the most important aspects of the dentinal structure is the presence of tubules. This unique compositional feature results from odontoblastic activity during dentin formation. The tubules traverse from the dentinoenamel junction (DEJ) to the pulp, and the density and location of the tubules differ from location to location within the tooth. An example of dentinal tubule structure is shown in Fig. 1.2.

In permanent teeth, the tubule density decreases from the pulp to DEJ, and inside the tubules are odontoblastic processes and fluid (Marshall et al., 1997). Pashley (1989) reported that the percentage of tubule area including tubule diameters differs from place to place within the permanent tooth. For example, the diameter of the dentinal tubules ranges from 2.5 μm adjacent to the pulp to 0.8 μm near the DEJ. Similarly, the percentage of dentin area occupied by tubules varies from 22% near the pulp to 1% at the DEJ. Dentinal area occupied by intertubular dentin has been reported to be 12% in proximity of the pulp and 96% near the DEJ. The area occupied by peritubular dentin ranges from 3% close to the pulp to 60% at the DEJ. Numerous studies on permanent teeth have reported that the mean numerical density of tubules increases from the DEJ to the pulp (Garberoglio and Brannstrom, 1976; Fosse et al., 1992).

Tubules are lined with peritubular (intratubular) dentin consisting of a layer of highly mineralized matrix material made primarily of apatite crystals. The intertubular dentin, which lies between the tubules, is a less-calcified matrix that consists of some apatite crystals embedded within a collagen matrix. The influence of peritubular and intertubular dentin on successful dentin bonding has been postulated by numerous investigators (Nör et al., 1997; Sumikawa et al., 1999; Hosoya, 2006). Numerous studies suggest that when traversing from the DEJ to the pulp, in primary and permanent teeth, the dentinal tubule diameters increase and the peritubular thickness decreases (Allred, 1968; Ten Cate, 1994).

A critical factor in the clinical success of composite resins is the adhesive bond formed at the restorative material/tooth surface interface. Although acid etching provides effective mechanical bonding between the composite restoration and treated enamel in permanent teeth, breakdown at the dentin surface continues to challenge the long-term viability of these restorations. Current theories on dentin bonding suggest that two fundamental processes are involved in bonding an adhesive to dentin. First, the mineral phase must be extracted from the dentin substrate without altering the collagen matrix, and second, the voids left by the mineral must be filled with adhesive resin that undergoes complete in situ polymerization, ie, the formation of a resin-reinforced or hybrid layer. The ideal hybrid layer (Fig. 1.3) would be characterized as a three-dimensional polymer/collagen network that provides both a continuous and stable link between the bulk adhesive and dentin substrate (Nakabayashi et al., 1991;

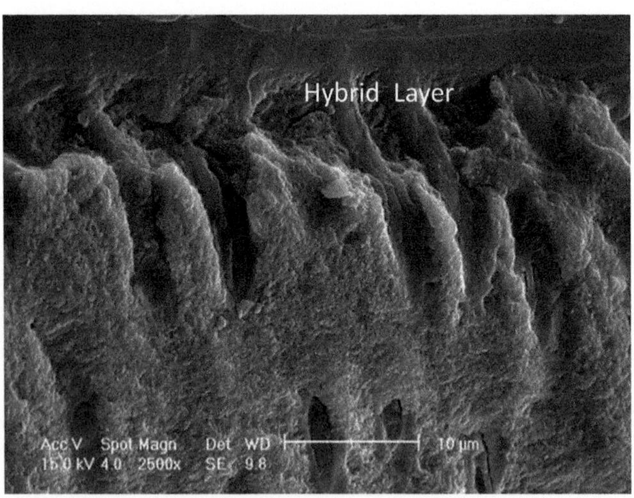

Figure 1.3 Scanning electron micrograph of the hybrid layer.

Eick et al., 1993). There is substantial evidence to suggest that this ideal objective is not achieved. Instead of serving as a stable connection between the bulk adhesive and subjacent intact dentin, the hybrid layer has been called the weakest link in the dentin/adhesive (d/a) bond (Sano et al., 1999; Spencer and Wang, 2002).

A poor-quality hybrid layer can leave unreinforced and exposed collagen at the composite margin and/or beneath the restoration (Spencer and Swafford, 1999; Spencer et al., 2000; Wang and Spencer, 2002). This zone of exposed collagen is susceptible to breakdown after only 3 years storage in aqueous media (Burrow et al., 1996). Poor-quality hybrid layers translate to sites of incomplete adhesive penetration, sites where the adhesive is unstable because of inadequate monomer/polymer conversion, or sites where the adhesive fails to form a cross-linked polymer (Wang and Spencer, 2005a,b; Spencer et al., 2006) Because of the profound effect the seal at the d/a interface has on the clinical performance of composite restorations, it is very likely that a weak hybrid layer threatens the serviceability of the composite. This relationship may be particularly relevant at the gingival margin of Class II composite restorations where there is little enamel available for bonding. Clinical studies have reported that as many as half of the failures in class II composite restorations are due to recurrent caries at the gingival margin (Nordbo et al., 1988; Purk et al., 2007).

Clinical failure of Class II composite restorations are demonstrated in Figs. 1.4 and 1.5. These figures show the gingival margins of an in vivo Class II resin restoration in a permanent tooth and the gingival margin of a Class II resin restoration in an extracted primary tooth. Both show marked demineralization and recurrent caries at the gingival margin of the restoration.

An additional component of tooth preparation that influences the potential success or failure of ideal hybridization is the presence or absence of debris left behind during tooth preparation. Whenever dentin is cut to prepare a tooth to receive any type of restoration, the residual organic and inorganic components of the cut dentin leave a "layer" of debris on the surface. This debris is called the smear layer (Eick et al., 1970). The smear layer complicates the bonding process by acting as a physical

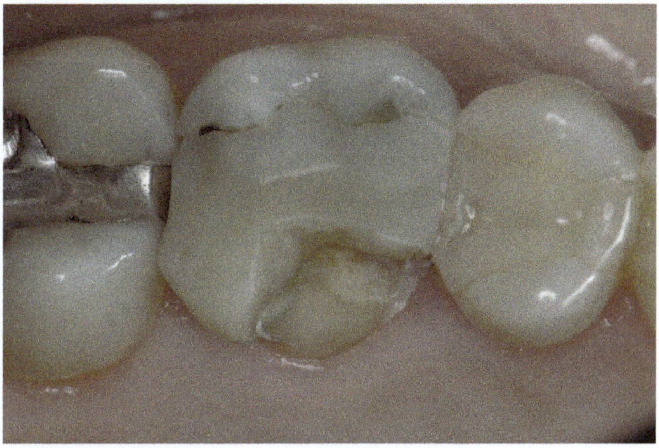

Figure 1.4 Class II resin failure in permanent tooth.

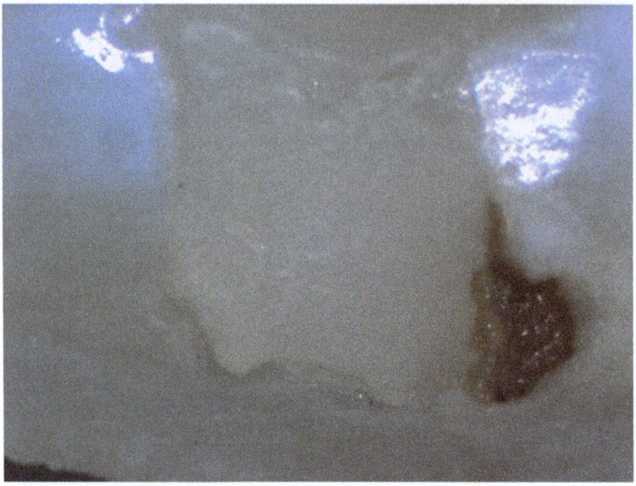

Figure 1.5 Class II resin restoration from recovered primary tooth.

barrier to bonding agent penetration (Brannstrom, 1984). Although there may be some advantages in keeping the smear layer intact, the majority of the literature supports the idea that the smear layer must be either removed or rendered permeable so that the bonding agent can penetrate the tooth substrate directly (Pashley et al.1988, 1991; Perdigao, 2007; Spencer et al., 2001; Wang and Spencer, 2002).

1.3 Clinical performance of resin restorations

Resin composite is the most common alternative to dental amalgam, however, numerous studies report that composite restorations have more recurrent caries, higher failure rates, and increased frequency of replacement (Simecek et al., 2009; Malhotra et al., 2011). Simecek et al. (2009) reviewed the dental records of more than 3000 patients and concluded that there was a significantly higher risk of replacement for posterior composite restorations when compared with dental amalgam. A study of composite and amalgam restorations in the pediatric population indicated that the need for additional treatment was 50% greater in children receiving composite restorations (DeRouen et al., 2006).

Although the concern for developing resin materials that function better and last longer in the mouth continues, there have been documented improvements in restoration longevity as reported in a 2014 study by Pallesen et al. The study by Pallesen and colleagues suggested that resin composite restorations placed in children younger than 18 years had an annual failure rate of 2% (Pallesen et al., 2014). Clinical studies do not, however, consistently report high success rates with posterior composite restorations, particularly Class II composite restorations in patients with high caries risk, and thus, the Dental Materials and Biomaterials Program at the National Institutes of Dental and Craniofacial Research continues to emphasize the need for materials that will increase the service life of resin dental composite restorations (National Institute of Health Funding).

The use of composite to restore form and function to posterior teeth damaged by disease, age, or trauma continues to gain wide acceptance by the dental community, and indeed, there are many dental amalgam–free practices. A myriad of factors can influence the clinical success of composite resin restorations. Clinical parameters include patient selection, tooth preparation, and techniques used in restoration placement.

1.4 Patient selection

The popularity and demand for resin-based posterior restorations have been increasing steadily since the introduction of these materials in the mid-1950s. The societal focus on esthetics as well as the worldwide move to eliminate dental amalgam has contributed to this phenomenon (Murray et al., 2002). Unfortunately, the success and/or failure of resin-based composite restorations depend on variables that may be difficult for the operator to control. For example, restorations placed in patients with high caries risk have higher restoration failure rates than those placed in patients with low caries risk (Hunter et al., 1995; Blum and Lynch et al., 2014). These findings have been documented in adult as well as pediatric dental patient populations (Soncini et al., 2007; Bernardo et al., 2007). Clinical data indicate that regardless of which preparation design is adopted or the which type of posterior resin-based restoration is utilized, the practitioner must give careful consideration to the caries status of the patient and adjust recommendations for restorative materials accordingly.

1.5 Tooth preparation, form, and function

Posterior resin restorations have been indicated for Class I, Class V, and Class II tooth preparations (Figs. 1.6–1.9). In particular, resins are utilized to maximize the esthetics and minimize the loss of tooth structure during preparation. Due to the location of the caries and thus the need to restore proximal surfaces in Class II restorations, a number of tooth preparation designs have been advocated. The underlying goal of all these designs is a reduction in the loss of sound tooth structure.

The "tunnel" technique, as reported by Hunt (1984) and Knight (1992) has been used to remove proximal caries while leaving the marginal ridge intact. Although potentially promising, the lack of long-term clinical studies limits wide adoption of this technique (Wiegand and Attin, 2007). Of course, the ability to access and restore an interproximal carious lesion directly represents the most conservative proximal restorative technique available. This technique is relatively successful in preserving intact tooth structure.

The ability to access proximal carious lesions directly is usually limited. Minibox or "slot" preparations for the restoration of proximal lesions in posterior teeth have

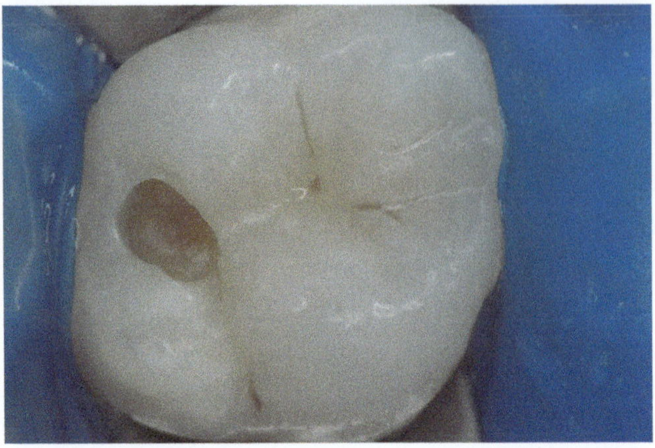

Figure 1.6 Class I tooth preparation.

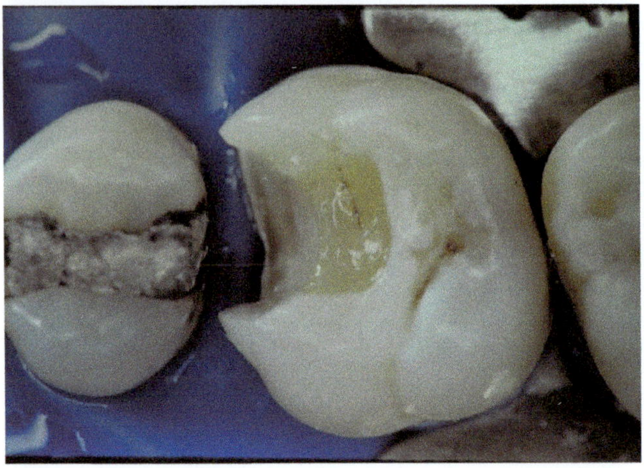

Figure 1.7 Class II tooth preparation.

also been recommended by clinicians and researchers. These preparation designs have been described as minimally invasive and relatively successful with a reported 70% success rate over an average of 7 years (Tyas et al., 2000; Peters et al., 2001).

The aforementioned tooth preparation designs successfully limit the removal of sound tooth structure and take advantage of appropriate etching techniques in bonding to intact enamel and dentin. In general, the cavity preparation design is dictated by the location and extent of the disease. Thus, depending on the location and extent of the caries, extensive preparation designs, which involve access through the marginal ridge and removal of infected enamel and dentin, may be required. These more invasive preparations and restorations are indicated in these clinical situations and are well documented in the literature (Fig. 1.9). (Lopes et al., 2004) Whenever possible, conservative, structure-sparing preparation techniques should be used to restore proximal surfaces with resin-based composite.

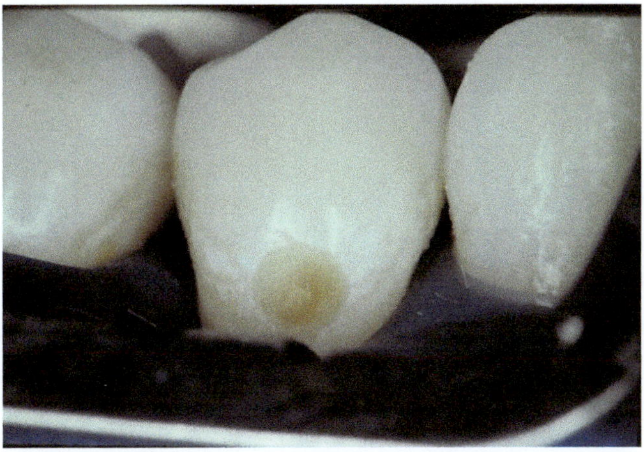

Figure 1.8 Class V tooth preparation.

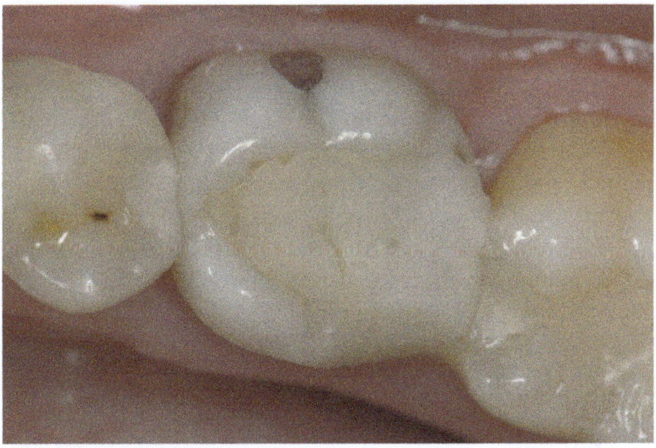

Figure 1.9 Extensive Class II resin restoration.

Considerable attention has been devoted to the relationship between cavity type, cavity size, number of surfaces restored, and the risk of restoration failure. As the number of restored surfaces increases, the risk of restoration failure also increases (DaRosa et al., 2006, 2011). For example, it is reported that single-surface and Class I restorations are less likely to fail when compared with multisurface restorations, extensive cavities, and Class II restorations (Correa et al., 2012). Conservative Class I composite restorations are not, however, immune to failure as demonstrated in Fig. 1.10.

To minimize restoration failure and mitigate the effects of bonding multiple tooth surfaces, most clinical strategies have focused on methods to decrease the ratio between the bonded surface area to the nonbonded surface area, also described as the cavity configuration or C-factor. The higher the C-factor, the less the chance for relaxation of polymerization shrinkage. Some studies have indicated that the increase in C-factor is also associated with decreased bond strength (El-Sahn et al., 2011; Shirai, 2005).

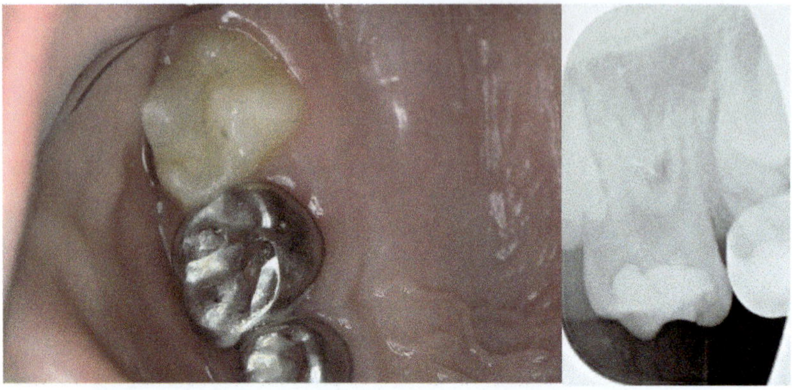

Figure 1.10 Clinical presentation of Class I resin restoration with periapical lesion.

Recent investigations have suggested that this finding may not be valid for the newer low-shrink resin-based composites (Van Ende et al., 2012).

Along with preparation design and extent of tissue removal, the position of the tooth in the mouth directly influences the overall clinical performance and longevity of the restoration. Studies suggest that restorations placed in premolars fail less often than similar restorations placed in molars (DaRosa et al., 2006, 2011). Intuitively, this finding makes sense in that the masticatory forces and stresses placed on restorations in molar teeth are higher than those placed in premolars. Nonetheless, the findings, in terms of tooth position and number of restored surfaces, indicate that clinicians should utilize posterior resin composites in areas where esthetics is deemed essential and should maintain as much tooth structure as possible.

1.6 Restoration placement techniques

The techniques used to fill and cure resin-based composites, particularly in areas of high masticatory stresses, have received considerable attention. The debate among researchers as well as practitioners regarding bulk cure versus incremental cure continues. Incremental filling (Fig. 1.11) techniques have long been recommended due to the polymerization shrinkage associated with dental composites. Reducing the volume of composite that is polymerized at each stage of the restorative procedure minimizes shrinkage and maximizes the conversion of monomers to polymer. This is achieved, in part, by decreasing the attenuation of the curing light (Kujis et al., 2003). Although incremental filling techniques have been taught and utilized for decades, some studies indicate that incremental filling of resin-based composites produces higher shrinkage stress (Kujis et al., 2003; Abbas et al., 2003). In direct contrast, more recent studies report that incremental filling produces lower shrinkage stress when compared with bulk filling techniques (Lee et al., 2007; Park et al., 2008). These diverse and contradictory conclusions are likely due to the different testing methods (Kwon et al., 2012).

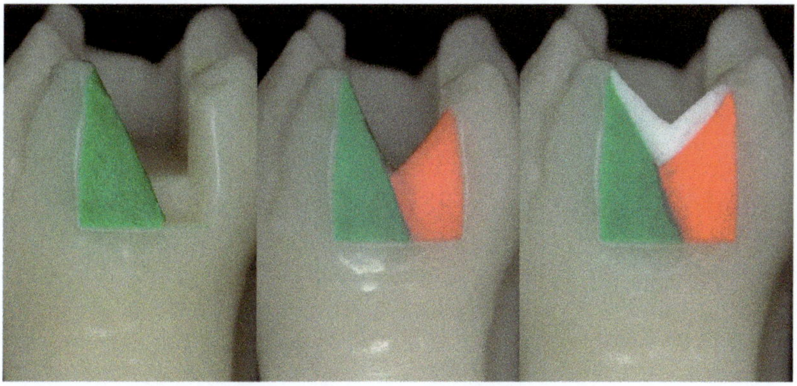

Figure 1.11 Incremental fill technique for resin restorations.

Currently, manufacturers are striving to produce resin-based composite systems that have less polymerization shrinkage (<2%) and more importantly, reduced polymerization shrinkage stress. Strategies to improve shrinkage include utilizing new low-shrinking monomers or those with an increased molecular weight (Van Ende et al., 2013). As the low-shrinking composite resins improve, incremental filling and curing of posterior composites may no longer be recommended. However, until the long-term clinical success of the low-shrinking composite resin systems is confirmed, using an incremental filling technique in deep cavity preparations is recommended (Van Ende et al., 2013).

The influence of matrix type on the quality of the proximal contact and the ease of placement of Class II resin restorations has also been evaluated. The ability to reproduce an appropriate, functional interproximal contact with a Class II resin restoration is important to minimize food impaction and thus, maintain healthy periodontal tissues. In addition, a poorly adapted and finished proximal restoration may have an "open margin" through which oral fluids, eg, saliva, enzymes, water, and cariogenic bacteria may penetrate. This marginal leakage can lead to recurrent caries; recurrent caries is the primary reason for composite restoration failure (Simecek et al., 2009; Malhotra et al., 2011; Opdam et al., 2007, 2014).

Manufacturers have introduced various types of matrices with the goal of affecting or influencing the direction of composite shrinkage during polymerization (Cenci et al., 2006). The literature no longer supports the concept of "directional polymerization" (Versluis et al., 1998), but these matrices still exist. Although there are a myriad of different shapes and sizes, the majority of matrices fall into one of two basic types: (1) metal matrices, which are straight or circumferential/precontoured and (2) transparent matrices, which are either straight or circumferential/precontoured. Despite the theory that transparent matrices will enhance polymerization at the gingival margin, the literature suggests that the choice of matrix does not influence the clinical success of Class II posterior resins (Cenci et al., 2006).

In addition to matrix type, there are numerous tooth separation (wedging) products and techniques. These include wooden wedges and separation rings. The literature suggests that the type of matrix material/wedge does not influence the clinical performance of Class II composite restorations (Cenci et al., 2006). The literature does, however, indicate that no matrix/wedge combination can accurately reproduce an intact proximal surface contact at the precise location of the natural intact tooth (Kampouropoulis et al., 2010).

1.7 Clinical challenges and composite restoration failures

Researchers and industry continue their efforts to modify composite resin restorative materials to improve their handling characteristics, mechanical and physical properties, and clinical performance. The majority of the current resin composites have mechanical properties that make them suitable for use in all areas of the mouth. The functionality of these restorations, however, in areas of high masticatory stress is still a concern. Resin restorations that are placed in areas of high function are more prone to exhibit excessive wear and/or marginal fracture despite the advances in composite materials. Clinicians must exercise caution when placing large resin-based composite restorations in areas of high function. The longevity of posterior resin restorations placed in patients who have a history of clenching or grinding may be particularly limited (Kampouropoulis et al., 2010).

Although resin composition, tooth preparation design, and matrix systems may influence the lifetime of posterior composite restorations, the primary factor in the clinical failure of moderate to large composite restorations is secondary caries at the margins of the restorations (Mjor et al., 2000; Bernardo et al., 2007). An increase in secondary caries at the margins of composite restorations suggests that the seal at the composite/tooth interface is not adequate to resist the physical, chemical, and mechanical stresses that are present in the mouth. The failure of moderate to large composite restorations has been linked to degradation of the bond at the tooth surface/composite material interface (Koshiro et al., 2005; Mair et al., 1998; Mjor et al., 2002; Van Meerbeek et al., 2005) and an increase in the concentration of the cariogenic bacterium, *Streptococcus mutans*, at the perimeter of these materials (Santerre et al., 2001; Hansel et al., 1998; Svanberg et al., 1990). Degradation of the bond at the interface between the tooth and composite has been associated with the failure of adhesives to form an impervious seal with the dentin (Spencer et al., 2005, 2006; Wang et al., 2005a, 2005b). Failure of the dentin/adhesive (d/a) bond leads to open pores at the composite/tooth interface; bacterial enzymes, oral fluids, and even bacteria can penetrate these pores. Data from in vivo and in vitro studies indicate that the infiltration of these agents into these void spaces between the tooth and composite will lead to recurrent caries, hypersensitivity, and pulpal inflammation (Van Meerbeek et al., 2005; Hashimoto et al., 2001; Brannstrom, 1984). Results from clinical studies indicate loss of retention, poor marginal adaptation, and marginal discoloration when the d/a interface is exposed to the oral cavity (Breschi et al., 2008). Effective mechanical bonding between the composite restoration and treated enamel has been achieved using appropriate acid-etching protocols, but failure of the bond at the d/a interface threatens the long-term clinical survival of moderate to large posterior composite restorations (Van Meerbeek et al., 2005; Andersson-Wenckert et al., 2004).

Bonding failures have been commonly tracked to the gingival margin of Class II composite restorations (Bouillaguet et al., 2001). A separation between the composite material and tooth surface has been noted at the gingival margin (Van Dijkin et al., 2000). In Class II composite restorations there is generally very little enamel available for bonding at the gingival margin; therefore, the bond at this site depends on the integrity of the seal formed with dentin. Gaps at the gingival margin have been attributed to unreliable dentin bonding (Roulet, 1997). Furthermore, the "wet bonding" techniques, currently used to maintain a porous demineralized dentin matrix during resin infiltration, add another layer of challenges to creating an impervious d/a bond under clinical conditions.

Wet bonding techniques were introduced in the early 1990s to counteract the problems noted with collagen collapse following drying of the demineralized dentin matrix (Gwinnett, 1994; Kanca, 1992). Wet bonding means that the demineralized dentin matrix is fully hydrated throughout the bonding protocol. Using this procedure, the channels between the demineralized dentin collagen fibrils are filled with water, solvent, conditioner, and/or oral fluids (Pashley et al., 1993; Kato et al., 1998). It is expected that adhesive will diffuse into the fluid-filled spaces of the substrate and along the collagen fibrils. Ideally, the solvent in combination with hydrophilic monomers, eg, hydroxyethyl methacrylate (HEMA) conditions the collagen to remain expanded during adhesive infiltration. However, HEMA, a primary component in many single-bottle commercial dentin adhesives, can dramatically reduce the evaporation of water (Pashley et al., 1998). Hydrophobic monomers, such as Bis-GMA, would resist diffusing into these sites where there is residual water (Wang and Spencer, 2003).

In the in vivo situation, there may be little control over the amount of water left on the tooth. Thus, it is possible to leave the dentin surface so wet that the adhesive physically separates into hydrophobic- and hydrophilic-rich phases (Spencer et al., 2002; Ye et al., 2011, 2012). Under clinical conditions, dentists must routinely attempt to bond to naturally wet substrates, eg, caries-affected dentin (Ito et al., 2005) or deep dentin (Wang et al., 2003). The water content of caries-affected dentin is 2.7 times greater than that of normal dentin (Ito et al., 2005). Exposed tubules account for 22% of the surface area in deep dentin. In contrast, exposed tubules account for 1% of the surface area of dentin close to the DEJ (Pashley et al., 1989). The large increase in exposed tubules in deep dentin means that the pulpal fluid will contribute additional moisture to that already present within the demineralized dentin matrix. With the sensitivity of our current adhesives to excess moisture, it is obvious that bonding to these clinically relevant substrates is a significant challenge (Spencer et al., 2006; Wang and Spencer, 2005a, 2005b; Wang et al., 2007a, 2007b). This difficulty highlights the potential limitations in utilizing resin-based composites to restore large, deep carious lesions.

1.8 Effects of function, fatigue, and degradation

When measured immediately, dentin–composite bonds are generally considered adequate to tolerate conditions in the mouth, but these bonds deteriorate with time. The two major mechanisms of deterioration are fatigue and hydrolysis (Staninec et al., 2008). Fatigue has been linked to stresses transmitted to the bond by occlusal forces, thermal expansion and contraction, and polymerization shrinkage of the composite. Chronic deterioration of the dentin–composite bond is also related to hydrolysis and leaching of the adhesive that has infiltrated the tooth structure (Wang et al., 2003; Spencer et al., 2006).

Fatigue investigations have indicated that the overall time-dependent behavior of the composite–tooth interface is a complex function of the individual material phases. For example, finite element analyses have shown that each material phase at the d/a interface experiences different stress concentration at functional loads (Misra et al., 2004, 2005). The overall failure behavior of the bond at the d/a interface is not determined by the weakest component, but by the component whose stress concentration is closest to its failure strength. Similarly, the overall fatigue life of the d/a interface is governed by the material component with the shortest fatigue life under a given loading condition (Singh et al., 2011).

Under function, the material components at the composite–tooth interface are subjected to both chemical and mechanical stresses. The interplay between these stresses can result in the deterioration of the properties of the material over time. The breaking of covalent bonds by addition of water to ester bonds is considered one of the primary reasons for deterioration of the adhesive at the interface between the composite and tooth (Tay et al., 2003). Interestingly, degradation of methacrylate ester groups produces carboxylic acids—the same functional group that is the culprit in lactic acid–induced dental caries (Spencer et al., 2010, 2014). The change in mechanical properties of the materials can be attributed to a variety of mechanisms that include proliferation of surface and subsurface flaws (Staninec et al., 2008; Misra et al., 2005; Katz et al., 2007; Singh et al., 2010; Belli et al., 2010). These flaws in combination with the chemical and biochemical stresses that are present in the mouth can then lead to restoration failure (Hashimoto et al., 2001).

In summary, the d/a bond can be the first defense against substances that may penetrate and ultimately undermine the gingival margin in composite restorations in vivo. It has been hypothesized that in vivo degradation of the d/a interfacial bond follows a cascade of events that begins when the dentin is acid etched (Pashley et al., 2004; Sano et al., 1999). Disruption of the tooth structure by acid etching exposes and activates proteolytic enzymes, eg, matrix metalloproteinases, which can degrade the exposed collagen component of the hybrid layer. The following factors inhibit the formation of a durable bond at the d/a interface: (1) water sorption and hydrolysis of the adhesive resin, (2) inadequate monomer/polymer conversion of the infiltrating adhesive, (3) incomplete resin infiltration of the demineralized dentin matrix, (4) incomplete solvent evaporation, and (5) enzymatic challenges within the cavity preparation through exposure to oral fluids (Kostoryz et al., 2009; Ye et al., 2007, 2009a, 2009b, 2012). Although durable d/a bonds are critical for maintaining a seal at the tooth/composite interface, the properties of the materials are only one part of an extremely complex problem (Drummond et al., 2008).

References

Abbas G, Fleming GJ, Harrington E, Shortall AC, Burke FJ. Cuspal movement and microleakage in premolar teeth restored with a packable composite cured in bulk or in increments. J Dent 2003;31(6):437–44.

Allred H. The differential staining of peritubular and intertubular matrices in human dentine. Arch Oral Biol 1968;13(1):1–12.

Andersson-Wenckert IE, van Dijken JW, Kieri C. Durability of extensive Class II open-sandwich restorations with a resin-modified glass ionomer cement after 6 years. Am J Dent 2004;17(1):43–50.

Belli R, Sartori N, Peruchi LD, Guimaraes JC, Araujo E, Monteiro Jr S, et al. Slow progression of dentin bond degradation during one-year water storage under simulated pulpal pressure. J Dent 2010;38(10):802–10.

Bernardo M, Luis H, Martin MD, Leroux BG, Rue T, Leitao J, et al. Survival and reasons for failure of amalgam versus composite posterior restorations placed in a randomized clinical trial. J Am Dent Assoc 2007;138(6):775–83.

Blum IR, Lynch CD. Repair versus replacement of defective direct dental restorations in posterior teeth of adults. Prim Dent J 2014;3(2):62–7.

Bouillaguet S, Ciucchi B, Jacoby T, Wataha JC, Pashley D. Bonding characteristics to dentin walls of class II cavities, in vitro. Dent Mater 2001;17(4):316–21.

Bowen RL, Eick JD, Henderson DA, Anderson DW. Smear layer: removal and bonding considerations. Oper Dent Suppl 1984;3:30–4.

Bowen RL. Properties of a silica-reinforced polymer for dental restorations. J Am Dent Assoc 1963;66:57–64.

Brannstrom M. Smear layer: pathological and treatment considerations. Oper Dent Suppl 1984;3:35–42.

Breschi L, Mazzoni A, Ruggeri A, Cadenaro M, Di Lenarda R, De Stefano Dorigo E. Dental adhesion review: aging and stability of the bonded interface. Dent Mater 2008;24(1):90–101.

Buonocore MG. A simple method of increasing the adhesion of acrylic filling materials to enamel surfaces. J Dent Res 1955;34(6):849–53.

Burrow MF, Satoh M, Tagami J. Dentin bond durability after three years using a dentin bonding agent with and without priming. J Mater 1996;12:302–7.

Carvalho RM, Santiago SL, Fernandes CA, Suh BI, Pashley DH. Effects of prism orientation on tensile strength of enamel. J Adhes Dent 2000;2(4):251–7.

Cenci MS, Lund RG, Pereira CL, de Carvalho RM, Demarco FF. In vivo and in vitro evaluation of Class II composite resin restorations with different matrix systems. J Adhes Dent 2006;8(2):127–32.

Chen MH. Update on dental nanocomposites. J Dent Res 2010;89(6):549–60.

Correa, MB, Peres MA, Peres KG, Horta BL, Barros AD, Demarco FF. Amalgam or composite resin? Factors influencing the choice of restorative material. J Dent 2012;40(9):703–10.

Da Rosa Rodolpho PA, Cenci MS, Donassollo TA, Loguercio AD, Demarco FF. A clinical evaluation of posterior composite restorations: 17-year findings. J Dent 2006;34(7):427–35.

Da Rosa Rodolpho PA, Donassollo TA, Cenci MS, Loguercio AD, Moraes RR, Bronkhorst EM, et al. 22-Year clinical evaluation of the performance of two posterior composites with different filler characteristics. Dent Mater 2011;27(10):955–63.

Demarco FF, Cenci MS, Lima FG, Donassollo TA, Andre Dde A, Leida FL. Class II composite restorations with metallic and translucent matrices: 2-year follow-up findings. J Dent 2007;35(3):231–7.

DeRouen TA, Martin MD, Leroux BG, Townes BD, Woods JS, Leitao J, et al. Neurobehavioral effects of dental amalgam in children: a randomized clinical trial. JAMA 2006;295(15):1784–92.

Drummond JL. Degradation, fatigue, and failure of resin dental composite materials. J Dent Res 2008;87(8):710–9.

Eick JD, Wilko R, Anderson CH, Sorenson S. Scanning electron microscopy and electron microprobe analysis of cut tooth surfaces. J Dent Res 1970;49:1359–68.

Eick JD, Robinson S, Chappel RP, Cobb CM, Spencer P. The dentinal surface: its influence on dentinal adhesion. Part III. Quintessence Int 1993;24:265–73.

El-Sahn NA, El-Kassas DW, El-Damanhoury HM, Fahmy OM, Gomaa H, Platt JA. Effect of C-factor on microtensile bond strengths of low-shrinkage composites. Oper Dent 2011;36(3):281–92.

Ferracane JL. Current trends in dental composites. Crit Rev Oral Biol Med 1995;6(4):302–18.

Ferracane JL. Resin composite–state of the art. Dent Mater 2011;27(1):29–38.

Fosse G, Saele PK, Eide R. Numerical density and distributional pattern of dentin tubules. Acta Odontol Scand 1992;50(4):201–10.

Garberoglio R, Brannstrom M. Scanning electron microscopic investigation of human dentinal tubules. Arch Oral Biol 1976;21(6):355–62.

Gwinnett AJ, Matsui A. A study of enamel adhesives. The physical relationship between enamel and adhesive. Arch Oral Biol 1967;12(12):1615–20.

Gwinnett AJ. Dentin bond strength after air drying and rewetting. Am J Dent 1994;7(3):144–8.

Hansel C, Leyhausen G, Mai UE, Geurtsen W. Effects of various resin composite (co) monomers and extracts on two caries-associated micro-organisms in vitro. J Dent Res 1998;77(1):60–7.

Hashimoto M, Ohno H, Kaga M, Endo K, Sano H, Oguchi H. Resin-tooth adhesive interfaces after long-term function. Am J Dent 2001;14(4):211–5.

Hosoya Y. Hardness and elasticity of bonded carious and sound primary tooth dentin. J Dent 2006;34(2):164–71.

Hunt PR. A modified class II cavity preparation for glass ionomer restorative materials. Quintessence Int Dent Dig 1984;15(10):1011–8.

Hunter AR, Treasure ET, Hunter AJ. Increases in cavity volume associated with the removal of class 2 amalgam and composite restorations. Oper Dent 1995;20(1):2–6.

Ilie N, Hickel R. Silorane-based dental composite: behavior and abilities. Dent Mater J 2006;25(3):445–54.

Ito S, Saito T, Tay FR, Carvalho RM, Yoshiyama M, Pashley DH. Water content and apparent stiffness of non-caries versus caries-affected human dentin. J Biomed Mater Res B Appl Biomater 2005;72(1):109–16.

Kampouropoulos D, Paximada C, Loukidis M, Kakaboura A. The influence of matrix type on the proximal contact in class II resin composite restorations. Oper Dent 2010;35(4):454–62.

Kanca 3rd J. Resin bonding to wet substrate. 1. Bonding to dentin. Quintessence Int 1992;23(1):39–41.

Kato G, Nakabayashi N. The durability of adhesion to phosphoric acid etched, wet dentin substrates. Dent Mater 1998;14(5):347–52.

Katz JL, Misra A, Spencer P, Wang Y, Bumrerraj S, Nomura T, et al. Multiscale mechanics of hierarchical structure/property relationships in calcified tissues and tissue/material interfaces. Mater Sci Eng A Struct Mater 2007;27(3):450–68.

Knight GM. The tunnel restoration–nine years of clinical experience using capsulated glass ionomer cements. Case report. Aust Dent J 1992;37(4):245–51.

Koshiro K, Inoue S, Sano H, De Munck J, Van Meerbeek B. In vivo degradation of resin-dentin bonds produced by a self-etch and an etch-and-rinse adhesive. Eur J Oral Sci 2005;113(4):341–8.

Kostoryz EL, Dharmala K, Ye Q, Wang Y, Huber J, Park JG, et al. Enzymatic biodegradation of HEMA/bisGMA adhesives formulated with different water content. J Biomed Mater Res B Appl Biomater 2009;88(2):394–401.

Kugel G, Ferrari M. The science of bonding: from first to sixth generation. J Am Dent Assoc 2000;131(Suppl.):20S–5S.

Kuijs RH, Fennis WM, Kreulen CM, Barink M, Verdonschot N. Does layering minimize shrinkage stresses in composite restorations? J Dent Res 2003;82(12):967–71.

Kwon Y, Ferracane J, Lee IB. Effect of layering methods, composite type, and flowable liner on the polymerization shrinkage stress of light cured composites. Dent Mater 2012;28(7):801–9.

Laswell HR, Welk DA, Regenos JW. Attachment of resin restorations to acid pretreated enamel. J Am Dent Assoc 1971;82(3):558–63.

Lee MR, Cho BH, Son HH, Um CM, Lee IB. Influence of cavity dimension and restoration methods on the cusp deflection of premolars in composite restoration. Dent Mater 2007;23(3):288–95.

Lopes GC, Vieira LC, Araujo E. Direct composite resin restorations: a review of some clinical procedures to achieve predictable results in posterior teeth. J Esthetic Restor Dent 2004;16(1):19–31. discussion 32.

Mair LH. Ten-year clinical assessment of three posterior resin composites and two amalgams. Quintessence Int 1998;29(8):483–90.

Malhotra N, Mala K, Acharya S. Resin-based composite as a direct esthetic restorative material. Compend Contin Educ Dent 2011;32(5):14–23. quiz 24, 38.

Marshall GW, Marshall SJ, Kinney JH, Balooch M. The dentin substrate: structure and properties related to bonding. J Dent 1997;25(6):441–58.

Misra A, Spencer P, Marangos O, Wang Y, Katz JL. Micromechanical analysis of dentin/adhesive interface by the finite element method. J Biomed Mater Res B Appl Biomater 2004;70(1):56–65.

Misra A, Spencer P, Marangos O, Wang Y, Katz JL. Parametric study of the effect of phase anisotropy on the micromechanical behaviour of dentin-adhesive interfaces. J R Soc Interface 2005;2(3):145–57.

Mjor IA, Dahl JE, Moorhead JE. Age of restorations at replacement in permanent teeth in general dental practice. Acta Odontol Scand 2000;58(3):97–101.

Mjor IA, Dahl JE, Moorhead JE. Placement and replacement of restorations in primary teeth. Acta Odontol Scand 2002;60(1):25–8.

Murray PE, Smyth TW, About I, Remusat R, Franquin JC, Smith AJ. The effect of etching on bacterial microleakage of an adhesive composite restoration. J Dent 2002;30(1):29–36.

Nakabayashi N, Nakamura M, Yasuda M. Hybrid layer as dentin bonding mechanism. Esthet Dent 1991;3:133–8.

National Institute of Health Funding. http://www.nidcr.nih.gov/GrantsAndFunding/See_Funding_Opportunities_Sorted_By/ConceptClearance/CurrentCC/DentalResinComposites.htms.

Nor JE, Feigal RJ, Dennison JB, Edwards CA. Dentin bonding: SEM comparison of the dentin surface in primary and permanent teeth. Pediatr Dent 1997;19(4):246–52.

Nordbo H, Leirskar J, von der Fehr FR. Saucer-shaped cavity preparations for posterior approximal resin composite restorations: observations up to 10 years. Quintessence Int 1988;29(1):5–11.

Opdam NJ, Bronkhorst EM, Roeters JM, Loomans BA. Longevity and reasons for failure of sandwich and total-etch posterior composite resin restorations. J Adhes Dent 2007;9(5):469–75.

Opdam NJ, van de Sande FH, Bronkhorst E, Cenci MS, Bottenberg P, Pallesen U, Gaengler P, Lindberg A, Huysmans MC, van Dijken JW. Longevity of posterior composite restorations: a systematic review and meta-analysis. J Dent Res 2014;30(10):943–49.

Pallesen U, van Dijken JW, Halken J, Hallonsten AL, Hoigaard R. A prospective 8-year follow-up of posterior resin composite restorations in permanent teeth of children and adolescents in Public Dental Health Service: reasons for replacement. Clin Oral Investig 2014;18(3):819–27.

Park J, Chang J, Ferracane J, Lee IB. How should composite be layered to reduce shrinkage stress: incremental or bulk filling? Dent Mater 2008;24(11):1501–5.

Pashley DH, Tao L, Boyd D, King GE, Horner JA. Scanning electron microscopy of the substructure of t smear layers in human dentine. Arch Oral Biol 1988;33:265–70.

Pashley DH, Ciucchi B, Sano H, Horner JA. Permeability of dentin to adhesive agents. Quintessence Int 1993;24(9):618–31.

Pashley EL, Zhang Y, Lockwood PE, Rueggeberg FA, Pashley DH. Effects of HEMA on water evaporation from water-HEMA mixtures. Dent Mater 1998;14(1):6–10.

Pashley DH, Tay FR, Yiu C, Hashimoto M, Breschi L, Carvalho RM, et al. Collagen degradation by host-derived enzymes during aging. J Dent Res 2004;83(3):216–21.

Pashley DH. Dentin: a dynamic substrate–a review. Scanning Microsc 1989;3(1):161–74. discussion 174–166.

Pashley DH. Clinical correlations of dentin structure and function. J Prosthet Dent 1991;66:777–81.

Perdigao J. New developments in dental adhesion. Dent Clin North Am 2007;51(2):333–57. viii.

Peters MC, McLean ME. Minimally invasive operative care. I. Minimal intervention and concepts for minimally invasive cavity preparations. J Adhes Dent 2001;3(1):7–16.

Puckett AD, Fitchie JG, Kirk PC, Gamblin J. Direct composite restorative materials. Dent Clin North Am 2007;51(3):659–75. vii.

Purk JH, Dusevich V, Glaros A, Eick JD. Adhesive analysis of voids in class II composite resin restorations at the axial and gingival cavity walls restored under in vivo versus in vitro conditions. Dent Mater 2007;23(7):871–7.

Roulet JF. Benefits and disadvantages of tooth-coloured alternatives to amalgam. J Dent 1997;25(6):459–73.

Sano H, Yoshikawa T, Pereira PN, Kanemura N, Morigami M, Tagami J, et al. Long-term durability of dentin bonds made with a self-etching primer, in vivo. J Dent Res 1999;78:906–11.

Santerre JP, Shajii L, Leung BW. Relation of dental composite formulations to their degradation and the release of hydrolyzed polymeric-resin-derived products. Crit Rev Oral Biol Med 2001;12(2):136–51.

Schmidt M, Kirkevang LL, Horsted-Bindslev P, Poulsen S. Marginal adaptation of a low-shrinkage silorane-based composite: 1-year randomized clinical trial. Clin Oral Investig 2011;15(2):291–5.

Sensi LG, Webley W. A simplified approach for layering composite resin restorations. Gen Dent 2007;55(7):638–45.

Shirai K, De Munck J, Yoshida Y, Inoue S, Lambrechts P, Suzuki K, et al. Effect of cavity configuration and aging on the bonding effectiveness of six adhesives to dentin. Dent Mater 2005;21(2):110–24.

Simecek JW, Diefenderfer KE, Cohen ME. An evaluation of replacement rates for posterior resin-based composite and amalgam restorations in U.S. Navy and marine corps recruits. J Am Dent Assoc 2009;140(2):200–9. quiz 249.

Singh V, Misra A, Marangos O, Park J, Ye Q, Kieweg SL, et al. Viscoelastic and fatigue properties of model methacrylate-based dentin adhesives. J Biomed Mater Res B Appl Biomater 2010;95(2):283–90.

Singh V, Misra A, Marangos O, Park J, Ye Q, Kieweg SL, et al. Fatigue life prediction of dentin-adhesive interface using micromechanical stress analysis. Dent Mater 2011;27(9):e187–195.
Soncini JA, Maserejian NN, Trachtenberg F, Tavares M, Hayes C. The longevity of amalgam versus compomer/composite restorations in posterior primary and permanent teeth: findings from the New England Children's Amalgam Trial. J Am Dent Assoc 2007;138(6):763–72.
Spencer P, Swafford JR. Unprotected protein at the dentin-adhesive interface. Quintessence Int 1999;30(7):501–7.
Spencer P, Wang Y. Adhesive phase separation at the dentin interface under wet bonding conditions. J Biomed Mater Res 2002;62(3):447–56.
Spencer P, Wang Y, Walker MP, Wieliczka DM, Swafford JR. Interfacial chemistry of the dentin/adhesive bond. Res Rep 2000;79(7):1458–63.
Spencer P, Wang Y, Walker MP, Swafford JR. Molecular Structure of acid-etched dentin smear layers- in situ study. J Dent Res 2001;80(9):1802–7.
Spencer P, Wang Y, Katz JL, Misra A. Physicochemical interactions at the dentin/adhesive interface using FTIR chemical imaging. J Biomed Opt 2005;10(3):031104.
Spencer P, Wang Y, Bohaty B. Interfacial chemistry of moisture-aged class II composite restorations. J Biomed Mater Res B Appl Biomater 2006;77(2):234–40.
Spencer P, Ye Q, Park J, Topp EM, Misra A, Marangos O, et al. Adhesive/Dentin interface: the weak link in the composite restoration. Ann Biomed Eng 2010;38(6):1989–2003.
Spencer P, Ye Q, Misra A, Goncalves SE, Laurence JS. Proteins, pathogens, and failure at the composite-tooth interface. J Dent Res 2014;93(12):1243–9.
Staninec M, Kim P, Marshall GW, Ritchie RO, Marshall SJ. Fatigue of dentin-composite interfaces with four-point bend. Dent Mater 2008;24(6):799–803.
Sumikawa DA, Marshall GW, Gee L, Marshall SJ. Microstructure of primary tooth dentin. Pediatr Dent 1999;21(7):439–44.
Svanberg M, Krasse B, Ornerfeldt HO. Mutans streptococci in interproximal plaque from amalgam and glass ionomer restorations. Caries Res 1990;24(2):133–6.
Tay FR, Pashley DH. Have dentin adhesives become too hydrophilic? J Can Dent Assoc 2003;69(11):726–31.
Ten Cate AR. Oral histology: development, structure, and function. St. Louis: Mosby; 1994.
Tyas MJ, Anusavice KJ, Frencken JE, Mount GJ. Minimal intervention dentistry–a review. FDI commission project 1-97. Int Dent J 2000;50(1):1–12.
Van Dijken JW. Direct resin composite inlays/onlays: an 11 year follow-up. J Dent 2000;28(5):299–306.
Van Ende A, Mine A, De Munck J, Poitevin A, Van Meerbeek B. Bonding of low-shrinking composites in high C-factor cavities. J Dent 2012;40(4):295–303.
Van Ende A, De Munck J, Van Landuyt KL, Poitevin A, Peumans M, Van Meerbeek B. Bulk-filling of high C-factor posterior cavities: effect on adhesion to cavity-bottom dentin. Dent Mater 2013;29(3):269–77.
Van Meerbeek B, Van Landuyt K, De Munck J, Hashimoto M, Peumans M, Lambrechts P, et al. Technique-sensitivity of contemporary adhesives. Dent Mater J 2005;24(1):1–13.
Versluis A, Tantbirojn D, Douglas WH. Do dental composites always shrink toward the light? J Dent Res 1998;77(6):1435–45.
Wang Y, Spencer P. Analysis of acid-treated dentin smear debris and smear layers using confocal Raman microspectroscopy. J Biomed Mater Res 2002;60(2):300–8.
Wang Y, Spencer P. Hybridization efficiency of the adhesive/dentin interface with wet bonding. J Dent Res 2003;82(2):141–5.
Wang Y, Spencer P. Continuing etching of an all-in-one adhesive in wet dentin tubules. J Dent Res 2005a;84(4):350–4.

Wang Y, Spencer P. Evaluation of the interface between one-bottle adhesive systems and dentin by Goldner's trichrome. Am J Dent 2005b;18(1):66–72.

Wang Y, Spencer P, Walker MP. Chemical profile of adhesive/caries-affected dentin interfaces using Raman microspectroscopy. J Biomed Mater Res A 2007a;81(2):279–86.

Wang Y, Spencer P, Yao X, Brenda B. Effect of solvent content on resin hybridization in wet dentin bonding. J Biomed Mater Res A 2007b;82(4):975–83.

Wiegand A, Attin T. Treatment of proximal caries lesions by tunnel restorations. Dent Mater 2007;23(12):1461–7.

Ye Q, Spencer P, Wang Y, Misra A. Relationship of solvent to the process, properties, and structure in model dentin adhesives. J Biomed Mater Res A 2007;80(2):342–50.

Ye Q, Park J, Topp E, Spencer P. Effect of photoinitiators on the in vitro performance of a dentin adhesive exposed to simulated oral environment. Dent Mater 2009a;25(4):452–8.

Ye Q, Wang Y, Spencer P. Nanophase separation of polymers exposed to simulated bonding conditions. J Biomed Mater Res B Appl Biomater 2009b;88(2):339–48.

Ye Q, Park J, Laurence JS, Parthasarathy R, Misra A, Spencer P. Ternary phase diagram of model dentin adhesive exposed to over-wet environments. J Dent Res 2011;90(12):1434–8.

Ye Q, Park J, Parthasarathy R, Pamatmat F, Misra A, Laurence JS, et al. Quantitative analysis of aqueous phase composition of model dentin adhesives experiencing phase separation. J Biomed Mater Res B Appl Biomater 2012;100(4):1086–92.

Reconstructions using alloys and ceramics

2

S.E.P. Gonçalves, E. Bresciani
São Paulo State University, São José dos Campos, São Paulo, Brazil

2.1 Introduction

A wide variety of materials are used in prosthetic dental reconstructions. These materials include metals such as gold, silver, palladium, chromium, cobalt, nickel, and titanium; ceramics, eg, feldspathic, lithium disilicate, aluminized, zirconia-based; resins; as well as various combinations of metal/ceramic or metal/resin [1]. There are a variety of properties that must be considered when selecting from this diverse spectrum of materials. The properties include hardness, fracture toughness, stress, wear resistance, and the ability to polish the material. These properties are important for even thin restorations (between 0.7 and 2.5 mm) [2,3]. Essential biological factors that must be considered include interactions with surrounding tissues, biocompatibility, and wear of the opposing dentition.

Metallic restorations offer advantages such as decreased tooth reduction, fracture resistance, adaptation, and polishing properties. Despite these advantages, patients frequently request metal-free reconstructions because of the superior esthetics. A similar shift has been noted in direct restorative procedures, eg, the frequent use of resin composite for posterior restorations as opposed to dental amalgam.

Prosthetic crown restorations can be bonded to the remaining tooth structure using various cements. The cements present highly variable compositions. Differences in cement line thickness, adhesion, biocompatibility, mechanical strength, sealing ability, and resistance to bacterial penetration at the crown/tooth interface are among the factors that must be considered when selecting a cement [4].

2.2 Overview of materials used in prosthetic restorations

João Maurício Ferraz – *Assistant Professor – Dental Materials and Prosthesis Department-Univ. Estadual Paulista – SP – Brazil – UNESP*

Choosing a material for prosthetic dental reconstructions depends on careful consideration of the benefits, advantages, and disadvantages associated with this choice [6].

Material-Tissue Interfacial Phenomena. http://dx.doi.org/10.1016/B978-0-08-100330-5.00002-9

2.2.1 Base metals

Base metal alloys do not present gold, silver, platinum, or palladium in their composition (Table 2.1) [7,8].

2.2.1.1 Nickel–chromium (Ni-Cr)

Nickel–chromium alloys gained importance in the 1930s due to the cost of gold. Ni-Cr alloys have adequate properties for use with ceramics. The hardness and elastic modulus of the Ni-Cr alloy allows for the use of a thinner cross-section of material; the thinner cross-section provides more space for porcelain veneering while still offering good resistance [9–12]. Another advantage is their linear thermal expansion coefficient, which is similar to that of veneering porcelain. The similarity in thermal expansion reduces the risk of cracks and fractures during processing [9,13,14]. Nickel sensitivity may be a concern with these alloys. The patient's sensitivity to nickel must be carefully and thoroughly evaluated when selecting these alloys.

2.2.1.2 Cobalt–chromium (Cr-Co)

Cobalt is the main component of Co-Cr alloys, while chromium improves strength and corrosion resistance, maintaining the alloy's brightness [15]. Chromium percentages greater than 30% lead to improper alloy casting and potentially, a brittle sigma phase, which will affect the alloy's properties [12,16]. Metals such as molybdenum, tungsten, and nickel may be added to Co-Cr alloys. The addition of these metals will change the properties of the Co-Cr alloys. Despite the similarity with Ni-Cr alloys, Co-Cr alloys present lower ductility and their thermal expansion coefficient is not compatible with porcelains [11,12,17–19].

2.2.1.3 Titanium (Ti)

Titanium-aluminum-vanadium (Ti-6Al-4V) is the most frequently used titanium alloy for dental and medical applications. With the exception of a lower modulus of elasticity, the Ti-6Al-4V alloy has properties that are similar to Ni-Cr and Co-Cr alloys. The low density of titanium results in lighter and more comfortable restorations [20]. Titanium alloys are resistant to corrosion and are considered highly biocompatible. These positive features and the absence of Ni and Cr make these alloys an excellent choice for patients who are sensitive or allergic to Ni and Cr [6,21].

2.2.2 Noble metals

Gold, platinum, palladium, ruthenium, iridium, and osmium are included in this category, with gold, palladium, and platinum being relevant to the dental castings (Table 2.2) [6].

2.2.2.1 Gold-platinum-palladium (Au-Pt-Pd)

Gold-platinum-palladium alloys were the first alloys used in metal–ceramic restorations. They were largely discontinued due to the introduction of cheaper alloys, with

Table 2.1 Features of base metal alloys

Material	Advantages	Disadvantages	Indications	Contraindications	Commercial brand
Nickel–chromium (Ni-Cr)	• Adequate hardness (400–1000 Mpa) • Elevated modulus of elasticity • Linear coefficient of thermal expansion similar to ceramics • Adequate resistance to corrosion • Low cost	• Hypersensitivity to nickel	• Single crowns • Partial fixed prosthesis • Infrastructures for partial fixed prosthesis	• Patients with hypersensitivity to nickel	Durabond, Resistal P, Nicrodent Fit Cast–SB Plus Ligga N
Chromium-cobalt (Cr-Co)	• Adequate resistance to corrosion • Adequate hardness (520–820 Mpa)	• Difficult casting • Lower ductility than Ni-Cr alloys • Linear coefficient of thermal expansion not similar to ceramics	• Single crowns • Partial fixed prosthesis • Infrastructures for partial fixed prosthesis • Patients allergic to nickel	• Technical quality	Fit Flex
Titanium (Ti)	• Light and comfortable to patients • Resistance to corrosion • Biocompatible	• High fusion temperature • Expensive casting process	• Metallic crowns • Metallic infrastructure • Implants • Allergic patients	• Cost–benefit ratio	Dan Ceramalloy

Table 2.2 **Features of noble metal alloys**

Material	Advantages	Disadvantages	Indications	Contraindications	Commercial brand
Gold–platinum–palladium (Au-Pt-Pd)	• Adequate marginal adaptation	• High cost • Low flexural strength (480–500 Mpa) • Low hardness	• Metallic crowns, • Metallic infrastructure for metal–ceramic crown	• Partial fixed prosthesis with more than 3 elements	P.S.LaCroix
Gold–palladium–silver (Au-Pd-Ag)	• Adequate flexural strength (650–680 Mpa) • Adequate hardness	• Silver might discolor the porcelain • High linear coefficient of thermal expansion	• Metallic crowns • Metallic infrastructure for metal–ceramic crown	• Anterior teeth	Aurobond
Gold–palladium (Au-Pd)	• Adequate resilience (700–730 Mpa)	• Linear coefficient of thermal expansion similar to some porcelains • Axial and circumferential strength on porcelain	• Metallic crowns • Metallic infrastructure for metal–ceramic crown	• Anterior teeth	Pioneer II
Silver–palladium (Pd-Ag)	• Economic option • Favorable modulus of elasticity among noble alloys • Flexural strength (530–750 Mpa)	• Ceramic discoloration	• Metallic crowns • Metallic infrastructure for metal–ceramic crown • Metallic posts	• Anterior teeth	Palliag, Albacast

improved mechanical properties and greater flexural strength. Gold is the most abundant metal within the alloy (88%), whereas concentrations of platinum and palladium are variable. Small amounts of base metals are also reported [8].

2.2.2.2 Gold-palladium-silver (Au-Pd-Ag)

Gold-palladium-silver alloys were introduced to overcome the disadvantages of Au-Pt-Pd, including high cost, low hardness, and low bending resistance. Silver and palladium percentages vary within the alloy. The alloys are categorized into those with high and low amounts of silver [6,22,23]. The limitations associated with sliver-containing alloys include porcelain discoloration and mismatch in terms of the coefficient of thermal expansion.

2.2.2.3 Gold-palladium (Au-Pd)

Gold–palladium alloys were developed to address limitations associated with the silver-containing alloys. The composition of Au-Pd alloys ranges from 44% to 55% gold and from 35% to 45% palladium. The major disadvantage is the thermal expansion ratio, which is incompatible with that of some porcelain. An incompatibility in the thermal expansion ratio results in axial and circumferential tension in the porcelain during cooling. To address this issue, Au-Pd alloys with a low concentration of silver (<5%) have been developed [22–25].

2.2.2.4 Silver-palladium (Ag-Pd)

Silver-palladium alloys were introduced in the mid-1970s. They represented the first noble metal alloy with no gold in their composition. These alloys offered a more economical option when compared with the gold alloys. They were designed to improve operational problems, namely, difficulty in casting and porcelain adhesion. There are currently two types of Ag-Pd alloys, one having 55–60% Pd, 28–30% Ag, indium, and/or tin and the other type having less Pd (50–55%), more silver (35–40%), tin, and little to no indium [22–24,26].

2.2.3 Ceramics

Dental ceramics present favorable properties like compressive strength and wear resistance, thermal conductivity, and optical similarity to dental tissues. They also offer advantageous properties such as radiopacity, marginal integrity, color stability, and biocompatibility. Many systems have been developed. The overarching objective of the development of these various systems is an improvement in properties that will ultimately provide increased durability and clinical lifetime for the ceramic restoration (Table 2.3).

2.2.3.1 Feldspathic

Feldspathic were pioneer ceramics fabricated by high fusion. They are composed of quartz, feldspar, and kaolin. They provide excellent esthetic properties, with adequate opacity and translucency obtained by alterations of the mixture components. They are

Table 2.3 **Ceramics**

Material	Advantages	Disadvantages	Indications	Contraindications	Commercial brand
Feldspathic ceramics	• Esthetic properties	• Low strength (50–90 Mpa)	• Covering porcelain in metal/ceramic crowns • Veneers	• Areas of great occlusal stresses	• VITABLOCS Mark II • VITABLOC TriLuxe bloc
Leucite-reinforced feldspathic ceramics	• Increased strength (180 Mpa)	• Required minimum thickness	• Veneers • Inlay/onlay • Single crowns	• High-strength scenarios • Partial fixed prosthesis • Bruxism	• IPS Empress I • IPS ProCAD
Lithium disilicate–reinforced feldspathic ceramics	• Strength between 400 and 440 MPa	• Glass phase less resistant, leading to microcracks over time	• Inlay/onlay • Single crowns • Veneers • 3-element partial fixed prosthesis—up to premolar	• Partial fixed prosthesis in premolar • Bruxism	• IPS Empress II • IPS e.max Press
Aluminized ceramics	• Greater strength than feldspathic ceramics (120–180 Mpa)	• Esthetics—translucency loss • Crack propagation	• Partial fixed prosthesis in areas of low tension	• Veneers • Partial fixed prosthesis in areas of high tension	• In-Ceram Alumina
Glass-infiltrated aluminized ceramics	• Improved strength	• Esthetics—light transmission • Crack propagation	• Single crowns and posterior or anterior partial fixed prostheses • Personalized abutments for implants	• Veneers • Areas of demanding translucency	• Procera

Zirconia-based ceramics	• High strength (700 Mpa) • Clinical longevity • Biocompatibility • Radiopacity	• Opacity	• Full crowns and posterior partial fixed prosthesis	• Anterior crowns and veneer • Areas of demanding translucency	• In-Ceram Zirconia
Yttria-stabilized zirconia ceramics (Y-TZP)	• High fracture strength (900–1200 Mpa) • Excellent mechanical properties • Esthetics • Biocompatibility, low modulus of elasticity	• Opacity	• Infrastructure for partial fixed prosthesis (3–8 elements) • Metallic bar for overdentures	• Anterior crowns and veneer • Areas of demanding translucency	• InLava • Cercon

currently widely used in extremely thin laminates during smile esthetic recovery, with this application the underlying tooth reinforces the laminate [27].

2.2.3.2 Feldspathic with lithium disilicate

These ceramics evolved from feldspathic by incorporation of interlocking lithium disilicate crystals dispersed in a glassy matrix. This change in the composition of the feldspathic ceramic led to an improvement in mechanical properties without compromising the optical properties. They are composed of quartz, lithium dioxide, phosphoric oxide, alumina, and potassium oxide [27].

2.2.3.3 Aluminized ceramics

Aluminized ceramics originated by the incorporation of metallic oxides. The fracture resistance of these ceramics is approximately double that of conventional ceramics. Light transmission is limited due to the alumina crystals, and resistance is not sufficient to indicate the use of these materials for posterior prostheses. Recently, glass-infiltrated aluminized ceramic with high content of alumina offered improved resistance, increasing their indication for both anterior and posterior regions as well as for fabrication of single crowns and partial fixed dentures. The possibility of custom abutment fabrication is also important [28–31].

2.2.3.4 Zirconia

Adding zirconium oxide to ceramics resulted in increased flexural strength, higher toughness values, and increased resistance to crack propagation. Zirconia-based ceramics contain 69% aluminum oxide and 31% zirconium oxide. Its indications are limited to posterior regions, for single crowns or three-element fixed prostheses. Zirconia is currently the best option for infrastructure of larger metal-free fixed prostheses, due to excellent mechanical properties, good clinical longevity, radiopacity, and biocompatibility.

2.2.3.5 Yttria-stabilized zirconia

Yttria-stabilized zirconia (Y-TZP) was developed to overcome crack propagation presented by aluminized ceramics. Yttrium dioxide is added to pure zirconia to stabilize the tetragonal phase at room temperature, resulting in a polyphasic material known as stabilized zirconia. The stabilized tetragonal phase is responsible for high fracture toughness and increased flexural strength (900–1200 MPa).

2.2.4 Cements

The success of indirect restorations relies on correct material selection, and also on the cement used to bond the restoration to tooth structure (Table 2.4).

2.2.4.1 Zinc phosphate

Zinc phosphate cements have been used for decades, with high success rates. For this reason, they are the standard cement for assessing clinical efficacy. Although the

Table 2.4 **Cements**

Material	Advantages	Disadvantages	Indications	Contraindications	Commercial brand
Zinc phosphate cement	• Standard cement • Longevity • High initial strength • Adequate compression strength • Low cost	• No chemical adhesion • Low tensile strength	• Metallic inlay/onlay • Metal–ceramic feldspathic full crowns • Metal prefabricated or customized post • Partial fixed prosthesis	• Low retentive preparations	• Zinc cement–SS white • Cement LS-Coltene
GIC	• Friendly handling • Fluidity • Adhesion to tooth structure and metals • Fluoride release and uptake • Adequate translucency • Adequate strength • Relative low cost	• Initial solubility • Sensibility to humidity	• Metallic crowns • Metal–ceramic crowns • High strength metal-free crowns (alumina and zirconia)	• Intraradicular posts • Partial fixed prosthesis in areas of high occlusal load	• Vidrion C – (SS White)
Resin-modified GIC	• Similar to GIC • Less soluble • Improved compressive and diametral strength	• Initial solubility • Sensibility to humidity	• Metallic restorations • Metal–ceramic and high-strength metal-free crowns (alumina and zirconia)	• Metal-free ceramic restorations, susceptible to erosion • Intraradicular post—due to hygroscopic expansion	• Vitremer • Vitrebond
Resin cements	• Versatility • Adequate tensile and compressive strength • Low solubility • Esthetics.	• Hard excess removal • Sensitive adhesive technique • High cost • If restorations removal is needed	• Metal-free and veneer restorations • Metal restorations, metal–ceramic crowns in low-retentive preparations • Glass posts	• Areas where light does not reach	• RelyX Unicem • Panavia • Variolink II • Variolink Veneer • Relyx ART

GIC, glass ionomer cement.

cement does not offer either covalent or ionic bonding to the tooth, mechanical retention and high initial strength makes these materials suitable for cementing indirect restorations. The properties of the zinc phosphate cements may be influenced by powder/liquid ratio, mixing temperature, and presence of moisture [32,33].

2.2.4.2 Glass ionomer

Glass ionomer (GI) cements are also an excellent choice for cementing indirect restorations. The positive properties of the GI cement could be negatively influenced by changes in powder/liquid ratio and contact with moisture. Excess moisture during the cementation process leads to marginal cement loss, whereas excessive dry conditions might result in microcracks [32,33].

2.2.4.3 Resin-modified glass ionomer

These cements are more promising for cementing indirect restorations due to the incorporation of a light-activated component. They are less soluble and present higher compressive and tensile strengths, resulting in a lower susceptibility to erosion during the initial phase of cementation. The adhesive and film thickness properties are similar to conventional GI cements. Moisture control should, however, be maintained to avoid marginal losses [32,33].

2.2.4.4 Resin cements

Resin cements were introduced in the 1950s. They form a polymeric matrix that could eventually fill and seal any gap at the tooth/restoration interface. Resin cementation helps to dissipate stresses and to reduce microcrack formation at the inner portion of ceramic restorations [34,35]. Initially, resin cements presented low adhesion to tooth structure due to substantial polymerization shrinkage. They also presented high coefficient of thermal expansion and water absorption, which contributed to greater chance of microleakage. The removal of excess cement was difficult. The primary advantage of these cements was their low solubility [36].

Resin cements can be classified according to the process of matrix formation and adhesive technique, ie, matrix formation: self-cured, light cured, and dual, and adhesive technique: total etch (acid+ adhesive + cement), one step (acid/adhesive+cement), and self-etching (cement). Overall, total etch cements show excellent results and are currently preferred. If the main substrate is dentin, one-step cements are the most suitable [32]. Self-etching cements can be used for cementing crowns, both ceramic (alumina and zirconia) and metalloceramic crowns.

2.3 Clinical indications: philosophical context

Clovis Pagani –*Professor – Restorative Dentistry Department – Univ. Estadual Paulista – SP – Brazil – UNESP*
Hilton Riquieri – *PhD student – Graduate Program – Univ. Estadual Paulista – SP – Brazil – UNESP*

Eduardo Galera da Silva – *Assistant Professor – Social and Pediatric Dentistry Department-Univ. Estadual Paulista – SP – Brazil – UNESP*
Guilherme Siqueira Ferreira Saavedra – *Assistant Professor – Dental Materials and Prosthesis Department – Univ. Estadual Paulista – SP – Brazil – UNESP*

Conventional indirect prostheses include metal or ceramic restorations that replace lost structures of anterior or posterior teeth. Tooth loss may be partial or total. The selected material must restore the natural appearance, shape, and function.

2.3.1 Material selection

A number of factors must be considered when selecting materials for indirect prostheses. Patient characteristics that must be considered include proper maintenance and efficient oral hygiene, size and location of the restoration, presence of parafunctional habits and masticatory loads, and systemic conditions, eg, ulcer/gastrointestinal bulimia, reflux, anorexia, and citric food consumption. Dental professionals must consider their technical knowledge from treatment planning to execution of operative and restorative protocols. Materials-related factors include biocompatibility, toughness, wear resistance, moisture tolerance, dimensional stability, adhesion properties, and color stability.

The increased demand for esthetics might be attributed to several factors, such as improved technology of resin composites, the development of adhesive systems, as well as the training and experience of dental professionals. Furthermore, esthetics has become important from social, emotional, and professional perspectives; eg a harmonious smile is fundamental for interpersonal relationships. Recent advances in dental materials led to the introduction of several ceramic systems: feldspar, leucite, lithium disilicate, lithium silicate reinforced by zirconia, and zirconia, among others. Ceramic restorations have increasingly replaced conventional restorations, mainly due to esthetics and possible adhesion to dental substrates.

The clinical predictability of ceramic restorations depends on several factors including tooth preparation. Preparation should follow tooth anatomical configuration with minimum required reduction. The uniformity of tooth reduction ensures greater resistance to fracture and increases the longevity of indirect restorations [37]. For metal indirect restorations, less tooth reduction is required; this is related to the resistance of metals even with low thicknesses (0.7–1.5 mm thickness in metallic restorations would be adequate depending on the position of the tooth in the mouth). For ceramics, tooth reduction should not be less than 1.5 mm in the posterior region, imposing greater wear for achieving resistance requirements of the employed material. Tooth preparation for anterior indirect ceramic restorations, eg, veneers and lumineers, allows more conservative reduction, ranging from 0.5 to 1 mm.

2.3.2 Metal and ceramic indirect restorations

The physiological behavior of sound natural tooth is the result of close and balanced relationships between biological, mechanical, functional, and esthetic parameters. Knowledge and understanding of enamel structure, a brittle tissue adhered to resilient dentin, allows for a greater appreciation and recognition of the property requirements for dental restorative materials [5].

In many clinical situations, partial or whole tooth may be restored, but a question remains: which technique and/or material offers the best choice based on the clinical conditions? Esthetic dentistry considers that, regardless of the esthetic coating used, a work that mimics the tooth structure, with imperceptible interface, is one of excellence [38]. A new restorative concept has emerged with the advent of adhesive systems, where restoration and remaining tooth become a monoblock [38].

Feldspar ceramic was always known as a very brittle material. At present, it is extensively used, even in small thicknesses. What has changed? Thin feldspathic porcelain veneers are bonded to tooth structures, acquiring characteristics of a monoblock. If we correlate this thought to tooth characteristics, where enamel is also very brittle but when adhered to resilient dentin provides adequate mechanical properties for the tooth, one can understand that adhesive dentistry associated with ceramics tries to mimic the mechanical and esthetic properties of natural tooth.

Lost-wax casting technique, widely used for metallic restorations, is also used to fabricate precision metal-free restorations (Fig. 2.1).

The development of computer-aided design/computer-aided manufacturing (CAD/CAM) technology has revolutionized the restoration replacement process using indirect techniques. The type of materials and laboratory processes used to manufacture especially crowns, fixed partial denture abutments, and implants has changed with the introduction of this technology. Restorative options for traditional metal–ceramic and all-ceramic prostheses obtained by injection have migrated to rehabilitation using restorations with infrastructure in zirconia. The tendency of this system is to spread and succeed, becoming a viable treatment modality for the future of the profession [37,39,40] (Figs. 2.2–2.5).

The industry suggests the selection of materials that integrate with automated equipment to shorten production time, simplify manufacturing, and reduce labor costs. The approach suggested by industry, ie, integration of material choices with automated equipment, offers advantages like milling accuracy and adaptation of restorations. Additionally, wax blocks are available for milling of individual crowns and partial fixed prostheses infrastructures. The wax burns without leaving residues.

Many companies are marketing multicolor ceramic blocks for milling. They present different layers of translucency to enhance the esthetics of the final restoration. Initially, the use of presintered monochromatic ceramic blocks was solely indicated for single posterior restoration (monochromatic) [31–41].

Ceramic materials used for CAD/CAM technology can be classified, based on their chemical composition, as feldspathic, aluminized or vitreous ceramics, or simply as ceramics for "milled crown and infrastructure." Different ceramic materials, namely, aluminized, presintered, and glass ceramics based on leucite, lithium disilicate, or lithium silicate with zirconia, are produced in sheets or blocks that are adaptable to various milling systems and the dimension of the prosthesis to be manufactured [5,42].

2.4 Implant-supported restorations

Maria Aparecida Neves Jardini – *Associate Professor Diagnosis and Surgery Department – Univ. Estadual Paulista – SP – Brazil – UNESP*

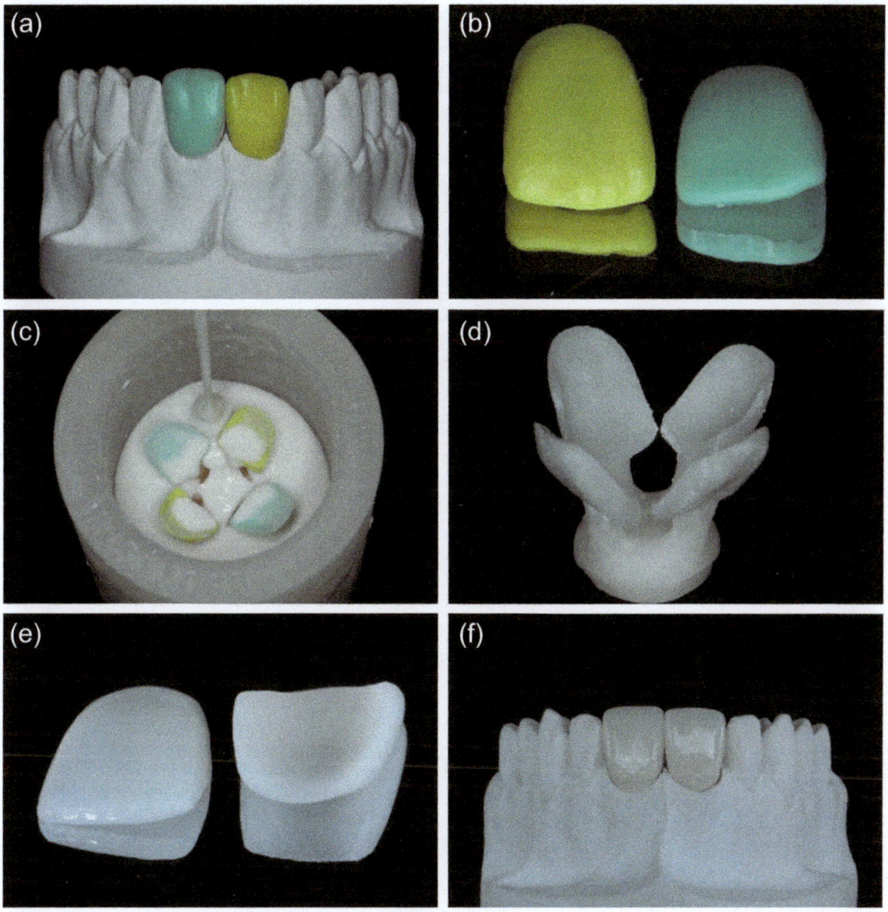

Figure 2.1 Functional waxing (a and b), laboratory stages (c and d) and final restorations (e and f) obtained by injection of lithium disilicate/e.max Press, Ivoclar Vivadent. Note the reproducibility of dental morphology achieved by the injection technique and computer-aided design/computer-aided manufacturing technology.

Antônio Braulino de Melo Filho – *Assistant Professor – Social and Pediatric Dentistry Department – Univ. Estadual Paulista – SP – Brazil – UNESP*

Osseointegration is generally described as a direct functional and structural connection between bone and implant surface [43]. This concept has offered benefits for patients receiving dental implants [44–48].

2.4.1 Implant indications: complete edentulous patients

Implants were initially indicated for completely edentulous patients. Previous rehabilitation for this condition was complete muco-supported prosthesis. The muco-supported prosthesis was often plagued by problems such as limited retention

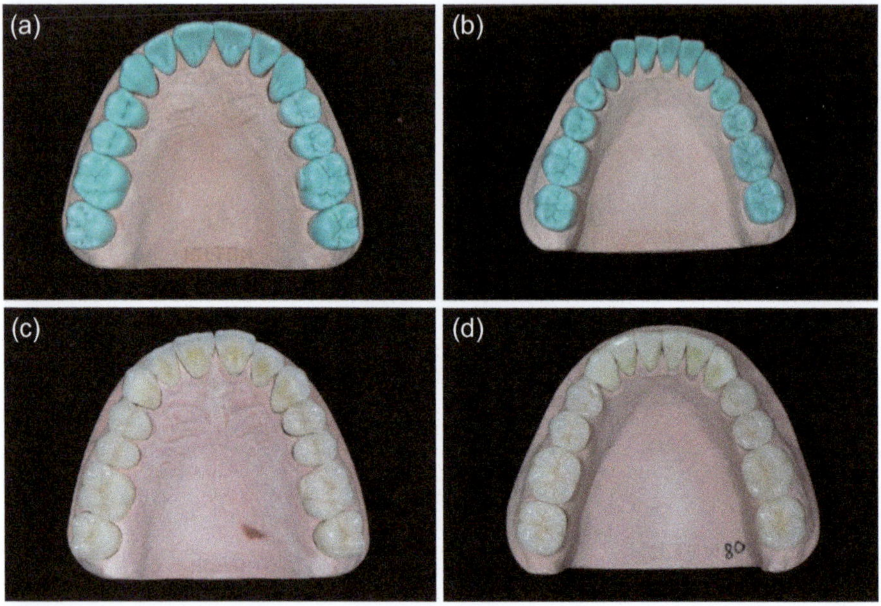

Figure 2.2 Functional waxing (a and b) and final restoration (c and d) of a complete rehabilitation. Note reproducibility of dental morphology achieved by the injection technique and CAD/CAM technology.

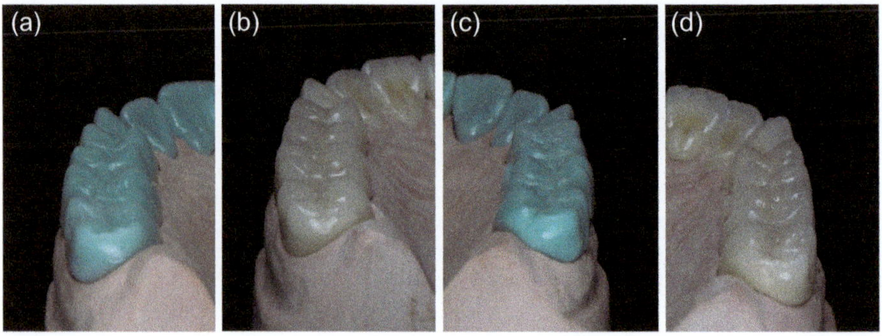

Figure 2.3 Cusp inclination, and anterior–posterior and laterolateral curves (a to d).

and stability. The prosthesis could be uncomfortable, and patients often expressed dissatisfaction with the muco-supported prosthesis.

The first implant cases, reported 20 years after implant development, used screw-shaped pure titanium implants that were 3.7 mm in diameter and 10 mm in length. Those characteristics allowed implants that could be used in the majority of edentulous jaws, regardless of the remaining bone volume and/or topography. A total of four–six implants were used with adequate support for prosthesis [49].

The implant technique evolved, due to scenarios requiring complex techniques, such as nerve transposition and bone grafts at the posterior region of the maxilla

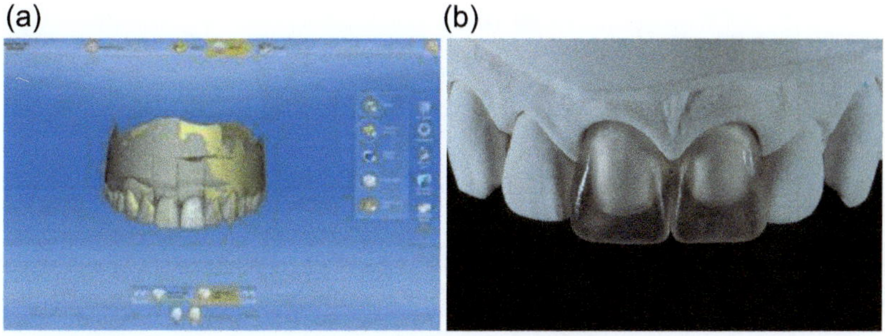

Figure 2.4 Planning using Software 4.2.5 in Lab (Sirona, Germany) (a) and indirect restorations milled in lithium silicate reinforced by precrystallized zirconia (b) (VITA, Germany).

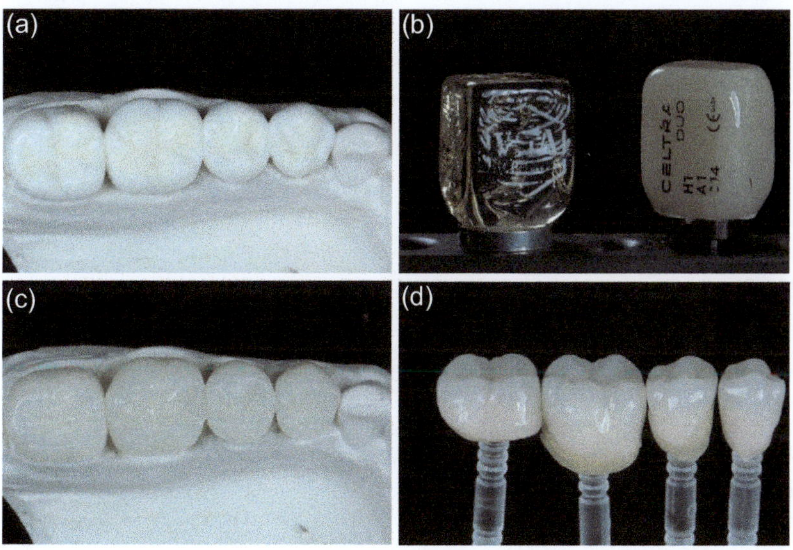

Figure 2.5 Functional waxing (a), restorative materials composed of lithium silicate reinforced by zirconia in different stages of crystallization (b) (Suprinity, VITA; and Celtra Duo, Dentsply), and final restorations before (c) and during the extrinsic pigmentation process.

and mandible. Currently, a solution for such situations is the "All-on-4" concept, developed by Paulo Malo [50]. This technique employs straight and angled microunit implants for immediate rehabilitation of edentulous patients. Four implants, two vertically placed at the anterior region and two placed at 45° inclination at the posterior region, are used. Angled implants lead to adequate bone anchorage with no interference with mental foramen in the mandible and sinus in the maxilla [50,51].

Zygomatic supported implants represent another option for posterior maxilla anchorage [52], with the advantage of maintaining sinus integrity and not requiring bone graft. Retrospective studies have reported 96–98% success rates at 12-year follow-up (Figs. 2.6–2.9) [53,54].

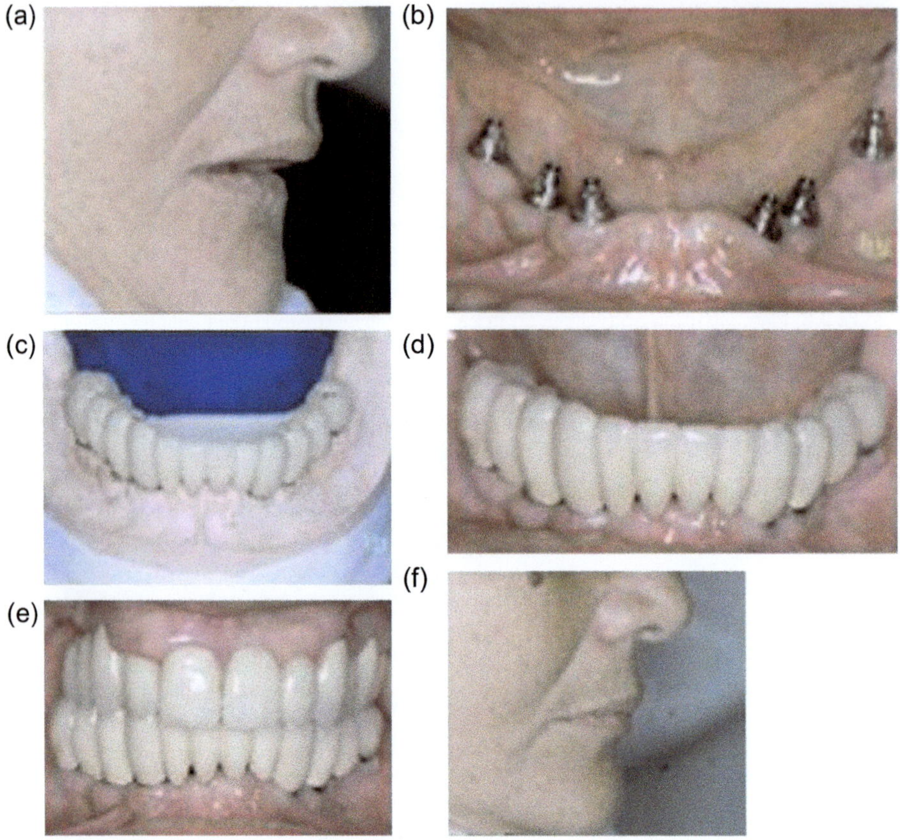

Figure 2.6 Mandible rehabilitation with implant-supported complete prosthesis (a to d), restoring function (e) and esthetics (f) for a 65-year-old patient.

2.4.2 Partially edentulous patients

Partially edentulous areas were restored with partial fixed or removable prostheses, according to the characteristics of abutment teeth. Most often, sound or minimally restored teeth were prepared and worn for prosthesis support.

Single or multiple edentulous spaces are currently rehabilitated with implant-supported prostheses. This scenario represents a new challenge for oral implantology. Occlusion, periodontal condition, spatial relationships, functional demands, and esthetics are some of the key requirements for implant rehabilitation success [45].

The great demand for implant rehabilitation has led to modifications of the installation arsenal of implants and prostheses, with focus on clinical practice. Similarly, additional examinations such as X-rays, computed tomography, and study models are being increasingly used to provide data for detailed treatment planning.

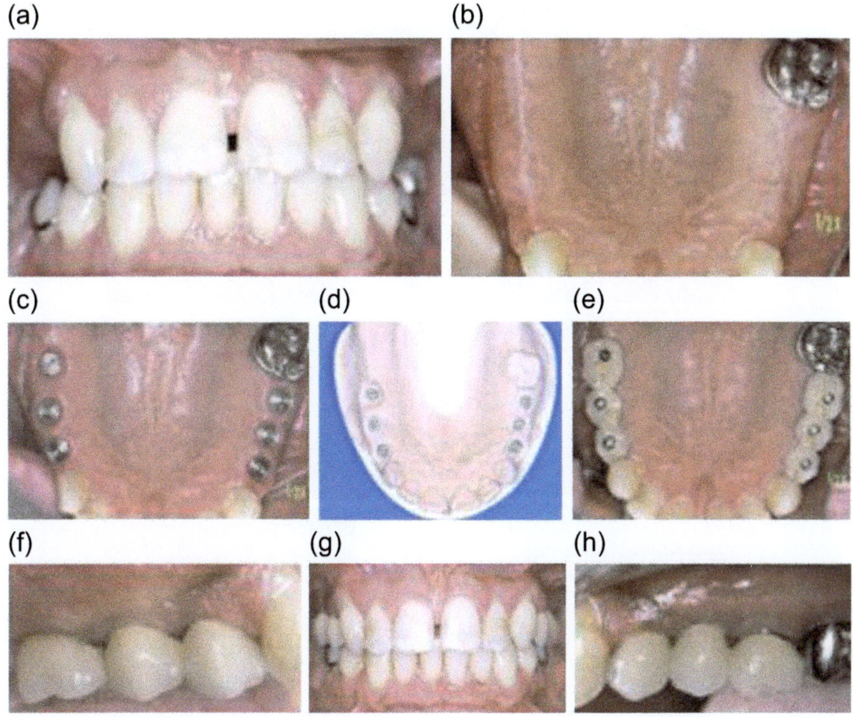

Figure 2.7 Patient with partial removable prosthesis, rehabilitated with implants (a to h).

2.4.3 Multiple teeth

The absence of several teeth, previously treated by partial fixed or removable prosthesis, might be rehabilitated with implant-supported prosthesis, with the major advantage being the maintenance of natural teeth [55]. Retrospective studies [56,57] evaluated the use of implants in partially edentulous anterior areas with encouraging results. The posterior region is reported to be more challenging as the presence of bone ridge resorption, inferior alveolar nerve or sinus, presence of cancellous bone and more intense occlusal forces might lead to impaired biomechanical long-term success of implant-supported restorations [58].

Lekholm et al. (2006) reported a 20-year follow-up study of posterior implants. The authors concluded that titanium implants work properly, even for extensively fixed reconstructions. The success rate in that study was around 91%.

2.4.4 Single tooth

Implant-supported prosthesis rehabilitation of a single tooth is indicated in cases of trauma, tooth longitudinal fracture and endodontic treatment failure. Single-tooth implant-supported prosthesis in the posterior region of the mouth

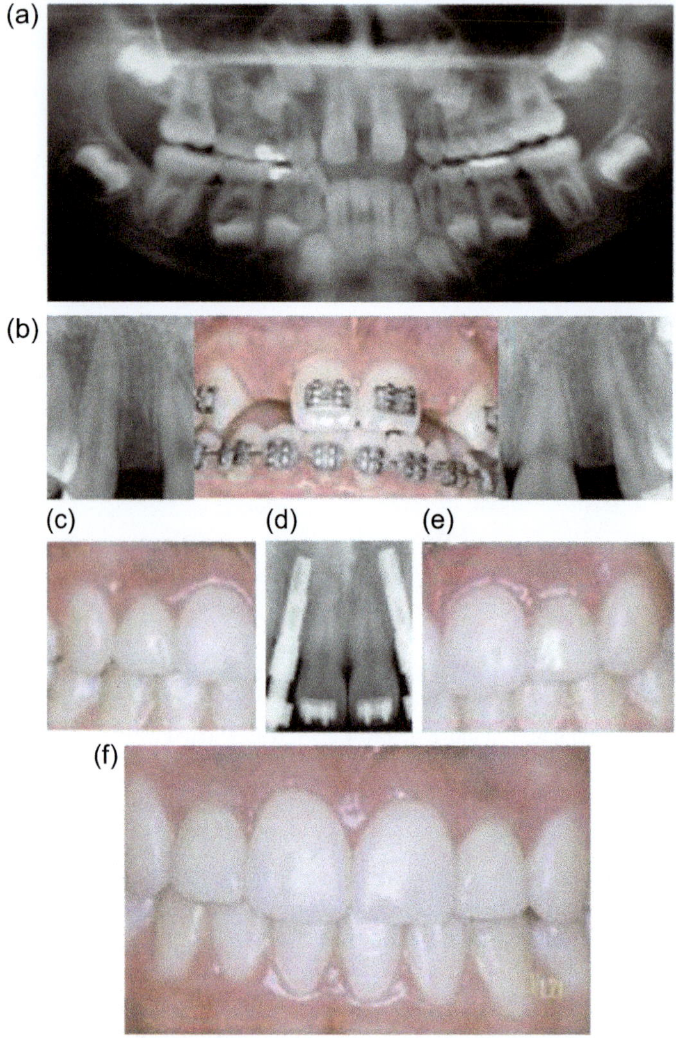

Figure 2.8 Anodontia of lateral maxillary incisors in a 9-year-old patient (a). Orthodontic treatment (b) and implant rehabilitation were performed. Implant placement and prostheses fabrication at the age of 19 years (c to f).

is subjected to more occlusal forces. Problems such as loosening of crowns or implant or the fracture of various components were initially reported. Changes in implant format, with larger diameters and/or internal fixation, addressed many of these problems.

Esthetics is a challenge for anterior single-implant rehabilitation. Factors like gingival smile line, bone width, periodontal biotype, and patients' expectations must be assessed. Henry et al. reported 96% success rate for single implants in the anterior area [59]. The placement of dental implants in the esthetic areas has little room for error.

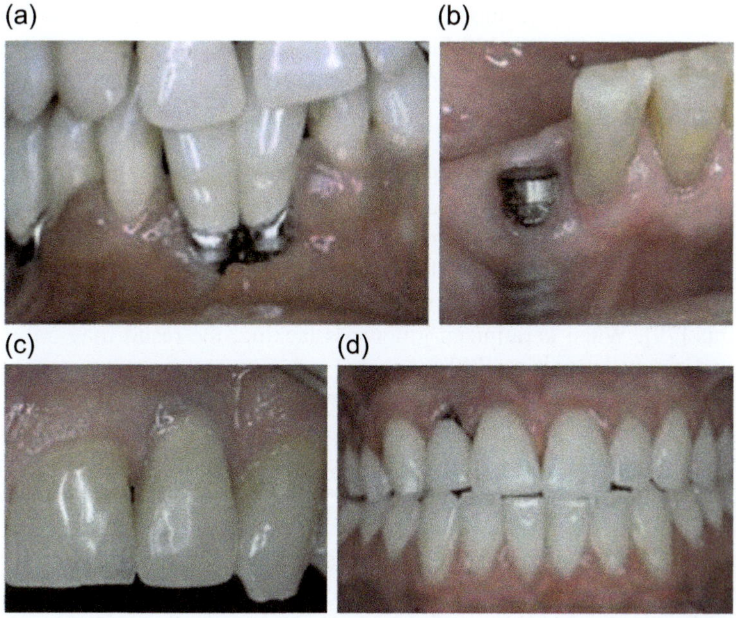

Figure 2.9 (a) Inadequate positioning of implants associated with inadequate biofilm control, resulting in peri-implantitis. (b) Inadequate positioning of implant with consequent metal exposure. (c) Alteration of color of mucosa resulted from implant positioning. (d) Presence of mucositis associated with gingival recession.

A subtle error in implant positioning or incorrect handling of soft or hard tissue might lead to esthetic failure and patient dissatisfaction [60–62].

2.4.5 Failures

Despite the high success index of osseointegrated implants, complications of a biologic, functional, or esthetic nature may occur [63–65]. Clinical studies [44,66] reported bone crest loss ranging on an average from 0.9 to 1.6 mm during the first year in service. Annual bone loss in subsequent years ranged from 0.05 to 0.13 mm. Thus, an average annual loss of bone crest lower than 0.2 mm might be one criterion for implant success [63].

Implant rehabilitation is currently the first choice, and the number of annually placed implants in the United States can reach 3 million (http://www.aaid.com). The diversification of implant-supported restorations such as single crowns, fixed partial denture, complete prosthesis, or overdentures possibly led to increased complications [63,67].

Biological complications, which are generally inflammatory in nature, impact the soft and hard tissues approximating the implants. Peri-implant diseases were defined during the First European Workshop on Periodontology [68] as inflammatory processes of tissues around dental implants. They are peri-implant mucositis, an inflammatory reaction in soft tissues around implants without bone loss, and peri-implantitis, an inflammation of implant-surrounded mucosa associated with bone loss [69].

Scientific evidence has demonstrated direct correlation between oral microbial flora and peri-implant diseases [70,71]. However, smoking and systemic diseases also appear to have a direct influence on peri-implant diseases [72]. Other factors such as diabetes, genetic factors, periodontal disease, and poor oral hygiene also contribute to peri-implantitis [73–76]. Treatment strategies should be developed based on careful and thorough consideration of these factors.

Esthetic complications involving the implant surrounding soft tissue, namely, gingival recession and lack of gingival papilla, have been reported [77]. Recent clinical studies reported that extended keratinized gingiva offers better preservation of soft and hard tissues [78] and provides more favorable long-term maintenance of dental implants [79]. When keratinized gingiva is lacking, the result may be poor oral hygiene and gingival recession [80].

Periodontal plastic surgery procedures can be performed at the second stage of implant procedure or after placing the prosthetic unit. This surgery may be done to improve the possibility of keratinized gingiva in proximity of the implant. Frequently, this will lead to better esthetic results regarding gingival color and presence of interdental papilla [81]. Results from clinical studies do not support the concept that thicker peri-implant gingiva leads to long-term success and survival rates.

Functional complications are related, in part, to the materials that are used. Material fatigue from repeated forces leads to implant and/or prosthesis fracture and prosthesis screw loosening.

Complications resulting from fracture of prosthesis materials, such as acrylic resin or ceramic, can be easily solved. On the other hand, implant fracture is the worst mechanical failure resulting in implant and prosthesis loss. Implant fracture is due to three main causes [82]: design and materials, nonpassive prosthesis fit, and physiological or biomechanical overload.

Esthetic complications are difficult to solve due to patient's expectation. They are mostly related to implant positioning, gingival recession with implant metal exposure, absence of interdental papilla, discrepancies in tooth shape, and mucosa discoloration [62,67].

2.4.6 Implant maintenance

A key factor for long-term success of dental implants is the maintenance of healthy peri-implant tissues, mainly by means of effective daily oral hygiene. There are effective strategies for cleaning the tissues surrounding the implant. The strategies include the use of soft, interproximal, and electric toothbrushes, as well as dental floss for proper cleaning of the less accessible areas. The adjunct use of antimicrobial agents, such as chlorhexidine, has been recommended [83].

Professional maintenance, associated with home care, should be performed periodically. Metallic instruments are not recommended for mechanical debridement, biofilm, and calculus removal from implant/abutment surfaces. The metallic instruments may damage the implant surface; this could lead to an increase in bacterial colonization of the implant surface. As opposed to metallic instruments, the recommended procedures include rubber cup polishing with abrasive paste, use of plastic or titanium curettes, and subgingival irrigation with antimicrobial agents [83].

2.5 Dental preparation, adaptation, and cementation of indirect restorations

Clovis Pagani –*Professor – Restorative Dentistry Department – Univ. Estadual Paulista – SP – Brazil – UNESP*
Hilton Riquieri – *PhD student – Graduate Program – Univ. Estadual Paulista – SP – Brazil – UNESP*
Eduardo Galera da Silva –*Assistant Professor – Social and Pediatric Dentistry Department- Univ. Estadual Paulista – SP – Brazil – UNESP*
Guilherme Siqueira Ferreira Saavedra – *Assistant Professor – Dental Materials and Prosthesis Department – Univ. Estadual Paulista – SP – Brazil – UNESP*

2.5.1 Preparation

Clinical planning by the dentist in conjunction with laboratory technician should be performed prior to the restorative phase. The clinical planning should follow the principles described by Shillingburg: preservation of tooth structure, retention and resistance, structural durability, marginal integrity, and periodontal preservation [84,85].

Mechanical (retention and stability) and biological (complex preservation of dentin pulp) principles should be considered for adequate tooth preparation. Due to advances in materials, which include more predictable adhesive bonding procedures, tooth preparation can be performed more conservatively. This leads to preservation of the tooth structure and maintenance of effectiveness and resistance of restoration [5].

The design and finish line of preparations vary according to baseline clinical condition, shape, and arrangement of sound hard tissues. Adequate finish line of preparation is determined by specific diamond burs, which also provide optimal shape and taper of preparations. Those characteristics are linked to adaptation and resistance of materials selected for metallic or ceramic prosthetic restorations. Metal restorations require beveled finish line, which allows a more precise adjustment in small thicknesses. Ceramic restorations require chamfer or right-angled terminations (Fig. 2.10).

2.5.2 Adaptation

As mentioned in the Table 2.2, gold remains the material providing better marginal fit, leading to considerable longevity. Metal alloys, like Ni-Cr, Ag-Pd, or even pure Ag, also provide adequate marginal fit with thin termination, ensuring good relationship with the surrounding soft tissues.

The adaptation of ceramics is more critical and generally, a very specialized laboratory is required for their fabrication. Adaptation often depends on the resin cement used for cementation, and this could risk restoration longevity. The cement line is the weak link between tooth structure and indirect restoration.

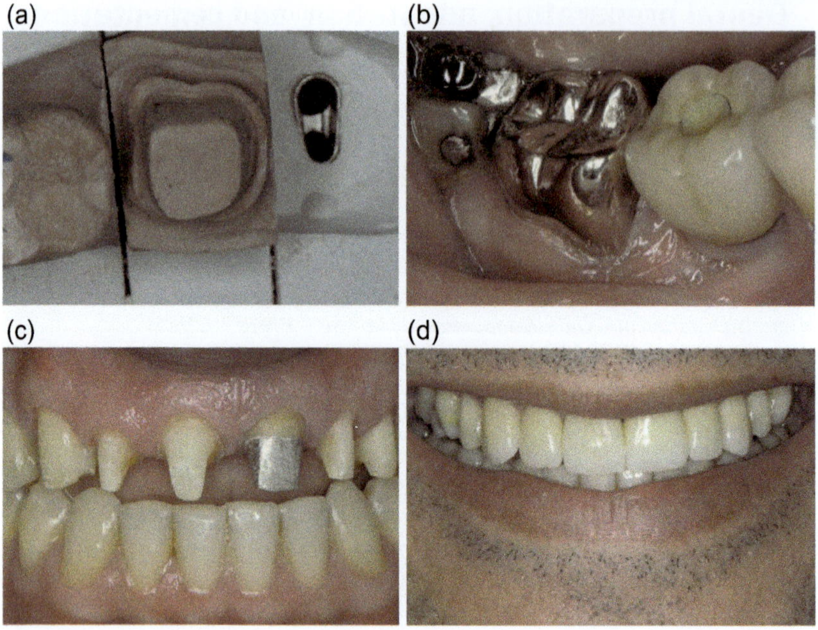

Figure 2.10 (a) A tooth preparation with beveled chamfer finishing line. (b) The adapted metal restoration in a clinical view. (c) Several preparations with chamfer finishing line, indicated for metal-free crowns. (d) The esthetic clinical aspect of cemented restorations.

2.5.3 Cementation

The development of metal-free materials led to the expression of different philosophies toward cementation. Zinc phosphate cement has been the gold standard for almost a century, with high success rates in metallic restorations, but limited success for esthetic restorations. When zinc phosphate cement is used, tensions are distributed at the restoration/tooth interface, which predisposes the restoration to fracture. It is thus important to select the cementing agent according to its characteristics.

The cementing procedure has been described as the "Achilles heel" in metallic, nonmetallic, and mixed indirect restorations. Cementation is often underestimated mainly due to the complexity of other steps and the apparent simple aspects of cementation.

Cementing is an extremely important factor among the steps of the whole restorative process, taking into consideration the success of indirect restoration and regardless of the chosen material. Materials used for cementation are responsible for adhesion between tooth structures (substrate) and restorative material (metallic and nonmetallic). For adequate clinical, functional, and esthetic performances and longevity of these restorations, the properties and type of cements should be considered. The choice for the right cement for a particular type of restorative material and clinical scenario is based on the characteristics of the ideal cement. According to Wilson et al.

[86], the ideal cementing agent should present the following features: high resistance to compressive, tensile and shear stresses; adhesion to both tooth structure and restoration; biocompatibility and cariostatic activity; low solubility in oral fluids; adequate working time and fast setting after the procedure; esthetics; low viscosity; and minimal film thickness.

Film thickness is a key property of cementing agent, as it will influence the fit and proper marginal adaptation of restorations. As a general principle, a lower thickness of the cement translates to a greater retention of the restoration. According to American Dental Association (ADA) specification No. 8, type 1 cements used for this purpose should allow a maximum thickness of 20 μm [87]. Still, lower film thickness, lower marginal infiltration, and greater longevity are reported.

Cements were reviewed in detail in the Section 2.2 of this chapter. For continuity, the cements are discussed briefly in this section.

Zinc phosphate cements and resin cements are among the most used cements in dentistry. Zinc phosphate cement is one of the most traditional cements used in dentistry. This material, however, does not bond the restoration to tooth structure, and cementation relies on mechanical retention. Resin cements were introduced in the 1950s and their initial composition was based on methyl methacrylate. Due to substantial polymerization shrinkage, difficulty in handling, pulp irritability, microleakage, and thick film formation, the use of methyl methacrylate resin cement was discontinued.

Recent self-curing, light curing, and dual curing resin cements, in association with oxygen inhibitors are the most used cements for esthetic restorations. Resin cements result in 13–20 μm film thickness. One factor to consider when choosing adhesive cements is the ability of the restorative material to transmit light. If restorative materials do not allow light transmission, chemically cured cement would be the choice. For intermediate scenarios, dual cured cement is indicated, whereas thin restorations of thickness less than 2 mm allow the use of light-cured cements. Adhesive cements should bond by hybridization to tooth surface, and bond to inner surfaces of ceramic restorations through selected surface treatments, ie, silanization, silica coating, and conditioning by hydrofluoric acid or aluminum oxide. Cement should present desirable physical, mechanical, and biological properties, including color stability and fluoride release. Current cements are milestone for esthetic dentistry, allowing esthetic, functional, and durable rehabilitations [88,89]. Accuracy of clinical and laboratory procedures is the only way to minimize marginal leakage after cementing procedures, regardless of the adhesive system that is utilized.

Proper marginal adaptation and sealing by cementation are factors that determine the longevity of prosthetic restorations. No cement is able to eliminate marginal leakage. Cements are the weak link in indirect restorations, being susceptible to oral environment moisture and mechanical loading from mastication. After the restoration is finished, imperfections may be noted initially or over time. Those imperfections, which represent the most common failures, are discussed in the Section 2.7. Imperfections include premature contacts, poor marginal adaptation, overexposure of cement, secondary caries, staining, chipping, postoperative sensitivity, and fractures.

2.6 Shape and function of indirect restorations

Clovis Pagani – *Professor – Restorative Dentistry Department – Univ. Estadual Paulista – SP – Brazil – UNESP*
Hilton Riquieri – *PhD student – Graduate Program – Univ. Estadual Paulista – SP – Brazil – UNESP*
Eduardo Galera da Silva – *Assistant Professor – Social and Pediatric Dentistry Department – Univ. Estadual Paulista – SP – Brazil – UNESP*
Guilherme Siqueira Ferreira Saavedra – *Assistant Professor – Dental Materials and Prosthesis Department – Univ. Estadual Paulista – SP – Brazil – UNESP*

2.6.1 Conventional

Although presenting an esthetic component, restorations should mainly present biological characteristics that allow harmony with other components, resulting in greater longevity. Therefore, it must be emphasized that dental restorations should present anatomical characteristics for greater biological tolerance.

Considering form and function of restorations, one should consider the determinants of dental morphology of tooth in function and its interaction with the stomatognathic system, highlighting the temporomandibular joint and the occlusal plane of teeth. The reestablishment of proximal, buccal, and lingual contours, as well as contact points and cervical finishing of restorations should be observed. In restorations lacking these anatomical features, there might be oral disease.

The rehabilitation treatment must ensure minimum conditions for biological and physiological reestablishment of natural structures, and also ensure the possibility of maintaining healthy status. Restored tooth should be balanced and in harmonious relationship regarding interproximal and occusal contacts. It is known that tooth morphology and its spatial position in the arch is influenced by the anatomy of the mandibular condyle, the joint cavity, and the trajectory of mandibular movements.

Current available metallic or ceramic materials for prosthesis fabrication represent adequate alternatives for restoring occlusal and proximal configuration of dental relationships. However, problems may be noted. These problems may involve wear of antagonistic teeth due to extremely hard ceramic, wear due to inadequate thickness of prostheses, and cusp fractures. It is clear that during the treatment planning stage, the dentist must comprehensively consider the patient's needs and characteristics.

2.6.2 Implant-supported prosthesis

Maria Aparecida Neves Jardini – *Associate Professor Diagnosis and Surgery Department – Univ. Estadual Paulista – SP – Brazil – UNESP*
Antônio Braulino de Melo Filho – *Assistant Professor – Social and Pediatric Dentistry Department– Univ. Estadual Paulista – SP – Brazil – UNESP*

The main purpose of dental restorations is to replace lost teeth, to restore severely damaged clinical crowns, to establish function, or to solve esthetic problems related to color, shape, and/or contour. According to the glossary of prosthetic terms [90], restoration is the general term for any material or prosthesis that restores or replaces lost tooth structure or the entire tooth. Dental restorations may be fixed or removable and partial or total, depending on the number and positioning of remaining teeth. Fixed prostheses are more stable, comfortable, and safe for patients. Limitations are related to the number and positioning of pillar teeth [91].

The recent wide availability of osseointegrated dental implants and scientifically proven excellent success rates led to increased number of pillar teeth, improving oral rehabilitation. Implant-supported prosthesis increase possibilities for solving partial or total tooth loss. It is, however, necessary to determine the ideal criteria of restoration function and esthetics, proper case selection, minimal morbidity risk, technical training, and costs [92].

Implant-supported prosthesis should start with careful and thorough treatment planning. Models are mounted on articulator, and diagnostic waxing is performed. The models in conjunction with radiographic examination lead to evaluation of local factors (relationship between arches, length of the prosthetic area, and proportions of crowns), to determine the position and number of required implants. Data on the quantity and quality of the remaining bone ridge, soft tissue quality, smile line height, vertical dimension, and lip support also influence the choice of prosthesis.

2.6.2.1 Biomechanical considerations

Biomechanical considerations are particularly important once teeth and implants are anchored in the bone. Understanding the biomechanics of implants is critical for the success of implant-supported prostheses. Excessive load might lead to mechanical failures, namely, fracture or loosening of screw and fracture of implant, or biological failures, related to the surrounding bone, leading to resorption and progressive bone loss [93,94].

The biomechanics of implant-supported prostheses is different from that of tooth-supported prostheses. The periodontal ligament allows movement of teeth, and thus, there is some ability to accommodate excessive loading. Dental implants do not possess a periodontal ligament. The connection between the implant and prosthesis is relatively rigid, and in the presence of excessive loads, could lead to fatigue or fracture, as well as have the potential of a detrimental impact on the supporting bone.

2.6.2.2 Immediate versus late loading

The oral implants protocol [95] was divided into two stages aiming to prevent infections during bone healing and immediate load. The development of implants system and technical progress led to the possibility of installing implant-supported prosthesis right after implant placement. This procedure is known as immediate implant loading [96,97]. Immediate implant loading should consider ideal conditions for implant primary stability, followed by installation of the prosthetic piece up to 48 h after surgery. Immediate implant loading is also possible due to the use of bioactive materials, due to treatments performed on the implant surface, due to the implant geometry that favors primary stability in the bone, and due to the constant improvements in surgical techniques.

Reduction in implant loading or delayed loading has been studied. Factors such as changes in implant disposition and shape of prostheses and prosthetic components have been considered. To date, there are unresolved questions regarding immediate and late loading of dental implants.

2.6.2.3 Cemented prosthesis versus screwed prostheses

The first implant-supported prostheses following Branemark's protocol (1965) used screwed abutment to implant, and the prosthesis was positioned and fixed to that abutment by means of gold or titanium screws [98]. Over the years, implant-cemented prostheses have emerged and are increasingly employed, leading to uncertainties among clinicians about which fixation system to use [99–101].

2.6.2.4 Advantages and disadvantages: passive adaptation

Neither system of implant-supported prosthesis represents a complete passive fit, leading to low-intensity tension on implants [102,103]. Passivity of screwed implant-supported prosthesis is more challenging due to dimensional discrepancies resulting from the manufacturing process. Those discrepancies usually do not influence implant-cemented prosthesis, as the cement film compensates for them. This particularity facilitates adaptation, ensuring that the forces are transferred along the entire bone–implant–prosthesis system [104–106].

2.6.2.5 Reversibility

Reversibility is the main advantage of screwed restorations. The convenience of prosthesis removal and repositioning facilitates repairs or modifications of restorations, favors hygiene maintenance, and allows monitoring of the peri-implant tissues.

Implant-cemented prostheses are reported to present fewer technical problems, but increased biological concerns, as implant failures and marginal bone loss [107]. On the other hand, screwed prostheses exhibit more technical issues like screw fracture or loosening [107]. For single crowns, both fixation methods are indicated but for extensive partial or complete fixed prostheses, the screwed system is preferred due to facilitated repair process, if needed.

2.6.2.6 Retention

Retention of implant-supported prosthesis is an important factor related to restoration longevity. Some authors [104,106,108] have reported prosthetic retention relies on several factors like preparation angle, surface area, surface roughness, height of pillar tooth, and type of cementing agent.

The main advantage of screw structure is the possibility of using a low retention profile abutment. In reduced interocclusal distances, cemented prosthesis requires abutments with height greater than 5 mm [109]. In cemented prostheses, the type of cement also influences retention. Definitive cements increase retention and provide good marginal sealing of the restoration, whereas provisional cements provide easy removal characteristics [99].

2.6.2.7 Esthetics

Cemented prostheses present improved esthetics when comparison with screwed ones [98,99,104,108,110,111]. Cemented prostheses allow improved implant placement considering tooth long axis, resulting in more natural anatomy of crowns. Cemented prostheses often allow correction of implant angulation. For screwed prostheses, that correction is obtained by using angled abutments, which may cause esthetic problems in the cervical region. Considering positioning, implants placed in the ideal position will allow proper esthetic results with either cemented or screwed prostheses [106].

Esthetics depends greatly on patient selection, type and amount of tissue surrounding the implants, and implant positioning. Implant positioning will simply determine the retention method. Cemented prosthesis has been preferred, whereas screwed ones are used when the screw access does not affect esthetics.

2.7 Clinical challenges and failures

Maria Filomena Rocha Lima Huhtala – *Assistant Professor – Restorative Dentistry Department – Univ. Estadual Paulista – SP – Brazil – UNESP*
Marcelo Gianini – *Associate Professor – Department – Piracicaba – UNICAMP*
Sergio Eduardo de Paiva Gonçalves – *Associate Professor – Restorative Dentistry Department – Univ. Estadual Paulista – SP – Brazil – UNESP*

2.7.1 Clinical challenges in dental prosthesis

After the restoration is finished, imperfections may be noted initially or over time. Those imperfections, which represent the most common failures, include premature contacts, poor marginal adaptation, overexposure of cement, secondary caries, staining, chipping, postoperative sensitivity, and fractures.

It is well established that there is a need for broad and deep knowledge of the mechanical and biological bases of the oral cavity, as well as the materials that could endure its challenging conditions [112]. The materials proposed for partial or total replacement of tooth loss face challenges including acid-producing pathogens, repeated mechanical loading, and a caustic wet environment that experiences temperature and pH fluctuations. On the other hand, the preparation of the tooth to receive these materials is also of great importance. These factors are leveraged alongside the science behind the knowledge on dental structure and its correlation with the oral environment and on the materials that are in contact with its various layers: external and internal [112]. With the new knowledge on the cause and mechanism of dental caries, these principles were adjusted to new scientific realities but, the search for a restoration that can replace the original strength, shape, and function of teeth, and simultaneously prevent the recurrence of new caries lesion is ongoing.

2.7.2 Selecting materials and techniques

The list of challenges that influence restoration longevity includes great variability among individuals regarding salivary composition, occlusal and oral habits, diet, and systemic conditions. There are a variety of alternatives for addressing specific clinical situations. The alternatives range from cast gold restorations, to nonprecious metal alloys, resins, and ceramics. Gold was the first metal chosen for the reconstruction of missing parts of teeth, and the techniques required to achieve success are well established in the literature [112–114]. A significant number of clinicians have considered gold as the ideal material, with the greatest longevity among the indirect restorative materials used in dentistry [115–118]. However, even for gold cast restorations, there are studies with disappointing results [119–121] (Fig. 2.11). This variability in the survival rate is explained as being related to different operators and to factors related to patients, such as diet, oral hygiene, susceptibility to decay, and parafunctional habits. In general, cast gold restorations remain in the mouth for periods ranging from 15 to 20 years [117,118,122] (Fig. 2.12).

The high cost of gold and the desire for esthetics, ie, a more natural appearance, have driven the search for alternative alloys. Thus, for several decades, various types of alloys were introduced into the dental market to be used as an alternative to gold. Seminoble alloys are an excellent alternative to gold-based ones for full-cast and metal–ceramic restorations. The following characteristics make them an excellent alternative

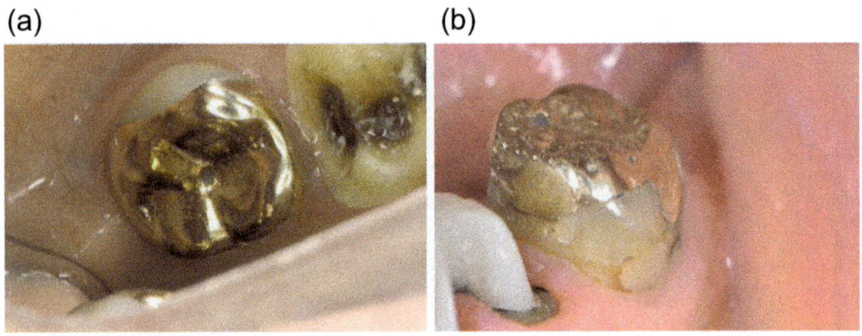

Figure 2.11 (a, b) Wear of gold cast restorations.

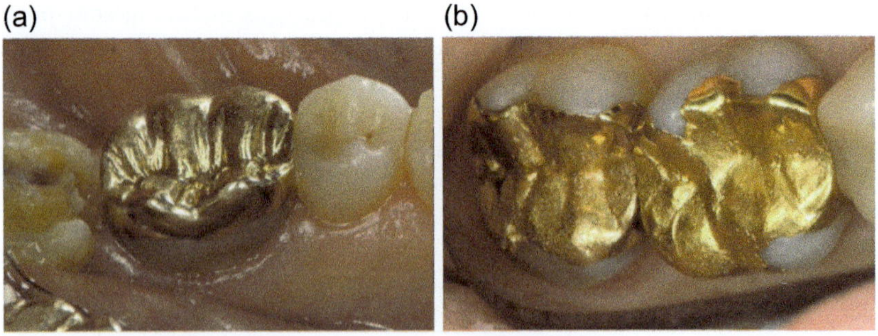

Figure 2.12 Cast gold restorations after 30 (a) and 40 (b) years.

to gold-based alloys: high resistance to corrosion [123,124], adequate porcelain adherence [123,125], and excellent mechanical properties. Alloys must be biocompatible and ideally, none of its components are released into the body [126]. The presence of a variety of alloys in the mouth can lead to galvanic effects, which enhances metal corrosion reactions (Fig. 2.13). Saliva has a great corrosive power on these oxides. These reactions release metal ions, which may provoke allergic or toxic responses in the tissues (Fig. 2.14). Sensitivity to nickel (Ni), cobalt (Co), and chromium (Cr) has been reported [123]. Dental alloys must meet several selection criteria. They should be biocompatible, be resistant to corrosion, be resistant to physical changes when in contact with oral fluids, withstand occlusal loads, adjust to individual characteristics of the patient, and not wear the antagonist tooth or deform the restoration surface (Fig. 2.14).

2.7.3 Marginal adaptation

Historically, prosthetic materials with the best marginal adaptation were gold alloys (Fig. 1). Characteristically, alternative or nonnoble metal alloys exhibit poorer marginal adaptation (Figs. 2.13(b), 2.15 and 2.16(a)). Due to their hardness and lack of malleability, they cannot be adjusted to the finish lines of the preparations. The optimal space between the prosthetic material and the finish line of the tooth preparation

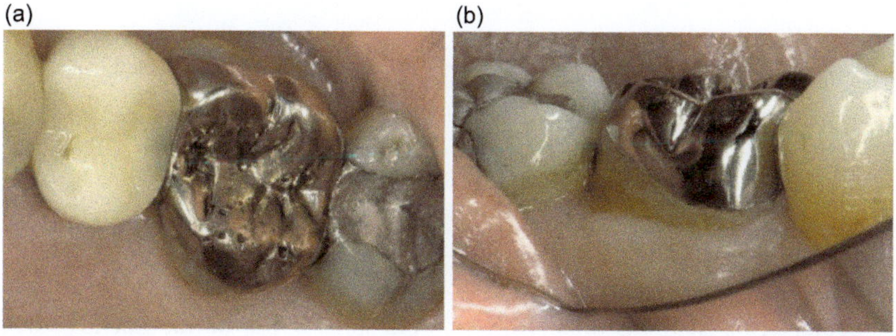

Figure 2.13 Surface degradation (a) and marginal adaptation (b) of a 30-year-old nickel–chromium restoration.

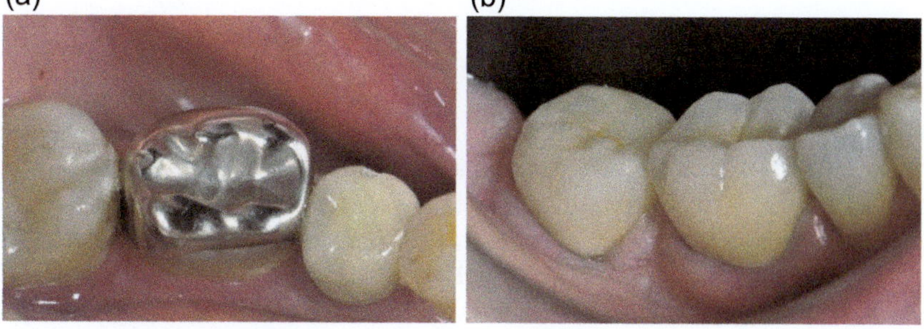

Figure 2.14 Nickel–chromium restoration surface deformation (a) and gingival alteration (b) of a porcelain fused to metal crown.

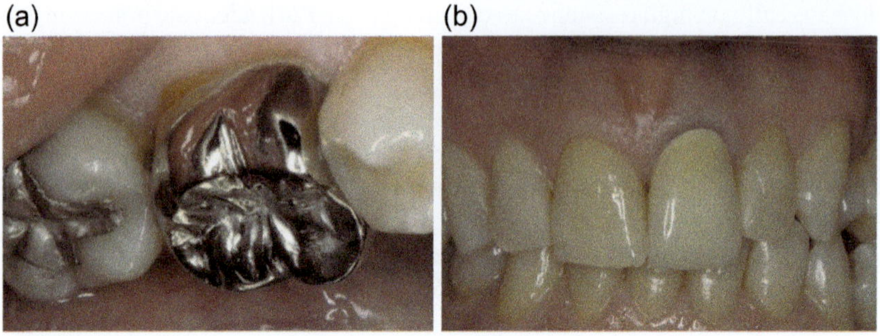

Figure 2.15 Nickel–chromium restoration marginal adaptation (a) and porcelain fused to metal crown (b).

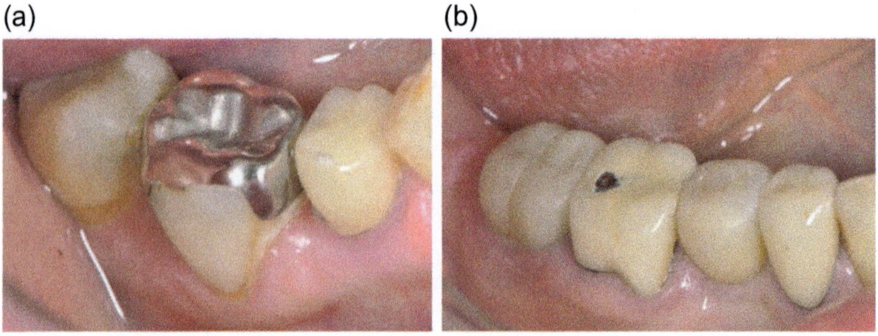

Figure 2.16 Marginal adaptation (a) and metal infrastructure exposure (b) of a 30-year-old nickel–chromium restoration.

should be between 30 and 40 μm, which may be filled by the cement. When the first ceramics were introduced, there was inadequate marginal adaptation, ie, adaptation approximating 200 μm was noted. In addition, the whole procedure was compromised by the cementation that was done with zinc phosphate. The development of dental ceramics and resin cements provided a significant improvement for this type of prosthesis. The marginal adaptation of current ceramics differs little among the various systems, and the marginal adaptation has been reduced by one-half.

2.7.4 Load to fracture, hardness, soft tissue relationships, biocompatibility

Some ceramic materials such as zirconium oxide, alumina, and lithium disilicate have shown load to fracture and hardness comparable with those of metal alloys. In general, the lack of resistance to occlusal forces of these esthetic materials is no longer a clinical problem. An exception is noted when there is a thin ceramic coating in a ceramic fused to metal crown (Figs. 2.16(b) and 2.17(b)). Zirconia-based ceramics have been clinically available as alternatives to metal framework for fixed dental prostheses (FDPs). A clinical complication with zirconia-based ceramics is chipping of the veneering porcelain. One of the reasons is the lack of a comprehensive understanding

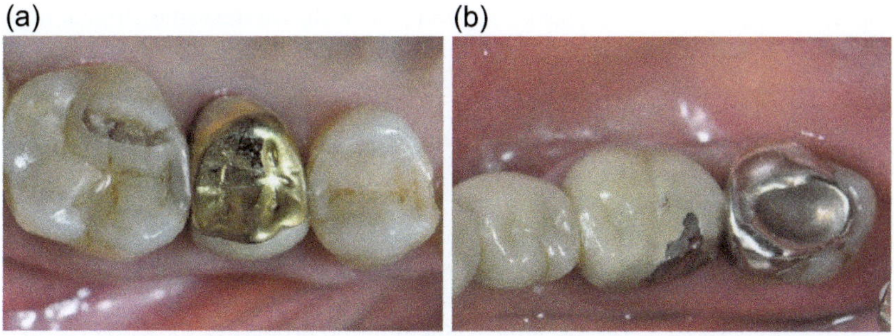

Figure 2.17 Surface degradation (a) and marginal adaptation (b) of a 30-year-old nickel–chromium restoration.

of the bonding mechanism between zirconia and the veneering ceramics. The bond between zirconia and porcelain is lower than that between metal and porcelain [127]. The surface smoothness of ceramic materials obtained by applying the "glaze" layer resembles enamel in texture as well as in terms of adhesion and buildup of biofilm [112]. Ceramic materials exhibit excellent biocompatibility with respect to periodontal tissues, although some patients may have allergy to the methacrylates in composite resins and resin cements.

2.7.5 Longevity

Restorations are exposed to saliva, masticatory loads, proteins, enzymes, food, bacteria, as well as temperature and pH fluctuations. Human saliva plays an important role in balancing the processes of demineralization and remineralization. An imbalance in this process can produce recurrent decay in the margins of restorations, especially when they are not perfectly sealed. Alternative and nonprecious metal alloys may corrode; corrosion is readily observed in the copper–aluminum, silver, and nickel–chrome alloys [11,128]. Esthetically, this corrosion is unfavorable because the oxidation products can impregnate tooth structure, and therefore impair future treatments with esthetic materials. Masticatory load along with prosthetic restorations' lifetime are the major causes of fractures and clinical failure of ceramic materials. However, fracture of the alloys is a rare phenomenon in dentistry. Metal ceramic crowns provided in private practice settings show good longevity (Fig. 2.17(b)). Bruxism appears to indicate a risk for metal-ceramic defects [129].

The fatigue that ceramic restorations are subjected to depends on each ceramic, wherein feldspathic porcelain, reinforced with alumina; leucite-based, lithium disilicate; and zirconia have different levels of fracture resistance and elastic modulus, and therefore show different clinical behavior in terms of fracture [130]. Some studies have reported that zirconia has better mechanical properties and superior resistance to fracture than the other conventional dental ceramics. Longevity will depend on the correct indication of the type of ceramic, tooth preparation, laboratorial technique, and cementing material (Fig. 2.17(a,b)). Of course, the patient's oral condition plays a role in the longevity of indirect restorations; however, in some studies modern all-ceramic prostheses cemented with resin-based materials have shown the same clinical longevity as conventional metal prostheses cemented with zinc phosphate [2].

2.8 Future directions

Eduardo Moreira da Silva – *Associate Professor – Analytical Laboratory of Restorative Biomaterials – LABiom-R – School of Dentistry – Federal Fluminense University*

Over the past two decades, the improvement in the properties of dental restorative biomaterials has led to substantial increases in clinical longevity of many types of restorations. However, even today, the conditions existing in the hostile oral environment, eg, temperature and pH changes, presence of microorganisms, and action of masticatory forces, still exert deleterious effects on restorations, irrespective of the biomaterial they are composed of. What are the future directions?

The reconstruction of the dental hard tissues lost by trauma or caries involves the use of clinically proven restorative biomaterials such as composites, alloys, titanium, ceramics, and cements. Because of improved clinical performance, some have gained more attention by clinicians. Since the extraordinary contribution of Branemark and colleagues [43], titanium and titanium alloys have been extensively studied and clinically used in implantology [131–135]. Due to corrosion resistance, excellent mechanical properties, and low density [136], this biomaterial performs superbly in bone-anchored dental prosthesis. Another important aspect of titanium for dental implants is its excellent biocompatibility, which is related to the spontaneous formation of a dense 4-nm layer of TiO_2 on its surface [137]. The oxide layer favors calcium deposition and adsorption of adhesive proteins, which are the earliest steps in the cascade of events leading to implant osseointegration [138]. Despite these properties that have led to the suggestion that titanium implants represent the most important innovation in dentistry [139], dental scientists continue to develop new technologies to improve the performance of oral rehabilitations supported by titanium implants [94,140]. The principal target for these efforts is to shorten the time between the surgical phase and the moment at which the oral rehabilitation starts. Hence, several investigations have focused on treating titanium implant surfaces with agents capable of promoting osteogenic differentiation. This purpose can be reached by approaches that create hierarchical topography at micrometer and nanometer scales at titanium implant surfaces [103,141,142], and/or through surface chemistry alterations to create multifunctional osteoconductive (Ca, Mg, Zn and P) ion-rich active implant surfaces [143–148]. Additionally and foremost, efforts to create titanium implant with antibacterial properties, highly osteoconductive and capable of killing adherent bacteria, thus avoiding biofilm formation and peri-implantitis, have also been made [149–151]. Together, all these properties are essential to accelerate wound healing and enhance implant–bone osseointegration.

The last advance on treating the surfaces of titanium implants is the biomimetic approach [140], which involves the functionalization of implant surfaces with biomolecules that present biological activities. The idea is to promote specific cell adhesion onto implant surfaces, eg, osteoblasts, thereby accelerating the bone formation and improving its remodeling process. Growth factors, such as bone morphogenetic proteins [152]; insulinlike growth factors, [153] peptides, such as arginine–glycine–aspartate sequence [154,155]; and extracellular matrix proteins, such as fibronectin [156,157] and collagen [158] have been tested with this goal. One of the future directions is to functionalize titanium implant surfaces with more than one of these biomimetic agents, to create multibioactive surfaces [159,160].

Besides titanium, another promising field of interest relies on implant fabrication with zirconia and polyetheretherketone (PEEK) [161–164]. These "white" implants claim to avoid unesthetic aspects linked to titanium such as dark shimmer of the peri-implant soft tissue in areas of gingival recession [165]. However, the literature has shown that the osseointegration capability of these implants could be inferior to those of titanium-based implants [166,167]. Irrespective of this limitation and taking into account the expectation of the patients for metal-free and highly esthetic oral rehabilitations, the development of surface treatment technologies to improve zirconia–bone and PEEK implants–bone osseointegration are also one of the future directions [167].

Patients frequently request rehabilitation with imperceptible restorations that mimic as closely as possible the natural features of dental hard tissues, ie, translucency, glossy nature, opacity, and adequate mechanical properties. Obviously, ceramic materials are the choice to deal with this esthetic appeal. The introduction of porcelain in dentistry [87], different ceramic materials, feldspathic, spinel, as well as aluminum-rich and glass ceramics, allow the dentists to generally satisfy the patients' demands regarding esthetics [168]. Today, however, the focus of scientists is on polycrystalline ceramics with high strength, the capability to eliminate metal frameworks, and the ability to achieve improved esthetic results, mainly in extensive edentulous areas [127,169]. Currently, the highest mechanical properties guaranteed by a *t-m* phase transformation toughening mechanism, biocompatibility, and good optical properties as well, yttrium stabilized polycrystalline zirconia (Y-TZP) pre-sintered blocks for CAD/CAM technology are the principal targets in this field. These blocks allow fabrication, with a high level of dimensional accuracy, of any kind of metal-free prosthetic restorations: single crowns, abutments, and frameworks for FPD [127,170].

Like many other restorative biomaterials, Y-TZP ceramics still present some shortcomings that must be overcome. These are, first, the inherent low-temperature degradation, which induces *t-m* phase transformation and may compromise its mechanical properties [171,172]; second, the poor bonding performance due to the absence of glass phase (silica) in its structure [173]; and finally, the common chipping of veneering porcelain sintered to Y-TZP framework [174]. Fortunately, some technologies involving the modification of Y-TZP ceramic structure [175], the modification of Y-TZP ceramic surface by using different phosphate primers [176], nonthermal plasma [177], silica nanofilm coating [178], and vitrification process [179], and the use of new methods to improve the compatibility between veneering porcelain and Y-TZP framework have been tested with promising results [180,181]. Certainly, these approaches point out the direction for where new investigations must be conducted.

A recent development that also deserves additional attention by the dental scientists is the "new" polymer-based milling blocks for CAD/CAM applications [182–184].

Overall, these restorative biomaterials, also named resin nanoceramic, flexible nanoceramic, and hybrid dental ceramic, are composed of 71–86 wt.% ceramic phase (silica nanofillers, barium glass, or porous ceramic scaffold) entangled or infiltrated by a reinforced methacrylate copolymer. From the mechanical behavior, these hybrid inorganic–organic bulks are able to develop less crack propagation under fatigue forces than brittle ceramics [185,186], besides presenting flexural properties (flexural strength and flexural modulus) similar to those of human dentin [182,187]. These features allow those materials to withstand more loading with thin layers [188], and undergo more elastic deformation before failure [182,189]. Also, being a resin composite in nature, these "new" materials present several clinical advantages when compared with dental ceramics such as repair friendly, easy occlusal adjustments, and lower abrasiveness to the antagonist teeth. These positive perspectives encourage future investigations toward the development of improved polymer-based CAD/CAM materials for indirect restorations, which would represent new materials with mechanical behavior approximating that of human hard dental tissues [169].

Finally, attention must also be given to the development of resin cements capable of maintaining the stability of bonding of hard dental tissue and restorative biomaterials over time, thereby increasing the long-term success of indirect restorative procedures. Due to the simplified protocol and clinical appeal, self-adhesive resin cements seem to be the choice for this goal [190]. However, new improvements are claimed to increase the reliability of adhesive interfaces produced with self-adhesive resin cements. This is represented by the development of monomers that are more hydrolytically stable, capable of bonding to the hydroxyapatite in the enamel and dentin, and present activity against matrix metalloproteinases and antibacterial properties [191]. These points are still the weak chain in bonding durability.

Beside all these new and interesting developments, dental scientists continue to pursue new discoveries that will lead to the development of optimum restorative materials. For example, the next frontier is the development of self-repair and bioresponsive or smart restorative biomaterials that possess the capability to respond, by themselves, to oral environment stimuli and alter one or more of their properties [24]. Of course, this is not an easy challenge, and these possibilities demand extensive laboratory research and in situ and, principally, clinical outcomes before they can be utilized on patients. There is no doubt that these advances will herald a new age in dentistry, and they mark directions that we must pursue to meet the needs of patients across the globe.

References

[1] Mundhe K, Jain V, Pruthi G, Shah N. Clinical study to evaluate the wear of natural enamel antagonist to zirconia and metal ceramic crowns. J Prosthet Dent 2015;114(3):358–63.

[2] Campos RE, Soares PV, Versluis A, de O Junior OB, Ambrosano GM, Nunes IF. Crown fracture: failure load, stress distribution, and fractographic analysis. J Prosthet Dent 2015;114(3):447–55.

[3] Sola-Ruiz MF, Agustin-Panadero R, Campos-Estelles C, Labaig-Rueda C. Post-fatigue fracture resistance of metal core crowns: press-on metal ceramic versus a conventional veneering system. J Clin Exp Dent 2015;7(2):e278–83.

[4] Spencer P, Ye Q, Misra A, Goncalves SE, Laurence JS. Proteins, pathogens, and failure at the composite-tooth interface. J Dent Res 2014;93(12):1243–9.
[5] Magne P, Belser U. Bonded porcelain restorations in the anterior dentition: a biomimetic approach. Chicago: Quintessence Publishing Company; 2002.
[6] Anusavice KJ. Phillips materiais dentários. Elsevier Brasil; 2013.
[7] Kelly JR, Rose TC. Nonprecious alloys for use in fixed prosthodontics: a literature review. J Prosthet Dent 1983;49(3):363–70.
[8] Roberts HW, Berzins DW, Moore BK, Charlton DG. Metal-ceramic alloys in dentistry: a review. J Prosthodont 2009;18(2):188–94.
[9] Roach M. Base metal alloys used for dental restorations and implants. Dent Clin North Am 2007;51(3):603–27. vi.
[10] Leinfelder KF. An evaluation of casting alloys used for restorative procedures. J Am Dent Assoc 1997;128(1):37–45.
[11] Wataha JC. Biocompatibility of dental casting alloys: a review. J Prosthet Dent 2000;83(2):223–34.
[12] Craig R, Powers J. Restorative dental materials. 11th ed. St Louis: Mosby; 2002.
[13] Tucillo JJ, Cascone PJ. The evolution of porcelain-fused-to-metal alloys systems in dental ceramics. Chicago: Quintessence; 1983.
[14] Jones TK, Hansen CA, Singer MT, Kessler HP. Dental implications of nickel hypersensitivity. J Prosthet Dent 1986;56(4):507–9.
[15] Paffenbarger GC, Caul HJ, Dickson MA. Base metal alloys for oral restorations. J Am Dent Assoc 1943;30:852–62.
[16] Hero H, Syverud M, Gjonnes J, Horst JA. Ductility and structure of some cobalt-base dental casting alloys. Biomaterials 1984;5(4):201–8.
[17] Lane JR. A survey of dental alloys. J Am Dent Assoc 1949;39(4):414–37.
[18] Morris HF, Manz M, Stoffer W, Weir D. Casting alloys: the materials and "the clinical effects". Adv Dent Res 1992;6:28–31.
[19] Asgar K, Peyton FA. Effect of microstructure on the physical properties of cobalt-base alloys. J Dent Res 1961;40:63–72.
[20] Lautenschlager EP, Monaghan P. Titanium and titanium alloys as dental materials. Int Dent J 1993;43(3):245–53.
[21] Wang RR, Fenton A. Titanium for prosthodontic applications: a review of the literature. Quintessence Int 1996;27(6):401–8.
[22] Naylor WP, Kessler JC, King AH. Introduction to metal ceramic technology. Quintessence Pub Co; 1992.
[23] O'Brien WJ. Dental materials and their selection. Quintessence; 2002. p. 204–7.
[24] Badami V, Ahuja B. Biosmart materials: breaking new ground in dentistry. Sci World J 2014;2014:986912.
[25] Mackert Jr JR, Ringle RD, Fairhurst CW. High-temperature behavior of a Pd-Ag alloy for porcelain. J Dent Res 1983;62(12):1229–35.
[26] Tucillo J, Cascone PJ. Composition and properties of noble and precious metal alloys. In: Smith DC, Williams DF, editors. CRC series in biocompatibility: biocompatibility of dental materials. Boca Raton, FL: CRC Press; 1982. p. 19–36.
[27] Gomes E, Assunção W, Rocha E, Santos P. Cerâmicas odontológicas: o estado atual. Cerâmica 2008;54(331):319–25.
[28] Donovan TE. Factors essential for successful all-ceramic restorations. J Am Dent Assoc 2008;139(Suppl.):14S–8S.
[29] Kina S. Cerâmicas dentárias. R Dent Press Estét 2005;2(2):112–28.
[30] Koutayas SO, Vagkopoulou T, Pelekanos S, Koidis P, Strub JR. Zirconia in dentistry: part 2. Evidence-based clinical breakthrough. Eur J Esthet Dent 2009;4(4):348–80.

[31] Bachhav VC, Aras MA. Zirconia-based fixed partial dentures: a clinical review. Quintessence Int 2011;42(2):173–82.
[32] Hill EE, Lott J. A clinically focused discussion of luting materials. Aust Dent J 2011;56(Suppl. 1):67–76.
[33] Lad PP, Kamath M, Tarale K, Kusugal PB. Practical clinical considerations of luting cements: a review. J Int Oral Health 2014;6(1):116–20.
[34] Christensen GJ. Reducing the confusion about resin cements. Clin Rep 2008;1:1–3.
[35] Hill EE. Dental cements for definitive luting: a review and practical clinical considerations. Dent Clin North Am 2007;51(3):643–58. vi.
[36] Phillips RW, Swartz ML, Norman RD. Materials for the practicing dentist. CV Mosby Co; 1969.
[37] Pagani C. Preparos Dentários: Ciência e Arte. Nova Odessa: Napoleão; 2014.
[38] Francci CE, Saavedra GSFA, Nishida AC, Luz JN. Harmonização do Sorriso. In: Pagani C, editor. Os desafios da clínica diária. 1st ed. Nova Odessa: Napoleão; 2014.
[39] Bottino MA, Faria R, Amaral JMBL, Saavedra GSFA. Tecnologia CAD/CAM na Reabilitação Protética. In: Albernaz Neto A, Barbosa LC, Barreto MA, Moreira AA, editors. Estética do Sorriso em Reabilitação Protética. 1st ed. Nova Odessa: Napoleão; 2014. p. 158–203.
[40] Kano P, Baratieri LN, Andretti F, Saito P, LAcerda E, Duarte Jr S. CAD/CAM: a whole new world of precision and excellence. In: Duarte Jr S, editor. Quintessence of dental technology 2015. Chicago: Quintessence; 2015. p. 127–44.
[41] Johnson P. Producti navigator. Inside Dent Technol 2012;3(10):01–92.
[42] Pagani C, Saavedra GSFA, Rocha DM, Carvalho RF. Previsibilidade Estética: a Utilização do Ensaio Restaurador (Mock Up) na Construção da Beleza do Sorriso. In: Callegari A, Dias RB, editors. Livro Especialidade em foco Vol1: Beleza do Sorriso. Nova Odessa: Napoleão; 2013. p. 66–108.
[43] Branemark PI, Adell R, Breine U, Hansson BO, Lindstrom J, Ohlsson A. Intra-osseous anchorage of dental prostheses. I. Experimental studies. Scand J Plast Reconstr Surg 1969;3(2):81–100.
[44] Adell R, Lekholm U, Rockler B, Branemark PI. A 15-year study of osseointegrated implants in the treatment of the edentulous jaw. Int J Oral Surg 1981;10(6):387–416.
[45] Lekholm U, Grondahl K, Jemt T. Outcome of oral implant treatment in partially edentulous jaws followed 20 years in clinical function. Clin Implant Dent Relat Res 2006;8(4):178–86.
[46] Buser D, Janner SF, Wittneben JG, Bragger U, Ramseier CA, Salvi GE. 10-year survival and success rates of 511 titanium implants with a sandblasted and acid-etched surface: a retrospective study in 303 partially edentulous patients. Clin Implant Dent Relat Res 2012;14(6):839–51.
[47] Weber HP, Crohin CC, Fiorellini JP. A 5-year prospective clinical and radiographic study of non-submerged dental implants. Clin Oral Implants Res 2000;11(2):144–53.
[48] Romeo E, Lops D, Margutti E, Ghisolfi M, Chiapasco M, Vogel G. Long-term survival and success of oral implants in the treatment of full and partial arches: a 7-year prospective study with the ITI dental implant system. Int J Oral Maxillofac Implants 2004;19(2):247–59.
[49] Fiorellini JP, Martuscelli G, Weber HP. Longitudinal studies of implant systems. Periodontol 2000 1998;17:125–31.
[50] Malo P, Rangert B, Nobre M. All-on-4 immediate-function concept with Branemark System implants for completely edentulous maxillae: a 1-year retrospective clinical study. Clin Implant Dent Relat Res 2005;7(Suppl. 1):S88–94.

[51] Galindo DF, Butura CC. Immediately loaded mandibular fixed implant prostheses using the all-on-four protocol: a report of 183 consecutively treated patients with 1 year of function in definitive prostheses. Int J Oral Maxillofac Implants 2012;27(3):628–33.
[52] Aparicio C, Ouazzani W, Hatano N. The use of zygomatic implants for prosthetic rehabilitation of the severely resorbed maxilla. Periodontol 2000 2008;47:162–71.
[53] Hirsch JM, Ohrnell LO, Henry PJ, Andreasson L, Branemark PI, Chiapasco M, et al. A clinical evaluation of the zygoma fixture: one year of follow-up at 16 clinics. J Oral Maxillofac Surg 2004;62(9 Suppl. 2):22–9.
[54] Kahnberg KE, Henry PJ, Hirsch JM, Ohrnell LO, Andreasson L, Branemark PI, et al. Clinical evaluation of the zygoma implant: 3-year follow-up at 16 clinics. J Oral Maxillofac Surg 2007;65(10):2033–8.
[55] Pylant T, Triplett RG, Key MC, Brunsvold MA. A retrospective evaluation of endosseous titanium implants in the partially edentulous patient. Int J Oral Maxillofac Implants 1992;7(2):195–202.
[56] Bragger U, Aeschlimann S, Burgin W, Hammerle CH, Lang NP. Biological and technical complications and failures with fixed partial dentures (FPD) on implants and teeth after four to five years of function. Clin Oral Implants Res 2001;12(1):26–34.
[57] De Boever AL, Keersmaekers K, Vanmaele G, Kerschbaum T, Theuniers G, De Boever JA. Prosthetic complications in fixed endosseous implant-borne reconstructions after an observations period of at least 40 months. J Oral Rehabil 2006;33(11):833–9.
[58] Blanes RJ, Bernard JP, Blanes ZM, Belser UC. A 10-year prospective study of ITI dental implants placed in the posterior region. I: clinical and radiographic results. Clin Oral Implants Res 2007;18(6):699–706.
[59] Henry PJ, Laney WR, Jemt T, Harris D, Krogh PH, Polizzi G, et al. Osseointegrated implants for single-tooth replacement: a prospective 5-year multicenter study. Int J Oral Maxillofac Implants 1996;11(4):450–5.
[60] Belser U, Buser D, Higginbottom F. Consensus statements and recommended clinical procedures regarding esthetics in implant dentistry. Int J Oral Maxillofac Implants 2004;19(Suppl.):73–4.
[61] Belser UC, Schmid B, Higginbottom F, Buser D. Outcome analysis of implant restorations located in the anterior maxilla: a review of the recent literature. Int J Oral Maxillofac Implants 2004;19(Suppl.):30–42.
[62] Buser D, Chen ST, Weber HP, Belser UC. Early implant placement following single-tooth extraction in the esthetic zone: biologic rationale and surgical procedures. Int J Periodontics Restor Dent 2008;28(5):441–51.
[63] Albrektsson T, Zarb G, Worthington P, Eriksson AR. The long-term efficacy of currently used dental implants: a review and proposed criteria of success. Int J Oral Maxillofac Implants 1986;1(1):11–25.
[64] Berglundh T, Persson L, Klinge B. A systematic review of the incidence of biological and technical complications in implant dentistry reported in prospective longitudinal studies of at least 5 years. J Clin Periodontol 2002;29(Suppl. 3):197–212. discussion 32–3.
[65] Lang NP, Wilson TG, Corbet EF. Biological complications with dental implants: their prevention, diagnosis and treatment. Clin Oral Implants Res 2000;11(Suppl. 1):146–55.
[66] Lindquist LW, Carlsson GE, Jemt T. Association between marginal bone loss around osseointegrated mandibular implants and smoking habits: a 10-year follow-up study. J Dent Res 1997;76(10):1667–74.
[67] Buser D, Martin W, Belser UC. Optimizing esthetics for implant restorations in the anterior maxilla: anatomic and surgical considerations. Int J Oral Maxillofac Implants 2004;19(Suppl.):43–61.

[68] Albrektsson T, Isidor F. Consensus report of session IV. In: Lang N, Karring T, editors. Proceedings of the 1st European workshop on periodontology. London: Quintessence; 1994. p. 365–9.
[69] Zitzmann NU, Berglundh T. Definition and prevalence of peri-implant diseases. J Clin Periodontol 2008;35(Suppl. 8):286–91.
[70] Salvi GE, Furst MM, Lang NP, Persson GR. One-year bacterial colonization patterns of *Staphylococcus aureus* and other bacteria at implants and adjacent teeth. Clin Oral Implants Res 2008;19(3):242–8.
[71] Vogel RE, Wheeler SL, Casellini RC. Restoration of congenitally missing lateral incisors: a case report. Implant Dent 1999;8(4):390–5.
[72] Tonetti MS, Schmid J. Pathogenesis of implant failures. Periodontol 2000 1994;4:127–38.
[73] Chaves ES, Lovell JS, Tahmasebi S. Implant-supported crown design and the risk for peri-implantitis. Clin Adv Periodontics 2014;4(2):118–26.
[74] Iacopino AM. Periodontitis and diabetes interrelationships: role of inflammation. Ann Periodontol 2001;6(1):125–37.
[75] Mombelli A, Lang NP. The diagnosis and treatment of peri-implantitis. Periodontol 2000 1998;17:63–76.
[76] Sorensen LT. Wound healing and infection in surgery. The clinical impact of smoking and smoking cessation: a systematic review and meta-analysis. Arch Surg 2012;147(4):373–83.
[77] Thoma DS, Brandenberg F, Fehmer V, Buchi DL, Hammerle CH, Sailer I. Randomized controlled clinical trial of all-ceramic single tooth implant reconstructions using modified zirconia abutments: radiographic and prosthetic results at 1 year of loading. Clin Implant Dent Relat Res 2016;18(3):462–72.
[78] Bouri Jr A, Bissada N, Al-Zahrani MS, Faddoul F, Nouneh I. Width of keratinized gingiva and the health status of the supporting tissues around dental implants. Int J Oral Maxillofac Implants 2008;23(2):323–6.
[79] Kim BS, Kim YK, Yun PY, Yi YJ, Lee HJ, Kim SG, et al. Evaluation of peri-implant tissue response according to the presence of keratinized mucosa. Oral Surg Oral Med Oral Pathol Oral Radiol Endod 2009;107(3):e24–8.
[80] Schrott AR, Jimenez M, Hwang JW, Fiorellini J, Weber HP. Five-year evaluation of the influence of keratinized mucosa on peri-implant soft-tissue health and stability around implants supporting full-arch mandibular fixed prostheses. Clin Oral Implants Res 2009;20(10):1170–7.
[81] Cornelini R, Barone A, Covani U. Connective tissue grafts in postextraction implants with immediate restoration: a prospective controlled clinical study. Pract Proced Aesthet Dent 2008;20(6):337–43.
[82] Balshi TJ. An analysis and management of fractured implants: a clinical report. Int J Oral Maxillofac Implants 1996;11(5):660–6.
[83] Esposito M, Worthington HV, Coulthard P, Thomsen P. Maintaining and re-establishing health around osseointegrated oral implants: a Cochrane systematic review comparing the efficacy of various treatments. Periodontol 2000 2003;33:204–12.
[84] Shillingburg HT, Hobo S, Whitsett LD, Jacobi R, Brackett SE. Fundamentals of fixed prosthodontics. St Louis: Mosby; 1979.
[85] Calamita MA, Coachman C, Sesma N. Preparos Dentais e moldagens na clínica restauradora Atual: o que precisamos fazer. In: Callegari A, Dias RB, editors. Especialidade em foco – Beleza do Sorriso. Nova Odessa: Napoleão; 2014.
[86] Wilson AD, Kent BE, Lewis BG. Zinc phosphate cements: chemical study of in vitro durability. J Dent Res 1970;49(5):1049–54.
[87] Anusavice KJ. Phillips' science of dental materials. St. Louis, MO: Saunders; 2003.

[88] Thompson JY, Stoner BR, Piascik JR, Smith R. Adhesion/cementation to zirconia and other non-silicate ceramics: where are we now? Dent Mater 2011;27(1):71–82.
[89] Breschi L, Mazzoni A, Ruggeri A, Cadenaro M, Di Lenarda R. De Stefano Dorigo E. Dental adhesion review: aging and stability of the bonded interface. Dent Mater 2008;24(1):90–101.
[90] The glossary of prosthodontic terms. J Prosthet Dent 2005;94(1):10–92.
[91] Zitzmann NU, Hagmann E, Weiger R. What is the prevalence of various types of prosthetic dental restorations in Europe? Clin Oral Implants Res 2007;18(Suppl. 3):20–33.
[92] Zarb GA, Lewis DW. Dental implants and decision making. J Dent Educ 1992;56(12):863–72.
[93] Brunski JB, Puleo DA, Nanci A. Biomaterials and biomechanics of oral and maxillofacial implants: current status and future developments. Int J Oral Maxillofac Implants 2000;15(1):15–46.
[94] Shibata Y, Tanimoto Y. A review of improved fixation methods for dental implants. Part I: surface optimization for rapid osseointegration. J Prosthodont Res 2015;59(1):20–33.
[95] Brånemark PI, Zarb G, Albrektsson T. Tissue-integrated prostheses: osseointegration in clinical dentistry. Chicago: Quintessence publishing Co; 1985.
[96] Aparicio C, Rangert B, Sennerby L. Immediate/Early Loading of Dental Implants: a Report from the Sociedad Espanola de Implantes World Congress Consensus Meeting in Barcelona, Spain, 2002. Clin Implant Dent Relat Res 2003;5(1):57–60.
[97] Cochran DL, Morton D, Weber HP. Consensus statements and recommended clinical procedures regarding loading protocols for endosseous dental implants. Int J Oral Maxillofac Implants 2004;19(Suppl.):109–13.
[98] Taylor TD, Belser U, Mericske-Stern R. Prosthodontic considerations. Clin Oral Implants Res 2000;11(Suppl. 1):101–7.
[99] Michalakis KX, Hirayama H, Garefis PD. Cement-retained versus screw-retained implant restorations: a critical review. Int J Oral Maxillofac Implants 2003;18(5):719–28.
[100] Siamos G, Winkler S, Boberick KG. Relationship between implant preload and screw loosening on implant-supported prostheses. J Oral Implantol 2002;28(2):67–73.
[101] Taylor TD, Agar JR. Twenty years of progress in implant prosthodontics. J Prosthet Dent 2002;88(1):89–95.
[102] Guichet DL, Caputo AA, Choi H, Sorensen JA. Passivity of fit and marginal opening in screw- or cement-retained implant fixed partial denture designs. Int J Oral Maxillofac Implants 2000;15(2):239–46.
[103] Kim MH, Park K, Choi KH, Kim SH, Kim SE, Jeong CM, et al. Cell adhesion and in vivo osseointegration of sandblasted/acid etched/anodized dental implants. Int J Mol Sci 2015;16(5):10324–36.
[104] Chee W, Jivraj S. Screw versus cemented implant supported restorations. Br Dent J 2006;201(8):501–7.
[105] Karl M, Taylor TD, Wichmann MG, Heckmann SM. In vivo stress behavior in cemented and screw-retained five-unit implant FPDs. J Prosthodont 2006;15(1):20–4.
[106] Shadid R, Sadaqa N. A comparison between screw- and cement-retained implant prostheses. A literature review. J Oral Implantol 2012;38(3):298–307.
[107] Sailer I, Muhlemann S, Zwahlen M, Hammerle CH, Schneider D. Cemented and screw-retained implant reconstructions: a systematic review of the survival and complication rates. Clin Oral Implants Res 2012;23(Suppl. 6):163–201.
[108] Hebel KS, Gajjar RC. Cement-retained versus screw-retained implant restorations: achieving optimal occlusion and esthetics in implant dentistry. J Prosthet Dent 1997;77(1):28–35.

[109] Misch CE, Bidez MW. Occlusal considerations for implant supported prostheses: implant protective occlusion. In: Misch CE, editor. Dental implant prosthetics. St Louis: Mosby; 2005.
[110] Avivi-Arber L, Zarb GA. Clinical effectiveness of implant-supported single-tooth replacement: the Toronto Study. Int J Oral Maxillofac Implants 1996;11(3):311–21.
[111] Gervais MJ, Hatzipanagiotis P, Wilson PR. Cross-pinning: the philosophy of retrievability applied practically to fixed, implant-supported prostheses. Aust Dent J 2008;53(1):74–82.
[112] Hannig C, Hannig M. The oral cavity–a key system to understand substratum-dependent bioadhesion on solid surfaces in man. Clin Oral Investig 2009;13(2):123–39.
[113] Donovan TE, Chee WW. Conservative indirect restorations for posterior teeth. Cast versus bonded ceramic. Dent Clin North Am 1993;37(3):433–43.
[114] Taggert WH. A new and accurate method of making gold inlays. Dent Cosm 1907;49:117.
[115] Mjor IA, Medina JE. Reasons for placement, replacement, and age of gold restorations in selected practices. Oper Dent 1993;18(3):82–7.
[116] Stoll R, Sieweke M, Pieper K, Stachniss V, Schulte A. Longevity of cast gold inlays and partial crowns–a retrospective study at a dental school clinic. Clin Oral Investig 1999;3(2):100–4.
[117] Studer SP, Wettstein F, Lehner C, Zullo TG, Scharer P. Long-term survival estimates of cast gold inlays and onlays with their analysis of failures. J Oral Rehabil 2000;27(6):461–72.
[118] Allan DN. The durability of conservative restorations. Br Dent J 1969;126(4):172–7.
[119] Crabb HS. The survival of dental restorations in a teaching hospital. Br Dent J 1981;150(11):315–8.
[120] Mjor IA, Jokstad A, Qvist V. Longevity of posterior restorations. Int Dent J 1990;40(1):11–7.
[121] Valderhaug JA. 15-year clinical evaluation of fixed prosthodontics. Acta Odontol Scand 1991;49(1):35–40.
[122] Donovan T, Simonsen RJ, Guertin G, Tucker RV. Retrospective clinical evaluation of 1314 cast gold restorations in service from 1 to 52 years. J Esthet Restor Dent 2004;16(3):194–204.
[123] Puskar T, Jevremovic D, Williams R, Eggbeer D, Vukelic D, Budak I. A comparative analysis of the corrosive effect of artificial saliva of variable pH on DMLS and cast Co–Cr–Mo dental alloy. Materials 2014;7(9):6486.
[124] O'Connor RP, Mackert Jr JR, Myers ML, Parry EE. Castability, opaque masking, and porcelain bonding of 17 porcelain-fused-to-metal alloys. J Prosthet Dent 1996;75(4):367–74.
[125] Goehlich V, Marek M. Corrosion behavior of Pd-Cu and Pd-Co alloys in synthetic saliva. Dent Mater 1990;6(2):103–10.
[126] Syrjanen S, Hensten-Pettersen A, Kangasniemi K, Yli-Urpo A. In vitro and in vivo biological responses to some dental alloys tested separately and in combinations. Biomaterials 1985;6(3):169–76.
[127] Miyazaki T, Nakamura T, Matsumura H, Ban S, Kobayashi T. Current status of zirconia restoration. J Prosthodont Res 2013;57(4):236–61.
[128] Viennot S, Lissac M, Malquarti G, Dalard F, Grosgogeat B. Influence of casting procedures on the corrosion resistance of clinical dental alloys containing palladium. Acta Biomater 2006;2(3):321–30.
[129] Reitemeier B, Hansel K, Kastner C, Weber A, Walter MH. A prospective 10-year study of metal ceramic single crowns and fixed dental prosthesis retainers in private practice settings. J Prosthet Dent 2013;109(3):149–55.

[130] Baladhandayutham B, Lawson NC, Burgess JO. Fracture load of ceramic restorations after fatigue loading. J Prosthet Dent 2015;114(2):266–71.
[131] Thomason JM, Lund JP, Chehade A, Feine JS. Patient satisfaction with mandibular implant overdentures and conventional dentures 6 months after delivery. Int J Prosthodont 2003;16(5):467–73.
[132] Hyland R, Ellis J, Thomason M, El-Feky A, Moynihan P. A qualitative study on patient perspectives of how conventional and implant-supported dentures affect eating. J Dent 2009;37(9):718–23.
[133] Branemark PI, Hansson BO, Adell R, Breine U, Lindstrom J, Hallen O, et al. Osseointegrated implants in the treatment of the edentulous jaw. Experience from a 10-year period. Scand J Plast Reconstr Surg 1977;16(Suppl.):1–132.
[134] Stenlund P, Omar O, Brohede U, Norgren S, Norlindh B, Johansson A, et al. Bone response to a novel Ti–Ta–Nb–Zr alloy. Acta Biomater 2015;20:165–75.
[135] Zhang Y, Zheng Y, Li Y, Wang L, Bai Y, Zhao Q, et al. Tantalum nitride-decorated titanium with enhanced resistance to microbiologically induced corrosion and mechanical property for dental application. PLoS One 2015;10(6):e0130774.
[136] Jorge JR, Barao VA, Delben JA, Faverani LP, Queiroz TP, Assuncao WG. Titanium in dentistry: historical development, state of the art and future perspectives. J Indian Prosthodont Soc 2013;13(2):71–7.
[137] Kato H, Nakamura T, Nishiguchi S, Matsusue Y, Kobayashi M, Miyazaki T, et al. Bonding of alkali- and heat-treated tantalum implants to bone. J Biomed Mater Res 2000;53(1):28–35.
[138] Coelho PG, Jimbo R, Tovar N, Bonfante EA. Osseointegration: hierarchical designing encompassing the macrometer, micrometer, and nanometer length scales. Dent Mater 2015;31(1):37–52.
[139] Wang G, Gao X, Lo EC. Public perceptions of dental implants: a qualitative study. J Dent 2015;43(7):798–805.
[140] Avila G, Misch K, Galindo-Moreno P, Wang HL. Implant surface treatment using biomimetic agents. Implant Dent 2009;18(1):17–23.
[141] Le Guehennec L, Soueidan A, Layrolle P, Amouriq Y. Surface treatments of titanium dental implants for rapid osseointegration. Dent Mater 2007;23(7):844–54.
[142] Qiao SC, Du J, Zhao JM, Shi JY, Gu YX, Lai HC. Effects of a hydroxyapatite-coated nanotube surface of titanium on MC3T3-E1 cells: an in vitro study. Implant Dent 2015;24(2):204–10.
[143] Cheng M, Qiao Y, Wang Q, Jin G, Qin H, Zhao Y, et al. Calcium plasma implanted titanium surface with hierarchical microstructure for improving the bone formation. ACS Appl Mater Interfaces 2015;7(23):13053–61.
[144] Shen X, Hu Y, Xu G, Chen W, Xu K, Ran Q, et al. Regulation of the biological functions of osteoblasts and bone formation by Zn-incorporated coating on microrough titanium. ACS Appl Mater Interfaces 2014;6(18):16426–40.
[145] Ong JL, Carnes DL, Bessho K. Evaluation of titanium plasma-sprayed and plasma-sprayed hydroxyapatite implants in vivo. Biomaterials 2004;25(19):4601–6.
[146] Yang CH, Li YC, Tsai WF, Ai CF, Huang HH. Oxygen plasma immersion ion implantation treatment enhances the human bone marrow mesenchymal stem cells responses to titanium surface for dental implant application. Clin Oral Implants Res 2015;26(2):166–75.
[147] Lugovskoy A, Lugovskoy S. Production of hydroxyapatite layers on the plasma electrolytically oxidized surface of titanium alloys. Mater Sci Eng C-Mater Biol Appl 2014;43:527–32.

[148] Ribeiro AR, Oliveira F, Boldrini LC, Leite PE, Falagan-Lotsch P, Linhares AB, et al. Micro-arc oxidation as a tool to develop multifunctional calcium-rich surfaces for dental implant applications. Mater Sci Eng C Mater Biol Appl 2015;54:196–206.
[149] Shibata Y, Suzuki D, Omori S, Tanaka R, Murakami A, Kataoka Y, et al. The characteristics of in vitro biological activity of titanium surfaces anodically oxidized in chloride solutions. Biomaterials 2010;31(33):8546–55.
[150] Shi C, Gao J, Wang M, Fu J, Wang D, Zhu Y. Ultra-trace silver-doped hydroxyapatite with non-cytotoxicity and effective antibacterial activity. Mater Sci Eng C Mater Biol Appl 2015;55:497–505.
[151] Wood NJ, Jenkinson HF, Davis SA, Mann S, O'Sullivan DJ, Barbour ME. Chlorhexidine hexametaphosphate nanoparticles as a novel antimicrobial coating for dental implants. J Mater Sci Mater Med 2015;26(6):5532.
[152] Lee JH, Ryu MY, Baek HR, Seo JH, Lee KM. Generation of an rhBMP-2-loaded beta-tricalcium phosphate/hydrogel composite and evaluation of its efficacy on peri-implant bone formation. Biomed Mater 2014;9(5):055002.
[153] Bhattarai G, Lee YH, Lee MH, Park IS, Yi HK. Insulin-like growth factor binding protein-3 affects osteogenic efficacy on dental implants in rat mandible. Mater Sci Eng C Mater Biol Appl 2015;55:490–6.
[154] Elmengaard B, Bechtold JE, Soballe K. In vivo study of the effect of RGD treatment on bone ongrowth on press-fit titanium alloy implants. Biomaterials 2005;26(17):3521–6.
[155] Fernandez-Garcia E, Chen X, Gutierrez-Gonzalez CF, Fernandez A, Lopez-Esteban S, Aparicio C. Peptide-functionalized zirconia and new zirconia/titanium biocermets for dental applications. J Dent 2015;43(9):1162–74.
[156] Gorbahn M, Klein MO, Lehnert M, Ziebart T, Brullmann D, Koper I, et al. Promotion of osteogenic cell response using quasicovalent immobilized fibronectin on titanium surfaces: introduction of a novel biomimetic layer system. J Oral Maxillofac Surg 2012;70(8):1827–34.
[157] Cei S, Karapetsa D, Aleo E, Graziani F. Protein adsorption on a laser-modified titanium implant surface. Implant Dent 2015;24(2):134–41.
[158] Marin-Pareja N, Salvagni E, Guillem-Marti J, Aparicio C, Ginebra MP. Collagen-functionalised titanium surfaces for biological sealing of dental implants: effect of immobilisation process on fibroblasts response. Colloids Surf B Biointerfaces 2014;122:601–10.
[159] Chen X, Sevilla P, Aparicio C. Surface biofunctionalization by covalent co-immobilization of oligopeptides. Colloids Surf B Biointerfaces 2013;107:189–97.
[160] Salvagni E, Berguig G, Engel E, Rodriguez-Cabello JC, Coullerez G, Textor M, et al. A bioactive elastin-like recombinamer reduces unspecific protein adsorption and enhances cell response on titanium surfaces. Colloids Surf B Biointerfaces 2014;114:225–33.
[161] Andreiotelli M, Wenz HJ, Kohal RJ. Are ceramic implants a viable alternative to titanium implants? A systematic literature review. Clin Oral Implants Res 2009;20(Suppl. 4):32–47.
[162] Schwitalla A, Muller WD. PEEK dental implants: a review of the literature. J Oral Implantol 2013;39(6):743–9.
[163] Spies BC, Sauter C, Wolkewitz M, Kohal RJ. Alumina reinforced zirconia implants: effects of cyclic loading and abutment modification on fracture resistance. Dent Mater 2015;31(3):262–72.
[164] Sarot JR, Contar CMM, da Cruz ACC, Magini RD. Evaluation of the stress distribution in CFR-PEEK dental implants by the three-dimensional finite element method. J Mater Sci Mater Med 2010;21(7):2079–85.
[165] Aydin C, Yilmaz H, Bankoglu M. A single-tooth, two-piece zirconia implant located in the anterior maxilla: a clinical report. J Prosthet Dent 2013;109(2):70–4.

[166] Kohal RJ, Bachle M, Att W, Chaar S, Altmann B, Renz A, et al. Osteoblast and bone tissue response to surface modified zirconia and titanium implant materials. Dent Mater 2013;29(7):763–76.

[167] Manzano G, Herrero LR, Montero J. Comparison of clinical performance of zirconia implants and titanium implants in animal models: a systematic review. Int J Oral Maxillofac Implants 2014;29(2):311–20.

[168] Conrad HJ, Seong WJ, Pesun IJ. Current ceramic materials and systems with clinical recommendations: a systematic review. J Prosthet Dent 2007;98(5):389–404.

[169] Denry I, Kelly JR. Emerging ceramic-based materials for dentistry. J Dent Res 2014;93(12):1235–42.

[170] Guess PC, Att W, Strub JR. Zirconia in fixed implant prosthodontics. Clin Implant Dent Relat Res 2012;14(5):633–45.

[171] Swain MV. Impact of oral fluids on dental ceramics: what is the clinical relevance? Dent Mater 2014;30(1):33–42.

[172] Lughi V, Sergo V. Low temperature degradation -aging- of zirconia: a critical review of the relevant aspects in dentistry. Dent Mater 2010;26(8):807–20.

[173] da Silva EM, Miragaya L, Sabrosa CE, Maia LC. Stability of the bond between two resin cements and an yttria-stabilized zirconia ceramic after six months of aging in water. J Prosthet Dent 2014;112(3):568–75.

[174] Fischer J, Stawarzcyk B, Trottmann A, Hammerle CH. Impact of thermal misfit on shear strength of veneering ceramic/zirconia composites. Dent Mater 2009;25(4):419–23.

[175] Kohorst P, Borchers L, Strempel J, Stiesch M, Hassel T, Bach FW, et al. Low-temperature degradation of different zirconia ceramics for dental applications. Acta Biomater 2012;8(3):1213–20.

[176] Miragaya L, Maia LC, Sabrosa CE, de Goes MF, da Silva EM. Evaluation of self-adhesive resin cement bond strength to yttria-stabilized zirconia ceramic (Y-TZP) using four surface treatments. J Adhesive Dent 2011;13(5):473–80.

[177] Valverde GB, Coelho PG, Janal MN, Lorenzoni FC, Carvalho RM, Thompson VP, et al. Surface characterisation and bonding of Y-TZP following non-thermal plasma treatment. J Dent 2013;41(1):51–9.

[178] Druck CC, Pozzobon JL, Callegari GL, Dorneles LS, Valandro LF. Adhesion to Y-TZP ceramic: study of silica nanofilm coating on the surface of Y-TZP. J Biomed Mater Res B Appl Biomater 2015;103(1):143–50.

[179] Vanderlei A, Bottino MA, Valandro LF. Evaluation of resin bond strength to yttria-stabilized tetragonal zirconia and framework marginal fit: comparison of different surface conditionings. Oper Dent 2014;39(1):50–63.

[180] Costa AK, Kelly RD, Fleming GJ, Borges AL, Addison O. Laminated ceramics with elastic interfaces: a mechanical advantage? J Dent 2015;43(3):335–41.

[181] Beuer F, Schweiger J, Eichberger M, Kappert HF, Gernet W, Edelhoff D. High-strength CAD/CAM-fabricated veneering material sintered to zirconia copings–a new fabrication mode for all-ceramic restorations. Dent Mater 2009;25(1):121–8.

[182] Awada A, Nathanson D. Mechanical properties of resin-ceramic CAD/CAM restorative materials. J Prosthet Dent 2015;114(4):587–93.

[183] Coldea A, Swain MV, Thiel N. Mechanical properties of polymer-infiltrated-ceramic-network materials. Dent Mater 2013;29(4):419–26.

[184] He LH, Swain M. A novel polymer infiltrated ceramic dental material. Dent Mater 2011;27(6):527–34.

[185] Kassem AS, Atta O, El-Mowafy O. Fatigue resistance and microleakage of CAD/CAM ceramic and composite molar crowns. J Prosthodont 2012;21(1):28–32.

[186] Ilgenstein I, Zitzmann NU, Buhler J, Wegehaupt FJ, Attin T, Weiger R, et al. Influence of proximal box elevation on the marginal quality and fracture behavior of root-filled molars restored with CAD/CAM ceramic or composite onlays. Clin Oral Investig 2015;19(5):1021–8.

[187] Della Bona A, Corazza PH, Zhang Y. Characterization of a polymer-infiltrated ceramic-network material. Dent Mater 2014;30(5):564–9.

[188] Chen C, Trindade FZ, de Jager N, Kleverlaan CJ, Feilzer AJ. The fracture resistance of a CAD/CAM Resin Nano Ceramic (RNC) and a CAD ceramic at different thicknesses. Dent Mater 2014;30(9):954–62.

[189] Duan Y, Griggs JA. Effect of elasticity on stress distribution in CAD/CAM dental crowns: glass ceramic vs. polymer-matrix composite. J Dent 2015;43(6):742–9.

[190] Ferracane JL, Stansbury JW, Burke FJ. Self-adhesive resin cements - chemistry, properties and clinical considerations. J Oral Rehabil 2011;38(4):295–314.

[191] Moszner N, Hirt T. New polymer-chemical developments in clinical dental polymer materials: enamel-dentin adhesives and restorative composites. J Polym Sci Part A Polym Chem 2012;50(21):4369–402.

Interfaces in fixed dental prostheses: challenges and opportunities

3

Y. Zhang[1], *A. Chughtai*[1], *M.S. Wolff*[1], *R. Trushkowsky*[1], *H. Chai*[2]
[1]New York University College of Dentistry, New York, NY, United States; [2]Tel Aviv University, Tel Aviv, Israel

3.1 Introduction

Restorative dentistry is undergoing a paradigm shift from the traditional metalloceramic system to a more esthetic all-ceramic restoration. The phenomenon is analogous to the transition from amalgam to composite direct restoratives that started in the mid to late 1980s and has continued through today.

Over the past decade, zirconia (in particular, yttria-stabilized tetragonal zirconia polycrystal or Y-TZP) and lithium disilicate glass ceramic have emerged as promising restorative materials for all-ceramic prostheses primarily because of their superior mechanical properties. Dental restorations are luted to prepared tooth structures or metal and even ceramic abutments (in the case of implant-supported restorations). Therefore, the durability of the resin–restoration bond holds the key to the clinical longevity of the final restoration. Glass ceramics can be simply acid etched and silanized to promote a strong and stable bond with resin cement [1,2]. Traditional etching silane chemistry is not effective with zirconia, as it is chemically inert and possesses a nonpolar surface [3,4]. There have been a number of surface-modification approaches to improve the resin cement bonding property of zirconia. These approaches may be categorized as mechanical, chemical, or a combination of both. Examples of mechanical surface-modification are grit blasting with alumina particles [5–7] and porous nanocrystalline alumina coating [8–10], whereas those for chemical treatments include thin silicate glass coatings [4,11] and surface functionalization using various chemical treatments [12,13]. Chemomechanical surface treatments have also been widely employed; a classical example is cojet grit blasting for surface silicatization [14]. More recently, a surface glass infiltration method has been developed to modify zirconia surface while preserving, if not, enhancing the mechanical properties of zirconia [15–18]. One of the most important aspects of surface glass infiltration is to create a glass-rich surface that allows the application of the conventional etching silane cementation technique.

Another limitation of the stronger ceramic restorative materials, especially zirconia and to a lesser degree lithium disilicate, is their relatively poor translucency with limited shade selections. New strategies have been implemented to improve the translucency and to expand the shade options of zirconia. To improve

Material-Tissue Interfacial Phenomena. http://dx.doi.org/10.1016/B978-0-08-100330-5.00003-0

the translucency, several manufacturers have introduced a more translucent (optically isotropic) cubic zirconia phase to an ordinarily tetragonal zirconia matrix (eg, CubeX^2, Dental Arts Laboratories, Peoris, IL; and Zpex smile, Tosoh, Tokyo, Japan). The problem is that the strength of these cubic/tetragonal hybrid zirconias is around 600–720 MPa, which is only about one-half to two-thirds that of tetragonal zirconia. To expand the shade selections, 3M ESPE has developed a dye infiltration technique, which also compromises the strength of zirconia [19]. Thus, for better esthetic outcomes, strong ceramics often require a porcelain overlay. In this case, the veneer/core interfacial bond strength becomes critical to clinical success. Porcelain bonding to zirconia is a challenge, due mainly to marked differences in the chemical, mechanical, and thermal properties of these materials. There have been several attempts to improve the adhesion of porcelain to zirconia. One such approach is to use a glass bonding layer to interface porcelain and zirconia. Unfortunately, this can only marginally, if at all, increase the interfacial fracture resistance. A much more effective strategy is to infiltrate zirconia veneering surface with glass prior to veneering. This way, the glass–zirconia graded interlayer provides durable bonds to both porcelain veneer and zirconia core.

Improving bond strength is one thing. To accurately determine a bond strength is another. Over the years, a number of testing methods have been developed to evaluate bond strength in prosthetic materials. The most commonly used in adhesive dentistry are the shear bond strength and microtensile bond strength (eg, Refs. [20–22]). Although relatively simple, such testing methods are flawed by large variations in the bond failure stress, attributed primarily to the inevitable stress concentration at the bond terminus [23,24].

In this chapter, we address the challenges in zirconia bonding, both with the porcelain veneer and resin cement, using a surface glass infiltration method. Such a glass infiltration treatment creates a glass-rich surface at both the veneering and cementation surfaces of a zirconia framework, facilitating a durable diffusion bond with the porcelain veneer via the conventional firing process [25] as well as a strong adhesive bond with resin cement through a standard etching silane technique [26]. The glass-infiltration technique can be readily interfaced with current soft-machining technology, where milled zirconia frameworks or restorations can be infiltrated with porcelain at the veneering and/or cementation surfaces. The glass-infiltrated structures can be glazed as monolithic restorations or veneered for better aesthetics.

We then address the challenges in assessing bond strength by proposing fracture mechanics test methods. The essence of these test methods is to introduce an initial crack starter, which in turn facilitates a smooth crack initiation and growth thus eliminating the sensitivity to stress gradients and flaws as well as reducing the effect of geometric misalignments.

3.2 Experimental

3.2.1 Fabrication of surface glass-infiltrated zirconia

To demonstrate the feasibility of surface glass infiltration of zirconia, a widely used yttria-stabilized zirconia ceramic was selected. Zirconia structures were fabricated from a commercial 3 mol% yttria-stabilized zirconia powder (TZ-3Y-E grade, Tosoh, Tokyo, Japan; average crystal size *d* ~28 nm). The powders were cold isostatically pressed (200 MPa) into green compacts, which were subsequently sintered at 1350°C for 1 h in air and set aside for glass infiltration. An in-house developed feldspathic porcelain composition with coefficient of thermal expansion (CTE) matching that of the zirconia was prepared for glass infiltration. The main composition of the feldspathic porcelain was SiO_2 (65.5 wt%), Al_2O_3 (11.7 wt%), K_2O (10.0 wt%), Na_2O (7.3 wt%), and CaO (3.0 wt%). The glass infiltration process began with the application of a uniform powdered feldspar slurry on the zirconia surface followed by infiltration and densification at 1450°C for 2 h in air. The resulting structure consisted of an outer surface residual glass layer, a glass–zirconia graded interlayer, which gradually transitioned to a dense zirconia interior. A cross-sectional scanning electron microscopic (SEM) (Hitachi 3500N, Japan) view of such a structure is shown in Fig. 3.1(a). As can be seen, the thickness of the residual glass layer is typically less than 50 μm, whereas that of the graded layer is ~120 μm. To elucidate the dependence of mechanical properties on microstructure, nanoindentations (3D Omni Probe TriboIndenter, Hysitron, Minneapolis, MN) were conducted from the outer surface residual glass layer, through the graded glass–zirconia layer, to the zirconia interior. The Young's modulus and hardness values increased from the residual glass layer, to the graded glass–zirconia layer, to the Y-TZP interior (Fig. 3.1(b) and (c)).

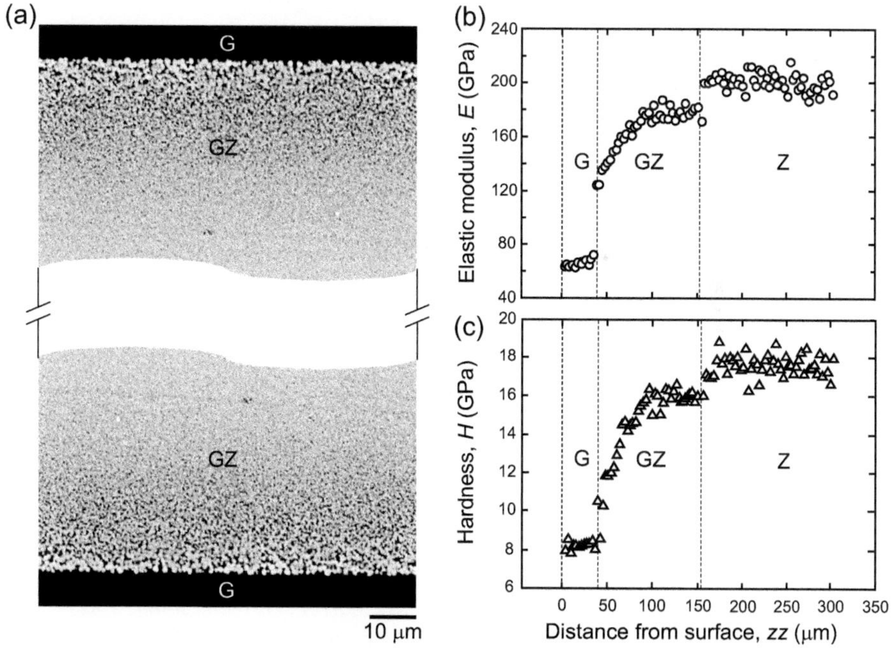

Figure 3.1 Structure and properties of surface glass-infiltrated zirconia. (a) SEM cross-sectional view of glass-infiltrated zirconia. Spatial dependence of (b) Young's modulus and (c) hardness in glass-infiltrated zirconia. *G*, residual glass; *GZ*, graded zirconia; *Z*, zirconia.

For comparison, zirconia monoliths were prepared using the same starting powder and sintered at 1450°C for 2h in air. The densified structure had an average grain size of ~0.5 μm and a 4-point flexure strength of 1400 MPa [27].

3.2.2 Determination of the veneer/core interfacial fracture resistance

To accurately determine the interfacial fracture resistance of porcelain-veneered zirconia structures, we adopted a 4-point-bend test configuration (Fig. 3.2) [26]. Fully sintered zirconia bars 30mm in length, 2.3mm in thickness, and 2.5mm in width were prepared. Two veneering protocols were applied: porcelain fused directly onto zirconia (P group, $n=10$) and porcelain fused to zirconia with a thin glass binder (B group, $n=10$). Prior to veneering, the zirconia surface was grit blasted with 50 μm Al_2O_3 particles at a pressure of 2 bars for 5 s and then steam cleaned. Porcelain was applied using a standard enameling method, where a powdered slurry (Heraceram Zirconia, leucite-reinforced porcelain, $CTE = 10.5 \times 10^{-6}\ K^{-1}$; Heraeus Kulzer GmbH, Hanau, Germany) was layered onto zirconia or zirconia with a glass binder (HeraCeram ZR-Adhesive paste, Heraeus Kulzer GmbH, $CTE = 10.5 \times 10^{-6}\ K^{-1}$) and fired at 870°C for 1 min. The thickness of the porcelain veneer was 0.4mm.

The graded Y-TZP bars were prepared as described in Section 3.2.1. All bending bars had a final dimension of $30 \times 2.7 \times 2.5\ mm^3$.

Fracture test was conducted using a 4-point-bend test with the porcelain veneer or the glass outer layer (in graded Y-TZP) loaded in tension. The distance between the lower and upper supporting pins, l and d, were 20 and 10mm, respectively. The tensile surface and side walls of the bar specimens were polished down to a 1 μm diamond suspension finish. A Vickers indentation was placed at the center of the tensile surface to produce a starter crack. For reference, some graded Y-TZP bars ($n=10$) were tested as fabricated. Flexural tests were performed on a conventional universal testing machine (Instron 5566, Norwood, MA) at a displacement rate of 0.1 mm/min. Crack evolution was monitored from the polished specimen side walls using a video camera (Canon EOS-7D) equipped with a high-power zoom lens (Optem, Inc.).

Under the current flexural loading configuration, the tensile stress, σ_p, at the porcelain surface (lower surface) of the porcelain-veneered zirconia bilayer is given by [28]

$$\sigma_p = 1.5P\,(l-d)\,/\,\left[bH^2\,(E_2/E_1 + 6h/H)\right] \tag{3.1}$$

where P is the fracture load, E is the Young's modulus, and subscripts 1 and 2 indicate porcelain and zirconia. H and b are the total thickness and width of the bar specimen, respectively, while h is the veneer thickness.

For the graded material, the tensile stress at the surface of the residual glass layer, σ_g, and at the adjacent zirconia surface, σ_y, can be estimated as in Ref. [25].

$$\sigma_g = 1.5P\,(l-d)\,E_1/\left(E_2bH^2\right) \tag{3.2a}$$

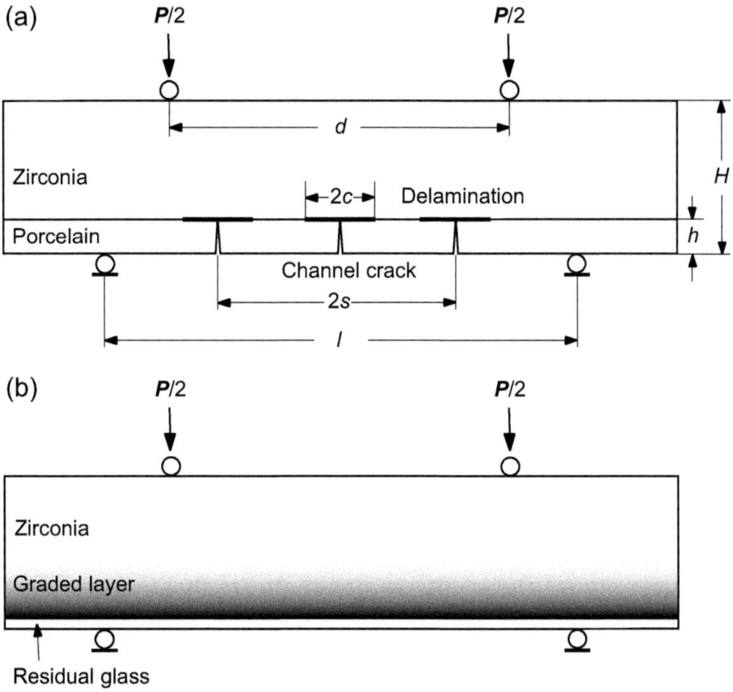

Figure 3.2 Four-point-bend flexural test for the interfacial fracture resistance measurement. (a) Porcelain-veneered zirconia and (b) glass-infiltrated zirconia bar specimens loaded in a four-point-bend fixture.

$$\sigma_y = 1.5P\,(l-d)\,/\,\left(bH^2\right) \tag{3.2b}$$

The energy release rate, G, for interfacial cracking in the porcelain-veneered zirconia bars was determined by numerical simulations using a commercial finite element analysis (FEA) code (Abaqus, Inc.) [25].

3.2.3 Determination of the zirconia–resin interfacial fracture resistance

To determine the fracture resistance at the zirconia–resin interface, we utilized a wedge-loaded double-cantilever beam test (Fig. 3.3). Fully sintered monolithic zirconia as well as glass-infiltrated zirconia bars 30 mm in length, 3 mm in thickness, and 3 mm in width were prepared. For reference, feldspathic ceramic bars 35 mm in length, 5 mm in thickness, and 3 mm in width were cut from commercial fine-structured feldspathic ceramic computer-aided design/computer-assisted manufacturing (CAD/CAM) blocks (VITABLOCS TriLuxe forte). The properties of the test specimens are shown in Table 3.1.

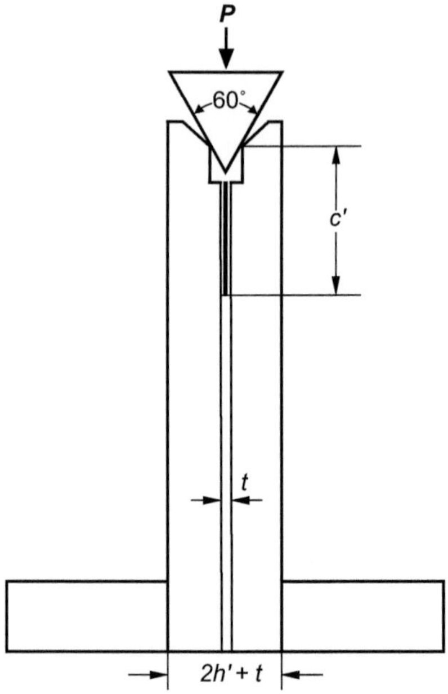

Figure 3.3 Wedge-loaded double-cantilever beam test for the interfacial fracture energy measurement.

Table 3.1 Young's modulus and Poisson's ratio for materials used in this study

Material	Young's modulus E (GPa)	Poisson's ratio ν
Monolithic zirconia	216[b]	0.30[b]
Glass-infiltrated zirconia	211[b]	0.32[b]
Feldspathic ceramic	63[a]	0.22[a]
Resin cement	7[a]	0.35[a]

[a]Manufacturers' data sheets.
[b]Measured using the ultrasonic method.

Test specimens were prepared by adhesive cementation of two identical ceramic bars with a commercial dental cement (Panavia F 2.0, Kuraray, Osaka, Japan). To enhance bond strength, the cementation surfaces of the ceramic bars were subject to grit blasting or acid etching [29–33]. Five groups of bonded specimens ($n=20$) were prepared: Groups 1, 2, and 3 being monolithic zirconia, glass-infiltrated zirconia, and feldspathic ceramic, respectively, grit blasted with 50 μm Al_2O_3 particles (1 bar for glass-infiltrated zirconia and feldspathic ceramic, and 2 bars for zirconia); Groups 4 and 5 being glass-infiltrated zirconia and feldspathic ceramic, etched with

5% hydrofluoric acid (VITA Ceramic Etch) for 2 and 1 min, respectively. Cementation was carried out following manufacturer's instructions; the thickness of the cement layer was controlled using a 50 μm-thick aluminum foil spacer. To examine the long-term durability of the cement bond, the cemented bars were subjected to two different conditioning treatments: (1) short-term incubation in distilled water at 37°C for 7 days and (2) long-term thermal cycling between 5°C and 55°C for 20,000 cycles followed by 60 days incubation at 37°C in distilled water.

The bonded specimens were loaded with a hardened steel wedge (60°) while their lower portions were clamped down by a vice. Load was applied with a constant displacement rate of 0.1 mm/min. The crack propagation was observed in situ from the polished specimen side using a video camera equipped with a high-power zoom lens. Critical load for the onset of rapid fracture was determined from the video footage. The fracture surfaces were examined with both optical microscope and SEM.

The energy release rate G from the interfacial cracking under wedge load can be described by Ref. [34]:

$$GEh' b^2/P^2 = f\left(c'/h'\right) \tag{3.3}$$

where P is the applied load and E is the Young's modulus of the test specimen. f is a function of c'/h', which can be obtained by FEA.

3.2.4 Statistical analysis

The interfacial fracture energy or energy release rate (G_C) data were analyzed by two-way analysis of variance (ANOVA) using a general linear model. Pairwise multiple comparisons were performed using the Tukey test. The significance level was set at $p = .05$ for all analyses.

3.3 Results

3.3.1 The veneer/core interface

3.3.1.1 Porcelain-veneered zirconia

Selective video frames revealing various stages of crack evolution are shown in Fig. 3.4. At a relatively low stress level, $\sigma_p = 93.1$ MPa, a channel crack popped in from the tensile surface of the porcelain veneer and ceased at the veneer/core interface (a). Close inspection revealed that this crack did not initiate from the Vickers indent, suggesting that the size of the defects in porcelain is of the same order as the indentation damage. Multiple channel cracks appeared at higher loads; the space between these cracks was approximately 3 times the layer thickness (b). At a higher stress level, $\sigma_p = 124.8$ MPa, cracks began to propagate along the porcelain/zirconia interface almost spontaneously from every channel crack (c). These interfacial cracks grew stably as the load further increased (d).

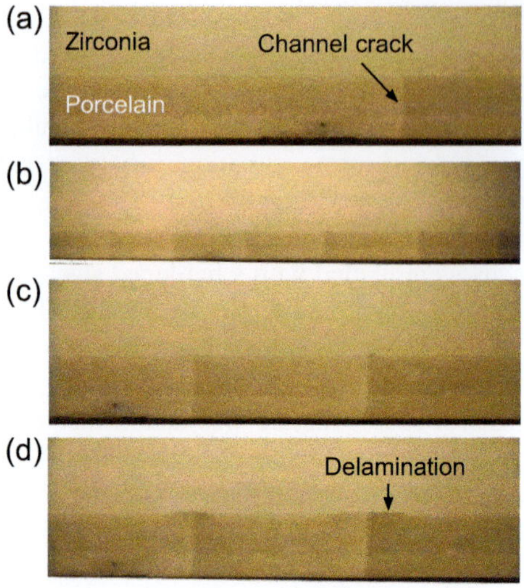

Figure 3.4 Selected video frames of porcelain-veneered zirconia bar specimens (Group P) loaded in a four-point-bend fixture. (a) Onset of a channel crack at σ=93.1 MPa. (b) A lower magnification view showing nearly evenly spaced channel cracks (σ=102 MPa). (c) Onset of delamination from the vertical cracks tips at σ=124.8 MPa. (d) Stable interfacial crack growth (delamination) at σ=184.8 MPa. σ defines the tensile stress at the lower surface of the porcelain veneer (~0.4 mm in thickness), as derived from Eq. (3.1).

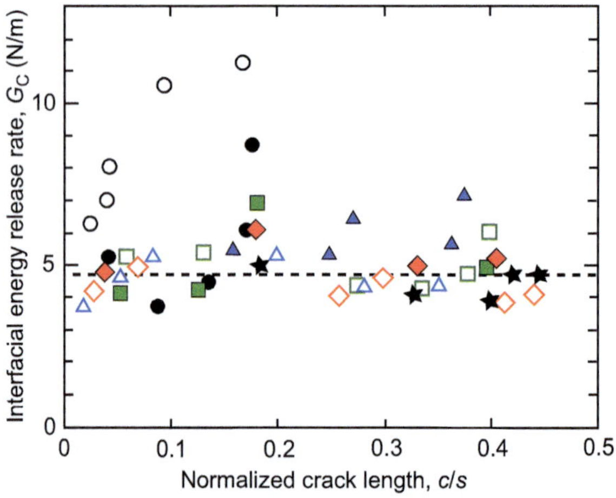

Figure 3.5 The dependence of the interfacial energy release rate on the normalized delamination length *c/s* for all porcelain-veneered zirconia bar specimens. The dashed line represents the mean fracture energy, whereas the open and filled symbols correspond to porcelain-veneered zirconia with (Group B) and without (Group P) a glass binder, respectively. Various symbols represent different specimens.

The relationship of critical interfacial energy release rate G_C with normalized crack length can be obtained using Eq. (3.3). The data are plotted in Fig. 3.5 with each test represented by a different symbol. There is no significant difference in the fracture energy for porcelain-veneered zirconia with (Group B, filled symbols) and without (Group P, unfilled symbols) a glass binder. In addition, there appears to be no apparent dependence of interfacial energy release rate G_C on crack length. It is important to note that the quantity G_C is a combination of nearly equal contribution from modes I and II [35]. The average ± standard deviation value of G_C was 4.8 ± 1.4 N/m, which is significantly lower than the literature value for pure mode I fracture of porcelain (11.0 N/m) [16].

3.3.1.2 Glass-infiltrated zirconia

All glass-infiltrated zirconia fractured by a characteristic single channel crack in flexure (Fig. 3.6(a)). A low-magnification view of the fractured bar revealed neither evidence of multiple channel cracks nor delamination of the glass overlay (Fig. 3.6(b)). Therefore, no quantitative evaluation of the G_C value was performed for this material system. A SEM image of the fractured surface of glass-infiltrated zirconia showed that the

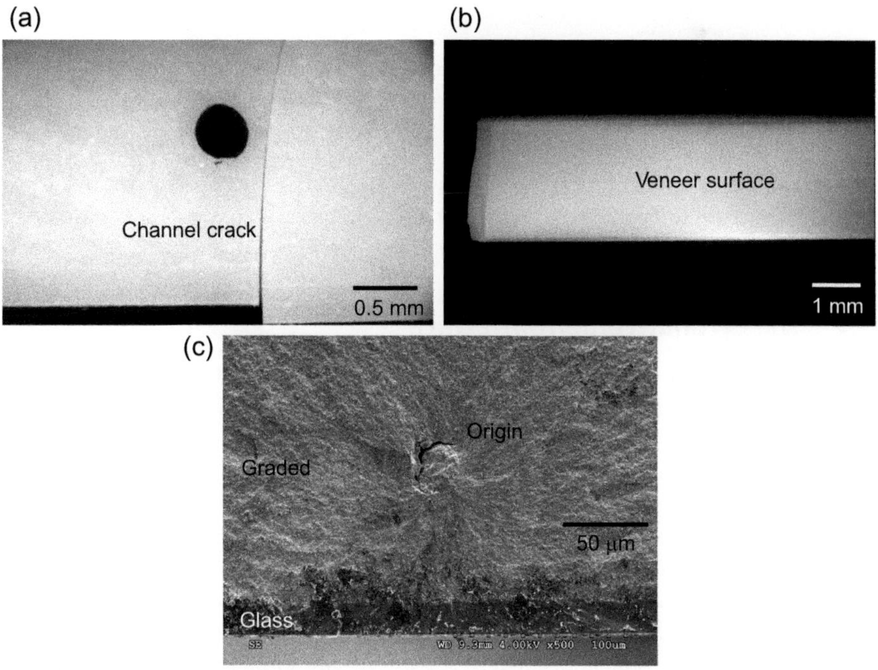

Figure 3.6 An optical micrograph revealing a characteristic single-channel crack mode in glass-infiltrated zirconia bar specimens (a). A low-magnification view of the fractured bar showing no evidence of multiple channel cracking as well as delamination of the glass overlay (b). An SEM image of the fracture surface in graded zirconia, showing that fracture initiates from the graded zirconia layer below the interface with the glass layer (c).

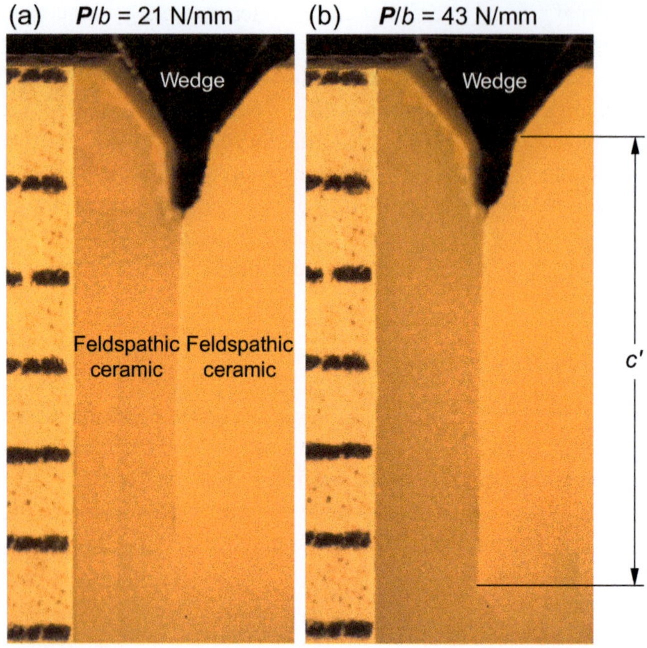

Figure 3.7 Selected video frames showing the interfacial crack configuration of feldspathic ceramic/cement/feldspathic ceramic double-cantilever beams loaded with a hardened steel wedge.

crack origin was located in the graded glass–zirconia zone, well below the interface with the glass overlay, suggesting that the graded layer was able to effectively transfer the maximum tensile stress from the surface to interior (Fig. 3.6(c)).

3.3.2 The ceramic/cement interface

Representative video frames of the crack configuration for feldspathic ceramic/cement/feldspathic ceramic specimen under the wedge load are shown in Fig. 3.7. The crack walls began to open upon loading, making the crack visible (see the bright line at the center of the specimen in Fig. 3.7(a)). With increasing load, the crack grew a small distance before rapid fracture took place (Fig. 3.7(b)).

The interfacial fracture energy G_C for each test group was computed using Eq. (3.3) in combination with FEA analysis and the elastic constants from Table 3.1. The crack length c_i was determined from postmortem inspection of the fractured surface using a stereomicroscope. The data are shown in Fig. 3.8, where the unshaded and shaded bars correspond to the mean and standard deviation values for baseline specimens and those subjected to thermocycling and aging treatments, respectively.

Quantitative comparison of the mean and standard deviation values from each specimen group with and without aging is shown in Table 3.2. Two-way ANOVA showed that both factors (time: $p = .044$; Groups: $p = .000$), and the interaction between them ($p = .000$), were significant.

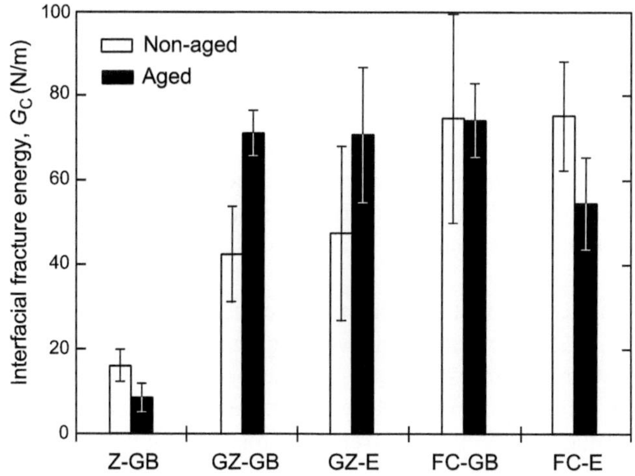

Figure 3.8 Bar chart of the interfacial fracture energy G_C (mean and standard deviation) for double-cantilever beam specimens with (shaded) and without (unshaded) thermocycling and aging treatments. *E*, acid etched; *FC*, feldspathic ceramic; *GB*, grit blasted; *GZ*, glass-infiltrated zirconia; *Z*, zirconia.

Table 3.2 The 95% confidence interval for the mean interfacial fracture energy

	Z-GB	GZ-GB	GZ-E	FC-GB	FC-E
Baseline	14.3–17.8^{cA}	34.8–49.7^{bB}	33.3–61.9^{abA}	58.5–84.6^{aA}	66.4–85.0^{aA}
Aged	6.2–10.7^{cB}	67.8–74.5^{aA}	60.3–81.3^{abA}	68.8–80.1^{aA}	47.7–61.5^{bB}

Superscript lowercase letters indicate significant difference among groups. Superscript uppercase letters indicate significant difference between baseline and thermocycled plus aged groups.
E, acid etched; *FC*, feldspathic ceramic; *GB*, grit blasted; *GZ*, glass-infiltrated zirconia; *Z*, zirconia.

Data from Fig. 3.8 and Table 3.2 revealed the following important findings:

First, glass-infiltrated zirconia exhibited a greater G_C relative to zirconia, approaching that of the feldspathic ceramic even after long-term thermocycling and wet storage. Second, thermal cycling and wet storage treatments only affected the G_C value of bonded zirconia specimens. Finally, no significant difference in G_C values was observed in grit-blasted and acid-etched specimen groups.

3.4 Discussion

3.4.1 Fracture resistance of veneer/core diffusion bonding

The fracture resistance of diffusion bonding between a thin porcelain layer and zirconia substrate with or without a glass binder has been determined using a 4-point-bend configuration with porcelain overlay loaded in tension. Upon loading, evenly spaced channel cracks initiated at the porcelain surface and extended to the porcelain/zirconia interface, where the cracks began to propagate along the veneer/core interface, resulting in delamination of the porcelain overlay. The space between the channel cracks was about 3 times the layer thickness. The measured interfacial energy release rate was $G_C = 4.8 \pm 1.4$ N/m for porcelain-veneered zirconia with or without an intermittent glass binder. The glass binder did not enhance the veneer/core interfacial bonding. This is because despite a good diffusion bond between the glass binder and the porcelain overlay, the bonding between the glass binder and zirconia framework remained weak.

It is interesting to note that the reported interfacial fracture G_C values on similar porcelain-veneered zirconia specimens were significantly higher than those observed in the present research. For instance, G_C values for porcelain-veneered zirconia bars made from four different commercial systems ranged between 8 and 17 N/m [36]. A similar G_C value (12.4 N/m) was reported for porcelain-veneered zirconia bars loaded in 4-point-bend flexure [37]. The discrepancy in G_C values between the current study and the previous studies may be attributed, in part, to the stress shielding effect afforded by the multiple channel cracks. Such channel cracks were not reported and analyzed in the previous studies [36,38]. Our FEA have shown that shielding provided by adjacent channel cracks has enhanced the interfacial fracture resistance, which has ultimately altered the critical interfacial energy release rate.

For glass-infiltrated zirconia specimens, fracture occurred from a single channel crack and the fracture stress was significantly higher than that of porcelain-veneered zirconia structures. Our findings have demonstrated that graded zirconia structures produced by surface glass infiltration can offer a remedy to prevent delamination at the veneer/core interface. In the case of dental restorations, interfacial cracks may form after occlusal surface–originated channel cracks propagate to the veneer/core interface. Once formed, these interfacial cracks may graze along the interface or deflect toward the free surface, resulting in delamination and/or chip [39]. Which route the crack may take depends on a number of factors, including the local geometry of the restoration and loading conditions, as well as residual stresses induced from CTE mismatch between the veneer and core [40–43], cooling rate [36], and veneer/core thickness ratio [44]. In addition, multiple channel cracks may also occur in regions where the veneer layer or glaze layer is relatively thin and are exposed to flexural tensile stresses, eg, the lower portion of connectors in multiunit fixed dental prostheses (Fig. 3.9).

3.4.2 Fracture resistance of ceramic/resin adhesive bonding

The interfacial fracture resistance of adhesively bonded zirconia-based restoratives relative to a bonded feldspathic ceramic has been examined using a wedge-loaded double-cantilever beam test. Upon loading, the preinduced initial crack at the cementation interface opens up. With increasing load the crack grows slowly a small distance before a rapid fracture occurs. The measured interfacial fracture energy G_C for grit-blasted and resin-bonded surfaces before long-term thermocycling and water storage treatments were 16.1 ± 3.9 N/m, 42.3 ± 11.4 N/m, 75.1 ± 24.9 N/m for zirconia, glass-infiltrated zirconia, and feldspathic ceramic, respectively. As can be seen, G_C for glass-infiltrated

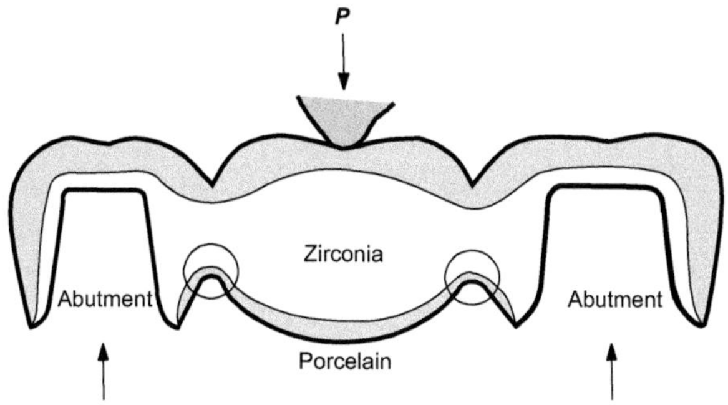

Figure 3.9 Illustration of a fixed dental prosthesis. The thin porcelain layer at the lower portion of the connectors experiences tensile stresses due to bending, which may lead to vertical cracks and delamination.

zirconia was significantly higher than that for zirconia. After the aging treatment, G_C for zirconia decreased to 8.4 ± 3.3 N/m, whereas that for glass-infiltrated zirconia increased to 71.1 ± 5.5 N/m, approaching the G_C value of 74.5 ± 8.6 N/m for feldspathic ceramic. In addition, both the glass-infiltrated zirconia and feldspathic ceramic surfaces can be acid etched (hydrofluoric acid, 5%) and silanized prior to resin bonding, a technique that is very familiar to the dental practitioner. Our data revealed that G_C for acid-etched and silanized glass-infiltrated zirconia before and after the aging treatment were 47.6 ± 20.6 N/m and 70.8 ± 16.0 N/m, respectively, again similar to those for their feldspathic ceramic counterparts 75.7 ± 13.4 N/m and 54.6 ± 11.1 N/m, respectively. Based on our findings, zirconia surface glass infiltration emerged as an effective technique to overcome the poor resin cement bonding properties of zirconia.

For adhesively bonded joints, the resistance to interfacial fracture is governed by several key factors: the adherend materials, cemention surface treatments, and stress states at the crack tip [45–49]. The current study examined the interfacial fracture resistance of zirconia-based and feldspathic ceramic structures bonded with a common adherend material under the same specimen and testing configurations. Thus, it provided a direct comparison of different cementation surface materials and treatments. For glass-infiltrated zirconia and feldspathic ceramic surfaces, the measured mode I fracture energy G_C was around 70 N/m, regardless of the surface treatment conditions (ie, acid etched or grit blasted). This finding suggests that it is the presence of the glass phase rather than the surface treatment condition that is responsible for the enhanced bond strength in glass-infiltrated zirconia. Previous studies investigated the mode I interfacial fracture energy G_C of epoxy resin–bonded aluminum alloys [46,47]. It was found that G_C values approached the intrinsic fracture resistance of a neat resin (~70 N/m) when the bond thickness $t<50\,\mu m$. Such a bond thickness range is most pertinent to the luting cement thickness used in restorative prostheses. Based on the this analysis, one may conclude that fracture in resin-bonded glass-infiltrated zirconia and feldspathic ceramic took place within the adhesive resin rather than the resin cement/glass interface. This is certainly not the case for resin cement–bonded zirconia, where the interfacial fracture energy G_C was much lower than that of the neat resin, suggesting that fracture occurred at the zirconia/resin cement interface.

The fact that thermocycling and water storage treatments tended to reduce the G_C for zirconia, whereas increase the G_C for glass-infiltrated zirconia and feldspathic ceramic warrants further discussion. Thermocycling between 5°C and 55°C water baths introduces stresses into the system owing to the difference in coefficient of thermal expansion between ceramic and cement. It is possible that the reduction in G_C of zirconia is due to the weakening of an already weak interface by cyclic thermal stressing. In addition, the weak interface permits incursion of water, which in turn can dramatically reduce the interfacial bond strength. The thermal stressing and water storage treatments become less effective in well-bonded glass-infiltrated zirconia and feldspathic ceramic. In fact, a slight increase in G_C was observed for these materials following thermocycling and water storage treatments. A previous study also reported a significant increase in the mean tensile bond strength of resin-bonded glass ceramics after thermocycling [50]. It was suggested that such an improvement may be attributed to postcuring of the resin cement owing to the elevated temperature utilized in the thermocycling treatment [50].

We acknowledge that the resin bond strength reported here was measured under pure mode I tensile loading. In a clinical setting, bonded dental restorations may be subjected to combined tensile and shear loading, which may significantly affect the interfacial fracture energy. A previous study showed that over the clinically acceptable cement thickness range (typically 20–100 μm), the fracture energy under shear loading (mode II) is much higher than that under tensile loading (mode I) [47]. In fact, to measure G_C in shear, one may need to apply such a high load that it can cause fracture of ceramic adherends before any growth of the interfacial crack. This is the reason why we have adopted a mode I tensile loading configuration in this study.

3.5 Conclusions

We have demonstrated that infiltration of glass into the zirconia veneering surface can effectively prevent veneer chipping and delamination, whereas glass infiltration at the cementation surface can increase the interfacial fracture energy of zirconia by over a factor of 3, to a level consistent with feldspathic ceramic. These qualities, together with the increased resistance to flexural fracture, occlusal contact damage, edge chipping, and delamination found in previous studies [17,51–54], suggest that glass-infiltrated zirconia is a promising dental restorative material. In addition, with much improved cement bond strength, the glass-infiltrated zirconia can now extend the clinical indications of zirconia to more conservative treatments, where adhesively bonded partial-coverage restorations are preferred over the traditional full-coverage crowns and fixed dental prostheses.

Acknowledgments

This work was sponsored by funding from the United States National Institute of Dental & Craniofacial Research, National Institutes of Health (P.I.Y. Zhang, Grant 2R01 DE017925) and the Israeli Science Foundation (P.I.H. Chai, ISF Grant no. 810/09).

References

[1] Tian T, Tsoi JK, Matinlinna JP, Burrow MF. Aspects of bonding between resin luting cements and glass ceramic materials. Dent Mater 2014;30:e147–62.
[2] Blatz MB, Sadan A, Kern M. Resin-ceramic bonding: a review of the literature. J Prosthet Dent 2003;89:268–74.
[3] Sanli S, Comlekoglu MD, Comlekoglu E, Sonugelen M, Pamir T, Darvell BW. Influence of surface treatment on the resin-bonding of zirconia. Dent Mater 2015;31:657–68.
[4] Piascik JR, Swift EJ, Thompson JY, Grego S, Stoner BR. Surface modification for enhanced silanation of zirconia ceramics. Dent Mater 2009;25:1116–21.
[5] Kosmac T, Oblak C, Jevnikar P, Funduk N, Marion L. The effect of surface grinding and sandblasting on flexural strength and reliability of Y-TZP zirconia ceramic. Dent Mater 1999;15:426–33.
[6] Zhang Y, Lawn BR, Malament KA, Van Thompson P, Rekow ED. Damage accumulation and fatigue life of particle-abraded ceramics. Int J Prosthodont 2006;19:442–8.
[7] Zhang Y, Lawn BR, Rekow ED, Thompson VP. Effect of sandblasting on the long-term performance of dental ceramics. J Biomed Mater Res B Appl Biomater 2004;71:381–6.
[8] Jevnikar P, Krnel K, Kocjan A, Funduk N, Kosmac T. The effect of nano-structured alumina coating on resin-bond strength to zirconia ceramics. Dent Mater 2010;26:688–96.
[9] Kocjan A, Dakskobler A, Kosmac T. Superhydrophobic nanostructured boehmite coatings prepared by AlN powder hydrolysis. Int J Appl Ceram Technol 2011;8:848–53.
[10] Srikanth R, Kosmac T, Della Bona A, Yin L, Zhang Y. Effects of cementation surface modifications on fracture resistance of zirconia. Dent Mater 2015;31.
[11] Queiroz JR, Benetti P, Massi M, Junior LN, Della Bona A. Effect of multiple firing and silica deposition on the zirconia-porcelain interfacial bond strength. Dent Mater 2012;28:763–8.
[12] Kern M, Wegner SM. Bonding to zirconia ceramic: adhesion methods and their durability. Dent Mater 1998;14:64–71.
[13] Oliveira-Ogliari A, Collares FM, Feitosa VP, Sauro S, Ogliari FA, Moraes RR. Methacrylate bonding to zirconia by in situ silica nanoparticle surface deposition. Dent Mater 2015;31:68–76.
[14] Blatz MB, Chiche G, Holst S, Sadan A. Influence of surface treatment and simulated aging on bond strengths of luting agents to zirconia. Quintessence Int 2007;38:745–53.
[15] Ren L, Janal MN, Zhang Y. Sliding contact fatigue of graded zirconia with external esthetic glass. J Dent Res 2011;90:1116–21.
[16] Zhang Y, Chai H, Lawn BR. Graded structures for all-ceramic restorations. J Dent Res 2010;89:417–21.
[17] Zhang Y, Lee JJ, Srikanth R, Lawn BR. Edge chipping and flexural resistance of monolithic ceramics. Dent Mater 2013;29:1201–8.
[18] Zhang Y, Sun MJ, Zhang DZ. Designing functionally graded materials with superior load-bearing properties. Acta Biomater 2012;8:1101–8.
[19] Shah K, Holloway JA, Denry IL. Effect of coloring with various metal oxides on the microstructure, color, and flexural strength of 3Y-TZP. J Biomed Mater Res B Appl Biomater 2008;87:329–37.
[20] Guess PC, Kulis A, Witkowski S, Wolkewitz M, Zhang Y, Strub JR. Shear bond strengths between different zirconia cores and veneering ceramics and their susceptibility to thermocycling. Dent Mater 2008;24:1556–67.
[21] Sano H, Shono T, Sonoda H, Takatsu T, Ciucchi B, Carvalho R, et al. Relationship between surface area for adhesion and tensile bond strength — evaluation of a micro-tensile bond test. Dent Mater 1994;10:236–40.

[22] Uhrenbacher J, Schmidlin PR, Keul C, Eichberger M, Roos M, Gernet W, et al. The effect of surface modification on the retention strength of polyetheretherketone crowns adhesively bonded to dentin abutments. J Prosthet Dent 2014;112:1489–97.
[23] Della Bona A, van Noort R. Shear vs. tensile bond strength of resin composite bonded to ceramic. J Dent Res 1995;74:1591–6.
[24] Van Noort R, Noroozi S, Howard IC, Cardew G. A critique of bond strength measurements. J Dent 1989;17:61–7.
[25] Chai H, Lee JJ, Mieleszko AJ, Chu SJ, Zhang Y. On the interfacial fracture of porcelain/zirconia and graded zirconia dental structures. Acta Biomater 2014;10:3756–61.
[26] Chai H, Kaizer M, Chughtai A, Tong H, Tanaka C, Zhang Y. On the interfacial fracture resistance of resin-bonded zirconia and glass-infiltrated graded zirconia. Dent Mater 2015;31.
[27] Tong H, Tanaka CB, Kaizer MR, Zhang Y. Characterization of three commercial Y-TZP ceramics produced for their high-translucency, high-strength and high-surface area. Ceram Int 2016;42:1077–85.
[28] Chai H, Fox J. On delamination growth from channel cracks in thin-film coatings. Int J Solids Struct 2012;49:3142–7.
[29] Della Bona A. Bonding to ceramics: scientific evidences for clinical dentistry. São Paulo Artes Médicas 2009.
[30] Kern M, Barloi A, Yang B. Surface conditioning influences zirconia ceramic bonding. J Dent Res 2009;88:817–22.
[31] Ozcan M, Kerkdijk S, Valandro LF. Comparison of resin cement adhesion to Y-TZP ceramic following manufacturers' instructions of the cements only. Clin Oral Investig 2008;12:279–82.
[32] Thurmond JW, Barkmeier WW, Wilwerding TM. Effect of porcelain surface treatments on bond strengths of composite resin bonded to porcelain. J Prosthet Dent 1994;72:355–9.
[33] Wolfart M, Lehmann F, Wolfart S, Kern M. Durability of the resin bond strength to zirconia ceramic after using different surface conditioning methods. Dent Mater 2007;23:45–50.
[34] Chai H, Ravichandran G. Transverse fracture in multilayers from tension and line-wedge indentation. Int J Fract 2007;145:299–312.
[35] Mei HX, Pang YY, Huang R. Influence of interfacial delamination on channel cracking of elastic thin films. Int J Fract 2007;148:331–42.
[36] Göstemeyer G, Jendras M, Dittmer MP, Bach FW, Stiesch M, Kohorst P. Influence of cooling rate on zirconia/veneer interfacial adhesion. Acta Biomater 2010;6:4532–8.
[37] Le Thanh R. Adhesion of veneering porcelain to zirconium dioxide ceramic as determined by the strain energy release rate. [Thesis: Doctor of Clinical Dentistry, Discipline of Prosthodontics 2009]. Sydney, Australia: The University of Sydney; Faculty of Dentistry; 2009.
[38] White SN, Miklus VG, McLaren EA, Lang LA, Caputo AA. Flexural strength of a layered zirconia and porcelain dental all-ceramic system. J Prosthet Dent 2005;94:125–31.
[39] Pang Z, Chughtai A, Sailer I, Zhang Y. A fractographic study of clinically retrieved zirconia-ceramic and metal-ceramic fixed dental prostheses. Dent Mater 2015;31:1198–206.
[40] Baldassarri M, Stappert CF, Wolff MS, Thompson VP, Zhang Y. Residual stresses in porcelain-veneered zirconia prostheses. Dent Mater 2012;28:873–9.
[41] Hermann I, Bhowmick S, Zhang Y, Lawn BR. Competing fracture modes in brittle materials subject to concentrated cyclic loading in liquid environments: trilayer structures. J Mater Res 2006;21:512–21.
[42] Mainjot AK, Schajer GS, Vanheusden AJ, Sadoun MJ. Influence of zirconia framework thickness on residual stress profile in veneering ceramic: measurement by hole-drilling. Dent Mater 2012;28:378–84.

[43] Meira JB, Reis BR, Tanaka CB, Ballester RY, Cesar PF, Versluis A, et al. Residual stresses in Y-TZP crowns due to changes in the thermal contraction coefficient of veneers. Dent Mater 2013;29:594–601.
[44] Swain MV. Unstable cracking (chipping) of veneering porcelain on all-ceramic dental crowns and fixed partial dentures. Acta Biomater 2009;5:1668–77.
[45] Cao HC, Evans AG. An experimental study of the fracture resistance of bimaterial interfaces. Mech Mater 1989;7:295–304.
[46] Chai H. On the correlation between the mode I failure of adhesive joints and laminated composites. Eng Fract Mech 1986;24:413–31.
[47] Chai H. Shear fracture. Int J Fract 1988;37:137–59.
[48] Swadener JG, Liechti KM. Asymmetric shielding mechanisms in the mixed-mode fracture of a glass/epoxy interface. J Appl Mech Trans ASME 1998;65:25–9.
[49] Wang JS, Suo Z. Experimental-determination of interfacial toughness curves using brazil-nut-sandwiches. Acta Metall Mater 1990;38:1279–90.
[50] Hooshmand T, van Noort R, Keshvad A. Bond durability of the resin-bonded and silane treated ceramic surface. Dent Mater 2002;18:179–88.
[51] Ren L, Liu L, Bhowmick S, Gerbig YB, Janal MN, Thompson VP, et al. Improving fatigue damage resistance of alumina through surface grading. J Dent Res 2011;90:1026–30.
[52] Zhang Y, Kim JW. Graded structures for damage resistant and aesthetic all-ceramic restorations. Dent Mater 2009;25:781–90.
[53] Zhang Y, Kim JW. Graded zirconia glass for resistance to veneer fracture. J Dent Res 2010;89:1057–62.
[54] Zhang Y, Ma L. Optimization of ceramic strength using elastic gradients. Acta Mater 2009;57:2721–9.

Part Two

Fundamental structure/ property characteristics

Fundamentals of the material-tissue interface in dental reconstructions: structure/property relationships and characterization

4

P. Spencer, A. Misra, Q. Ye
University of Kansas, Lawrence, KS, United States

4.1 Human teeth and the dentinoenamel junction

In nature, materials exhibit structure on more than one length scale, ie, the structural elements themselves have structure. This rich hierarchical organization is the genesis of extreme and unusual properties including damage tolerance and adaptability. Human bone and teeth are natural composites that exhibit rich hierarchical structure. The dentinoenamel junction (DEJ) is an example of a material system in which structural hierarchy contributes significantly to the performance of teeth (Chai et al., 2009; Goldberg et al., 2002; Imbeni et al., 2005; Marshall et al., 2001, 2003; White et al., 2000). Indeed, the durability of the tooth under repeated stress has been attributed to the inability of cracks in the enamel to propagate through the DEJ to the subjacent dentin (Dong and Ruse, 2003; Imbeni et al., 2005; Lin and Douglas, 1994).

Spanning the inner enamel to mantle dentin, the DEJ is a hierarchy of microstructures whose composition is derived from building blocks consisting of apatitic mineralite, collagen, and water (see Fig. 4.1 for structural hierarchy of dentin). Highly cross-linked collagen forms the DEJ matrix, and the matrix is infiltrated with variable amounts of mineralite, glycosaminoglycans (GAGs), and water. Many structures within biological systems are composed of similar materials yet display very different physicomechanical properties. These differences are likely related to the relative distribution of the components, their specific chemical structures, and their interactions.

The role of GAGs in the behavior and properties of the DEJ is of particular interest. GAGs are linear polymers composed of repeating disaccharide units (*N*-acetylgalactosamine and glucuronic acid), which are differentially modified with sulfate moieties (Fig. 4.2). These negatively charged groups both attract water and readily bind cations (Hunter et al., 1988; Rudd et al., 2007; Tanaka et al., 1989). In soft tissues, the sulfation density and specific modification pattern on GAGs control interfacial binding properties (Laurence et al., 2001; Varki, 2009). In the DEJ, this would affect hydration and mineral interactions. As such, GAG–mineral interactions in the DEJ may employ specific sulfation patterns to yield distinct structures with unique mechanical properties.

Material-Tissue Interfacial Phenomena. http://dx.doi.org/10.1016/B978-0-08-100330-5.00004-2

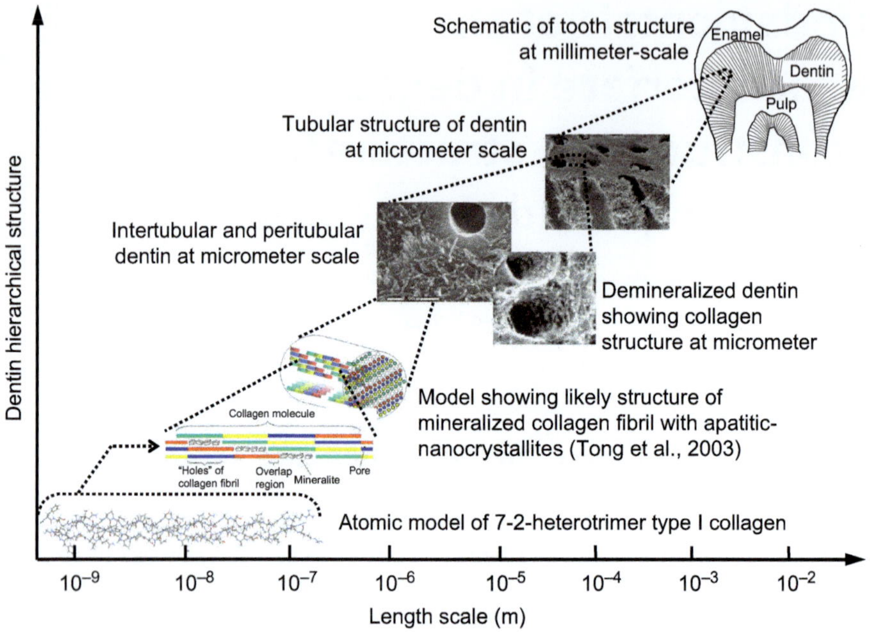

Figure 4.1 A schematic depiction of dentin hierarchical structure from molecular organization to the whole tooth.
Modified from Misra A, Marangos O, Parthasarathy R, Spencer P. Micro-scale analysis of compositional and mechanical properties of dentin using homotopic measurements. In: Biomedical Imaging and Computational Modeling in Biomechanics, Lecture Notes in Computational Vision and Biomechanics, vol. 4, 2013. pp. 131–141.

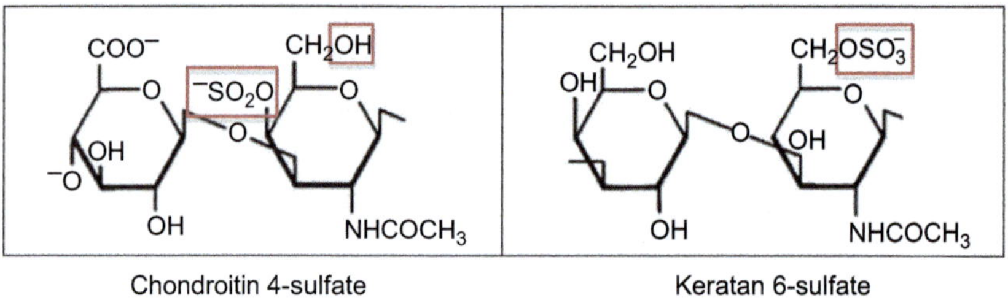

Figure 4.2 Chemical structures of the disaccharide units of chondroitin 4-sulfate and keratan 6-sulfate. The most common sulfation positions are in *red boxes*.

4.1.1 Dentinoenamel junction: mechanical properties

A number of high-resolution techniques have been applied to study the DEJ. These studies have provided valuable insight into the structure and composition of the DEJ (Gallagher et al., 2003; Goldberg et al., 2002; Hayashi, 1992; Kodaka et al., 1990; Lin et al., 1993; Marshall et al., 2003; Whittaker, 1978). Mechanical and fracture behavior of the DEJ have been determined using a variety of characterization techniques (Balooch et al., 2004; Dong and Ruse, 2003; Fong et al., 2000; Lin and Douglas, 1994; Marshall et al., 2001, 2003; Rasmussen, 1984; White et al., 2000). For example, hardness measurements across the DEJ have been performed using the Vickers indentation method (Imbeni et al., 2005; White et al., 2000). Hardness and elastic modulus measurements have also been performed using atomic force microscopy (AFM)-based indentation or nanoindentation and modulus mapping (Balooch et al., 2004; Fong et al., 2000; Marshall et al., 2003). These indentation measurements indicate the hardness and modulus transition from a high value in the bulk enamel to a low value in the bulk dentin. The thickness over which this transition occurs is a function of the indenter load and size; this relationship is not unexpected, as this zone possesses an abrupt variation of composition and structure (see Fig. 4.1). The DEJ width has been reported to vary from more than ~100 μm down to ~2–3 μm based on measurements with techniques of varying resolution (Balooch et al., 2004; Fong et al., 2000; Marshall et al., 2003; White et al., 2000).

Fracture toughness of the DEJ has been studied by investigating fracture propagation across the DEJ (Imbeni et al., 2005; Lin and Douglas, 1994; Rasmussen, 1984). The intent of these investigations has been to simulate the propagation of a fracture that emanates from the enamel, likely due to separation along enamel rods. These fractures are often blunted or arrested in the vicinity of the DEJ. Imbeni and colleagues (Imbeni et al., 2005) have investigated the fracture arrest/deflection process by following the propagation of fractures formed at the corners of the Vickers indents. Their examination of the fracture zones revealed that as the fracture propagates into dentin, a diffuse microfracture zone held together by bridging fibers forms ahead of the fracture tip. The results from other studies indicate a different mechanism for the resilience of the DEJ, ie, cracklike defects are inhibited from propagating due to stress shielding from neighboring cracks in the enamel (Chai et al., 2009). Morphologic features, eg, scallops at the DEJ, have also been described as a potential contributor to the fracture toughness of this interface (Shimizu and Macho, 2007).

4.1.2 Dentinoenamel junction: morphologic characteristics

Scallops whose characteristic size varies from 10 to 100 μm are key structural features of the DEJ (Fig. 4.3). Scallops vary in size and depth from cuspal to cervical locations (Doukoudakis et al., 1997). Findings from the work by Shimizu and Macho (Shimizu and Macho, 2007) suggest that the scalloped structure can significantly affect the stress distributions at the DEJ.

Based on high-resolution electron microscopy investigations, the morphology of the inner enamel in the vicinity of the DEJ has been classified into three zones (Kodaka et al. 1990, 1991). The innermost zone has been described as consisting of 5- to 10-μm-thick hypomineralized zone of disoriented crystallites that transitions through a 10- to 20-μm-thick intermediate zone to the outer enamel. Mantle dentin that underlies the optical DEJ is characterized by the absence of dentinal tubules and has been described to be somewhat less mineralized than primary dentin. The relative proportions of mineral and organic components in the DEJ region have also been investigated (Gallagher et al., 2003; Goldberg et al., 2002; Lin et al., 1993; Marshall et al., 2003).

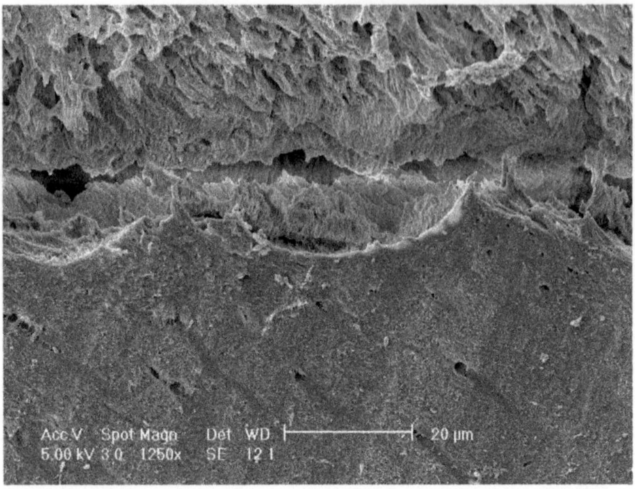

Figure 4.3 Scanning electron micrograph of DEJ showing ~20 µm interdigitated (scalloped) geometry.

Although there is general, qualitative agreement about the features of this region, there is also considerable conflicting information regarding the composition and structure, particularly with regard to the arrangement of crystallites in the inner enamel and the structure of mantle dentin.

In spite of the numerous qualitative explanations (Chai et al., 2009; Dong and Ruse, 2003; Goldberg et al., 2002; Imbeni et al., 2005; Lin and Douglas, 1994; Rasmussen, 1984; Shimizu and Macho, 2007; Zaslansky et al., 2006) as to why cracks in the enamel do not propagate as monolithic cracks into dentin, a quantitative interpretation of how the composition, structure, and properties of the DEJ lead to a robust interface between the stiff enamel and 2–4 times less stiff dentin is lacking. Completely understanding how these properties vary both across and along the DEJ requires multiscale characterization. As described in a later chapter, multiscale characterization must be integrated with modeling to understand how small features affect the overall mechanics of the tooth and more specifically, the DEJ.

4.2 Materials and systems: natural versus synthetic

The 1990s and the 2000s have seen a surge in the design, development, and use of new materials and systems for biomedical applications. In spite of the focus and need, few, if any, synthetic biomaterials in use today are as complex or robust as native biologic materials.

As opposed to materials that are synthesized using our current understanding and technologies, biologic materials are multifunctional and autonomic. In response to changing functional needs, biologic materials and systems have dynamic adaptations and flexibility at multiple hierarchical levels. Synthetic materials have not captured the advantages provided by properties such as adaptive structure, self-organization, and self-replication. The critical roadblock to achieving what Nature has accomplished is that the complexity in composition, structure, and function cannot be realized by simply superimposing the properties of the individual components. The limitations of synthetic materials are particularly evident in the composite and adhesive materials used in restorative dentistry.

Replacement of failed restorations accounts for nearly 70% of all restorative dentistry (Murray et al., 2002). This emphasis on replacement therapy will grow as the public's concern regarding mercury release from dental amalgam compels dentists to use alternative restorative materials. Resin composite is the most commonly used alternative to dental amalgam, but composite restorations have higher failure rates, more recurrent caries, and an increased frequency of replacement (Collins et al., 1998; DeRouen et al., 2006). The primary factor in the premature failure of composite restorations is recurrent caries at the composite/tooth interface. After nearly six decades of research, dental composites continue to show limited clinical service (Drummond, 2008; Opdam et al., 2010).

4.3 Interfacial engineering and composite restorations

4.3.1 Restorative dentistry: composites and adhesives

Resin-based composite is rapidly becoming the most popular material for direct restorative dentistry, and in 2006, 121 million composite restorations were placed (Kingman et al., 2012). Clinical results suggest that these restorations failed at 5.7 years (NIH, 2009) and that patients at the highest risk for decay are particularly susceptible to early failure (DeRouen et al., 2006; van de Sande et al., 2013). The primary reason for failure is recurrent decay (Opdam et al., 2010), and 80–90% of recurrent caries are located at the gingival margin of class II and V composite restorations (Li et al., 2014). Many clinical decisions to replace the composite restoration, even when caries have not yet developed, are based on defective margins—faulty margins may represent a breakdown in the bond between the composite and tooth (Gordan et al., 2009).

The viscous composite is not bonded directly to the tooth, instead the bond to the tooth is mediated by a low-viscosity adhesive. The adhesive connects the viscous composite to the tooth structure (enamel and dentin). It is intended that the adhesive will seal the tooth/material interface and act as a barrier between the restored tooth and the oral environment (Spencer et al., 2010). The results from numerous in vitro and in vivo investigations indicate that current adhesives do not provide a durable seal and that adhesive failure is a major problem with the use of composites in direct restorative dentistry (Spencer et al., 2010).

In vivo degradation and failure of the adhesive bond follows a cascade of events. These events are provoked by factors such as residual bacterial contamination of the cavity preparation. Cavity preparations are infected with residual *Streptococcus mutans*, one of the primary pathogens responsible for recurrent decay (Li et al., 2009). Bacterial and salivary enzymes as well as oral fluids degrade the adhesive (Delaviz et al., 2014). Matrix metalloproteinases (MMPs) degrade exposed collagen at the adhesive/dentin (a/d) interface.

The tooth is acid etched to remove the mineral, creating the porosity that is critical for adhesive infiltration, but acid etching also stimulates MMPs (Pashley et al., 2004). Caries-affected (c-a) dentin is frequently the clinical substrate that is bonded, and MMPs are abundant in c-a dentin (Vidal et al., 2014). The abundance of MMPs at the earliest stage of adhesive bonding incites an acute attack on the bond—exposed demineralized dentin (which is primarily collagen and water) that is not infiltrated by adhesive may be degraded by MMPs (Montagner et al., 2014). Remineralization impedes MMP activity (Tay and Pashley, 2008), but this technique alone merely shifts the site of failure elsewhere (Tjaderhane et al., 2013).

Chronic deterioration of the a/d bond, which includes the adhesive–collagen blend known as the hybrid layer, involves hydrolysis and leaching of the adhesive (Brackett et al., 2011). The breaking of covalent bonds by addition of water to ester bonds leads to degradation of the methacrylate resin within the hybrid layer (Tay et al., 2003; Tay and Pashley, 2003). With time, local domains of the methacrylate network become sufficiently degraded to permit access by esterases, which greatly accelerate ester bond hydrolysis (Finer and Santerre, 2004). Esterase activity from *S. mutans* also hydrolyzes the ester bonds in methacrylate adhesives (Bourbia et al., 2013). Establishing and maintaining the interfacial integrity of the a/d bond has been a critical roadblock to durable composite restorations (Spencer et al., 2014).

4.4 In situ structure/property characterization of the adhesive/dentin interface

The significant clinical need associated with composite restoration failure inspired our efforts to understand the interfacial phenomena controlling reactions at the composite/tooth interface. This quest also highlighted the limitations of popular techniques and approaches.

Traditionally, the mechanical behavior of the a/d interface has been investigated using bond strength tests. In a meta-analysis of bond strength published between 1992 and 1996, the authors concluded that although conventional tests are simple and fast, they have many drawbacks (DeRouen et al., 2006; Leloup et al., 2001). The bond strength tests measure a/d interfacial reactions primarily at the point of fracture. Bond strength tests treat the adhesive–dentin bond as an integrated entity. By their very nature, the bond strength investigations average the properties and structure across this complex construct (Fig. 4.4). Bond strength investigations incorporate the characteristics of dentin, exposed dentin collagen, collagen–adhesive composite (hybrid layer), the adhesive–dental composite interface, and the dental

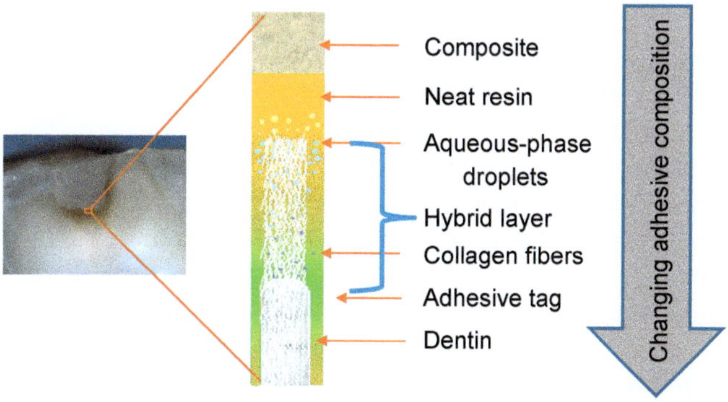

Figure 4.4 The adhesive/dentin interfacial bond is composed of dental composite, hybrid layer, demineralized dentin collagen, and adhesive.

composite (Armstrong et al. 1998, 2010; Roeder et al., 2011; Yiu et al., 2006). The bond strength tests seldom provide insight into the role played by each of the components that make up the a/d interfacial bond. They do not provide mechanical data at a resolution that would permit the identification of interfacial defects where failure likely initiates. Using conventional testing techniques, an investigator can neither identify the initial flaw nor directly correlate this flaw with the structure and chemistry of the substrate or the bonded assembly.

Understanding the role of the interface in a/d bond failure requires in situ structure and property characterization at spatial resolutions comparable to that of the hybrid layer, ie, a few micrometers. As described in our publications (Katz et al., 2001, 2002), by combining the unique capabilities of micro-Raman spectroscopy, scanning acoustic microscopy (SAM), and optical microscopy we can perform chemical, mechanical, and morphologic characterization over the same small region of the a/d interface. These complementary technologies provide direct nondestructive in situ detection of the interfacial molecular structure, micromechanics, and morphologic features of the bonded assembly. The data collected from these synergistic techniques provide added insight into the problems at the a/d interface. The a/d interface is the weak link in composite restorations (Spencer et al., 2010).

4.5 Raman spectroscopy

In the broadest sense the Raman effect involves the scattering of light as a result of its interaction with matter. When monochromatic light strikes a sample, most of the light is scattered elastically. This elastically scattered light is termed Rayleigh scattering. A small fraction of the light is scattered inelastically. The inelastically scattered light is termed Raman scattering (Stokes and anti-Stokes) and exhibits frequency shifts with respect to the incident light. The frequency shifts correspond to the vibrational energy transitions of the molecule. The Raman spectrum represents the intensity of the scattered photons as a function of the difference in frequency. It is similar to an infrared spectrum in that it provides a "fingerprint" of the molecules present within the sample and can be used for qualitative identification and quantitative determination (Chase, 1994; Turrell and Corset, 1996).

Raman spectroscopy permits structural analysis of samples by identifying specific light-induced molecular vibrations. Characteristic functional groups give rise to vibrational bands near the same frequency irrespective of the molecule in which they are found. Different molecules have different vibrational states and can therefore be distinguished with this technique. Information about the composition, secondary structure, and interaction of molecules, including the chemical microenvironment of molecular subgroups, can be determined through careful analysis of the positions, intensities, and widths of the Raman spectral bands. Raman spectroscopy is sensitive to the backbone conformation or secondary structure of proteins. This technique can provide critical data on triple helix to random coil transitions that may occur in dentin collagen as a result of heat, acid, or other degrading reagents. In the Raman spectra of collagen, bands associated with amide I and amide III are particularly sensitive to conformational changes in the triple helix (Tfayli et al., 2007).

Micro-Raman spectroscopy, which represents spectroscopy combined with microscopy, allows the investigator to detect and quantify the molecular chemistry of microscopic samples (Spencer et al. 2001, 2006; Wang and Spencer, 2002a; Wang and Spencer, 2002b; Wieliczka et al., 1997; Wieliczka et al. 1996). Using this technique, molecular information can be obtained at a spatial resolution comparable to optical microscopy. The spatial resolution of this technique is defined by the laser profile used to excite a particular part of the specimen. Functional groups are identified by their specific positions of wave numbers in the Raman spectrum, and the relative amounts of these groups are determined by the magnitude of intensity at each wave number. Samples can be analyzed directly, in air or water, at room temperature and pressure, and wet or dry, without destroying the sample. The capability of performing spatially resolved chemical analyses of microscopic regions of samples in situ has been applied to both material science and the biological sciences. Micro-Raman spectroscopy is an exceptional tool for investigating the chemistry of interfaces, because it does not rely on homogenization, extraction, or dilution, but rather each structure is analyzed in situ.

4.5.1 Raman and adhesive/dentin interface characterization

The molecular structure and micromechanical properties of the material/tooth interface have been largely overlooked during the development of new restorative dental materials. One reason this area has been neglected is because in situ chemical and mechanical characterization of the interface components is particularly challenging. To address these problems, our research team developed a novel technique using confocal Raman microspectroscopy to characterize and quantify reactions at the material/tissue interface (Spencer and Wang, 2007). The analysis is completed under normal atmospheric conditions, and the tissue is maintained in a "wet" environment throughout the process. The technique was used to determine, for the first time, the molecular structure of acid-etched smear layers (Spencer et al., 2001) and smear debris (Wang and Spencer, 2002a), to quantify the diffusion of single-bottle adhesives into the "wet" demineralized dentin matrix (Spencer et al., 2000; Wang and Spencer, 2002b, 2003, 2005c), to quantitate demineralization in hydrated dentin specimens (Spencer et al., 2001; Wang and Spencer, 2002a), and to determine the molecular structure at the material/tissue interface in class II composite restorations (Wang and Spencer, 2005c).

Micro-Raman spectroscopy was used in combination with histomorphology (Spencer and Swafford, 1999; Spencer et al., 2000) to reveal collagen exposed at the a/d interface. The specimen preparation protocol used in these studies and detailed in several of our publications (Lemor et al., 1999; Spencer and Swafford, 1999; Spencer et al., 2006; Spencer et al. 2004; Spencer and Wieliczka, 1999; Wang and Spencer, 2003, 2005b) proved particularly advantageous (Fig. 4.5). Using this specimen preparation protocol, separate but adjacent specimen blocks are available for analysis with complementary analytical techniques, including micro-Raman spectroscopy, scanning acoustic microscopy (SAM), Fourier transform infrared (FTIR) chemical imaging, and scanning electron microscopy.

As part of the histomorphologic method a conventional bone stain, ie, Goldner trichrome, was used to specifically identify exposed collagenous protein at the a/d interface (Fig. 4.6). Using this method, the mineralized dentin stains green, whereas the bulk adhesive frequently stains a pale yellow. The distinct red zone at the a/d interface represents exposed collagen. These results indicate that the adhesive did not penetrate the full depth of the demineralized layer, ie, it did not encapsulate the collagen fibrils throughout the width of the demineralized dentin (Wang and Spencer, 2003). Corresponding Raman spectra recorded from the intertubular area of the a/d interface (Fig. 4.7) and the sections from an optimum hybrid structure confirmed the morphologic observation (Wang and Spencer, 2003).

Since Raman microscopy is a nondestructive technique, the same a/d interface specimens can be analyzed using SAM. By combining the capabilities of Raman microscopy, FTIR spectroscopy, SAM, and optical microscopy (Fig. 4.8), our protocol permits complementary chemical, micromechanical, and optical analyses of not only the same specimen but also the same small region of the interface (Katz et al. 2001, 2003, 2005a, 2007).

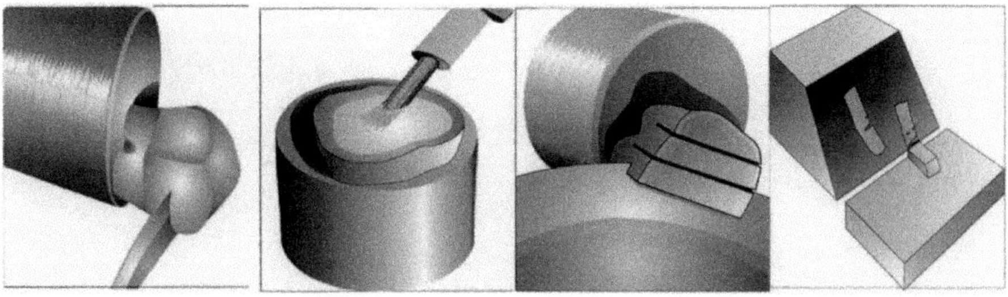

Figure 4.5 Specimen preparation protocol for histomorpologic analyses of the adhesive/dentin interface. Adjacent specimen blocks are available for analysis using various complementary techniques.

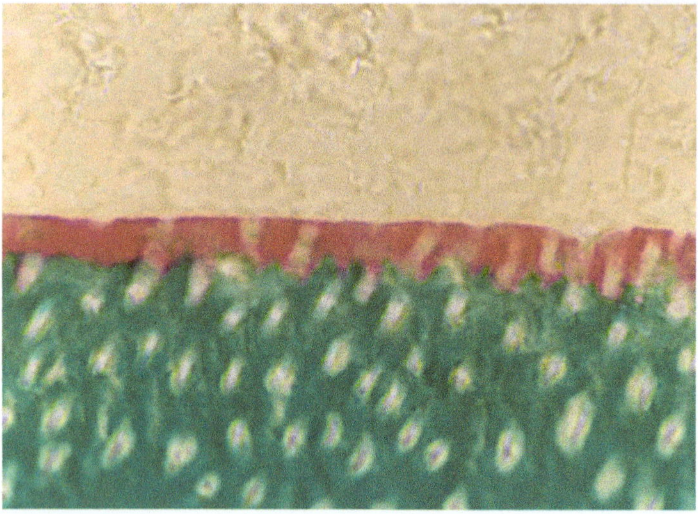

Figure 4.6 Goldner trichrome–stained section of the adhesive/dentin (a/d) interface. The mineralized dentin and bulk adhesive stain green and light yellow, respectively. Exposed collagen at the a/d interface stains red.

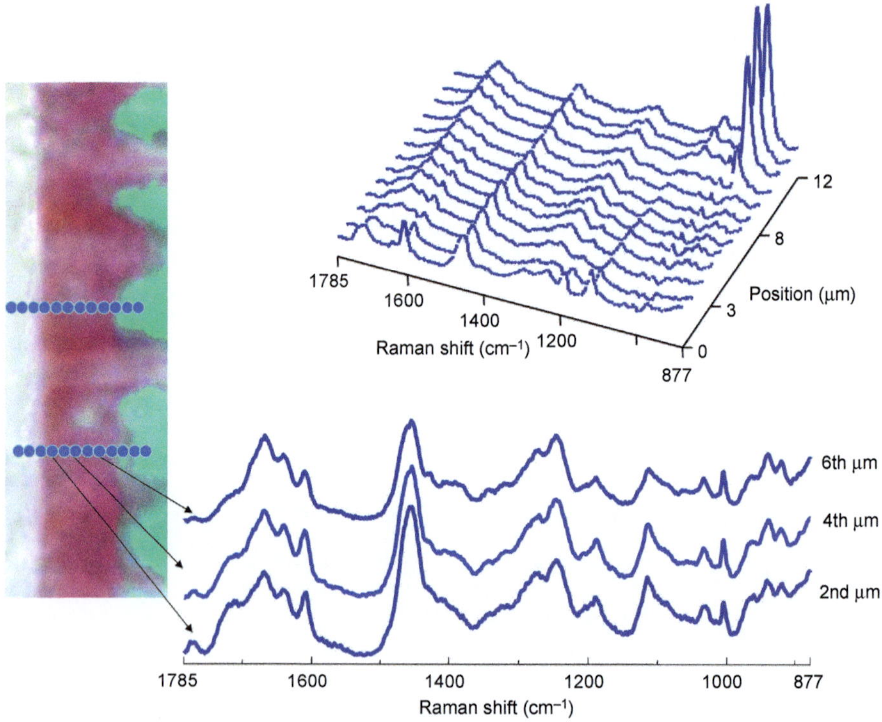

Figure 4.7 Goldner trichrome–stained section and corresponding Raman spectra recorded from the intertubular area of the adhesive/dentin interface.

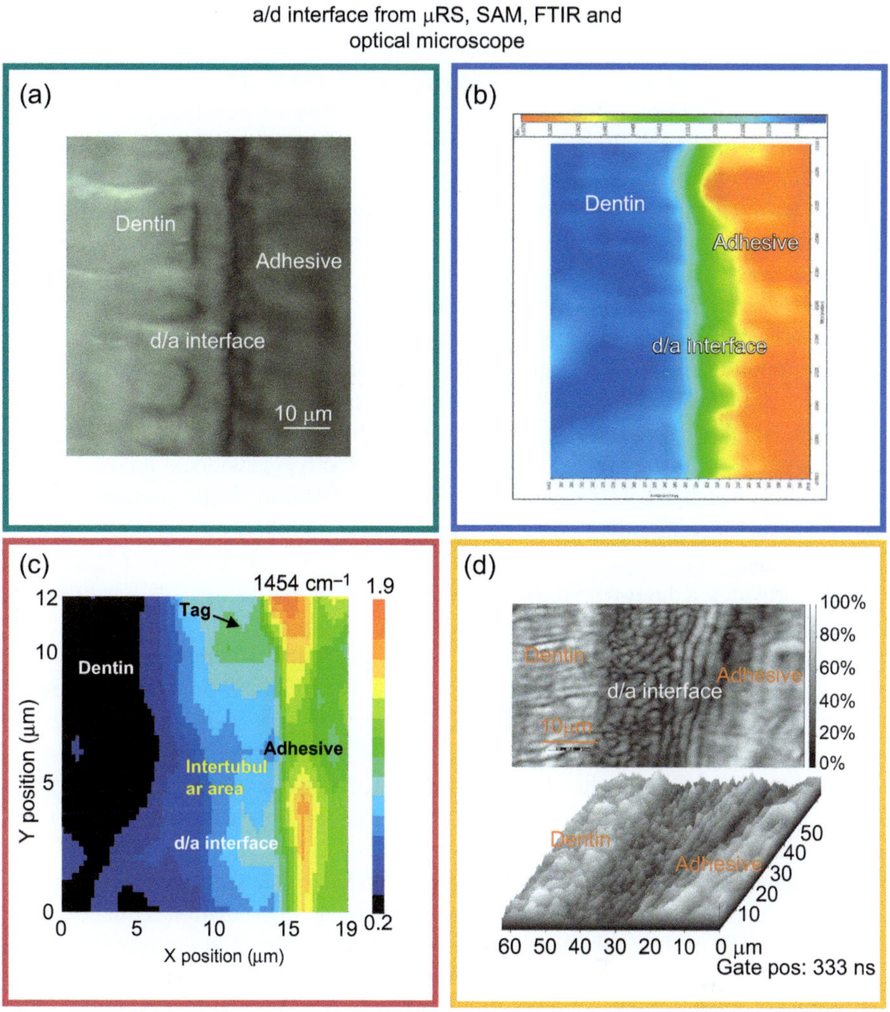

Figure 4.8 Images of the adhesive/dentin (a/d) interface using complementary analytical techniques, eg, optical microscopy, micro-Raman spectroscopy (μRS), Fourier transform infrared (FTIR) spectroscopy, and scanning acoustic microscopy (SAM).

4.6 Scanning acoustic microscopy

Introduced in the 1970s, SAM provided biomechanical property analysis of materials at much higher resolution than was achieved by the bulk ultrasonic technique (Katz et al., 2005b). The elastic properties of biological tissues and tissue/material interfaces have been measured at micrometer-level resolution using SAM (Bumrerraj and Katz, 2001; Katz et al., 2001, 2005a; Katz and Meunier, 1993; Katz et al., 1985, 2002, 2003, 2007; Lisy et al., 1994; Marangos et al., 2009, 2011;

Meunier et al., 1988; Spencer et al., 2003; Turner and Katz, 2000; Wang et al., 1998). The advantages of this technique include: (1) the ability to investigate the properties of internal and subsurface structures, (2) the ability to develop a property map of those samples that are optically opaque, (3) the capability of analyzing fresh and embedded specimens, and (4) the ability to keep the sample wet during all the measurements.

SAM uses acoustic waves to analyze the inherent properties of a material. The SAM images present the variations in acoustic signals that originate either from the intrinsic acoustic reflectivity of the material surface or through interference occurring between different surface and subsurface reflected signals. In surface imaging, the acoustic reflectivity variations are a result of the local changes in acoustic impedance (AI). The amplitude of the echo reflected back to the lens is a measure of the acoustic reflectivity of the surface at the point of focus. It is proportional to the reflection coefficient (r), which is directly related to the AIs of the liquid couplant and the investigated materials. AI is the product of the acoustic velocity, v, and local density, ϱ, and is usually denoted by Z, ie, $Z=\varrho v$. Converting AI (Z) data to elastic properties of the material requires some intermediate steps and calibration curves generated on standard materials.

SAM provides a high-resolution acoustic image of the sample, but it does not directly provide quantitative values of the acoustic property, ie, the reflection coefficient, r and thus of the AI value Z. One approach for obtaining quantitative values of Z and thus eventually of the Young's modulus, E, is to use a calibration method. Acoustic velocities and densities are measured for a set of known materials, eg, polyethylene, poly(methyl methacrylate) (PMMA), Durango apatite, aluminum, titanium, and stainless steel. The Young's modulus, E, is then calculated as $E=\varrho v^2$ (bar wave) or $E=9KG/(3K+G)$ (bulk wave) based on measurements of the densities and both the shear and dilatational longitudinal wave speeds for a similar set of known materials (Katz et al., 2003). The calibration materials are imaged with SAM to obtain their r values. Young's moduli for the experimental materials are obtained by an interpolation sequence using the Z vs E graphs of the calibration materials. A dark gray level in the acoustic image represents a lower value of AI (and thus of the Young's modulus, E) at the point being measured. Correspondingly, a bright gray level in the SAM image represents a higher AI value (and thus a higher value of E).

4.6.1 Scanning acoustic microscopy and adhesive/dentin interface characterization

Using SAM, Katz and colleagues (Katz et al., 2001) reported a modulus of elasticity for bulk dentin of 28 GPa. The modulus of elasticity of partially demineralized dentin as determined by SAM was 13 GPa and increased linearly to the in situ bulk property (Katz et al., 2001). The modulus at the a/d interface reflected the diffusion of the acid through the dentin substrate, thus there was a gradual decrease from the mineralized dentin to partial and complete demineralization. These relationships illustrated the capabilities of measuring the continuum of elastic properties at the material/tissue interface using the functional imaging power provided by SAM.

The modulus for demineralized dentin collagen was found to be 1.76 GPa based on extrapolation using calibration curves (Katz et al. 2002, 2003). The modulus of elasticity for demineralized dentin collagen infused with adhesive (optimum hybrid layer) was 1.84 GPa, and the modulus of elasticity of the infiltrated adhesive was 3.5 GPa. The lower modulus of the adhesive infiltrate when compared with the value recorded for the adhesive sample separately (5 GPa) may be related to several factors (Katz et al. 2002, 2003). As a result of residual solvent and/or water, the degree of monomer to polymer conversion of the adhesive infiltrate may have been less than that of the sample composed solely of adhesive. The lower modulus of elasticity of the infiltrate may reflect less polymerization and/or cross-linking of the material that infiltrated the wet demineralized dentin matrix when compared with the adhesive sample. The value for the adhesive infiltrate was, however, within the range reported by previous investigators. For example, using tensile stress–strain tests, Sano et al (Sano et al., 1995). obtained moduli of elasticity for resin-infiltrated demineralized dentin ranging between 2 and 3.6 GPa. With a modified AFM nanoindenter, investigators reported that the modulus of elasticity of Single Bond–infiltrated dentin was between 1.3 and 5.1 GPa, depending on the degree of hydration of the substrate (Schulze et al., 2002).

The structure of the a/d interface as well as the modulus of elasticity of the dental composite, the hybrid layer, the demineralized dentin collagen, and the adhesive profoundly affects the load transfer at the a/d interface. The in situ microstructural and micromechanical property measurements obtained from micro-Raman spectroscopy, SAM, and optical microscopy have been used in finite element analyses to predict stress concentration and distribution at the interface under tensile loading (Misra et al., 2004). Although the empirical data from Raman microspectroscopy and SAM provide the necessary guidance, the data are measured on the surface and cannot directly capture the three-dimensional multiaxial nature of the mechanical behavior. The nature and magnitude of the out-of-plane stress could change the failure initiation in a particular component of the a/d interface. As described in a later chapter, understanding these parameters requires the integration of mathematical modeling with analytical analyses.

4.7 Fourier transform infrared chemical imaging

When a molecule is exposed to an incident beam of light, energy can be absorbed by the molecule. The energy absorption can enable a transition among electronic, vibrational, and rotational energy levels. Thus, the basis for an infrared spectrum is the absorption of infrared light and the interaction of that absorption with the vibrational modes of a molecule. Infrared absorptions require that the molecular vibrations produce a change in the permanent dipole moment of the molecule. Raman spectroscopy similarly involves transitions among the vibrational energy levels of a molecule, but the energy exchange occurs in a completely different manner. Raman spectra result from vibrational motions that cause a change in the source-induced molecular dipole moment.

FTIR spectroscopic images are formed on the basis of the inherent contrast offered by the unique chemical bonds of the various components that make up the sample. Unique frequencies in the FTIR spectrum may be plotted as a function of spatial position and spectral intensity to provide a chemical image of each component. Each pixel within the image contains a specific infrared spectrum corresponding to that spatial position. A color scheme may be applied to the intensity values to create a "false-color composite" image. FTIR images can be acquired in minutes, but the spatial resolution is generally limited to about 10 μm.

4.7.1 Fourier transform infrared imaging and adhesive/dentin interface characterization

Understanding the structure of clinically relevant dentin substrates is vital to the development of improved dentin bonding agents and composite restorations, but efforts in this area have been fraught with problems (Spencer et al., 2005, 2013, 2010). The complexity of the biopolymer that forms at the adhesive interface with clinically relevant substrates, eg, caries-affected (c-a) or sclerotic dentin, presents a formidable challenge. Conventional techniques cannot adequately define the elements that initiate failure at this complex interface. Analytical techniques that allow direct nondestructive in situ detection of the variable composition and inhomogeneity across the length and breadth of the interface are required. By combining spectroscopy (infrared and Raman) with microscopy, molecular information can be obtained at a spatial resolution comparable to the optical microscope.

FTIR microspectroscopy has been used to determine the relative composition, degree of cure, and inhomogeneities across the length and breadth of the adhesive/c-a dentin interface (Spencer et al., 2005). Differences in the mineral/matrix ratio, crystallinity, and collagen organization were noted on comparing healthy and c-a dentin. For example, features associated with the organic component showed a dramatic loss of structure and intensity in the spectra recorded from the c-a dentin (Fig. 4.9–4.11). These results indicate disorganized and denatured collagen. There was also a dramatic reduction in monomer/polymer conversion when the adhesive was used on c-a dentin (Spencer et al., 2005; Wang et al., 2007).

In a separate but complementary study, morphologic investigation of adhesive bonding to c-a dentin from primary molars was noted to be sporadic and very irregular (Fig. 4.12) (Bohaty, 2010). It is postulated that the lack of adhesive penetration in the c-a dentin is due, in part, to a phase transition in the collagen; the collagen is disordered by caries (Spencer et al., 2005). Frequently, the initial step in the application of the adhesive is etching of the tooth with acid (the commercial product utilized in Fig. 4.12 required etching of the tooth with 37% phosphoric acid prior to applying the adhesive). Acid etching increases the porosity of the dentin by removing the mineral component to expose the collagen fibril network. Since c-a dentin may be characterized by zones of disorganized collagen, acid etching could promote phase transition of this disorganized collagen to a gel. The gel could inhibit adhesive infiltration.

Adhesive infiltration of the wet, demineralized c-a dentin could also be affected by adhesive phase separation (Spencer et al., 2004; Wang and Spencer, 2003, 2005a). As

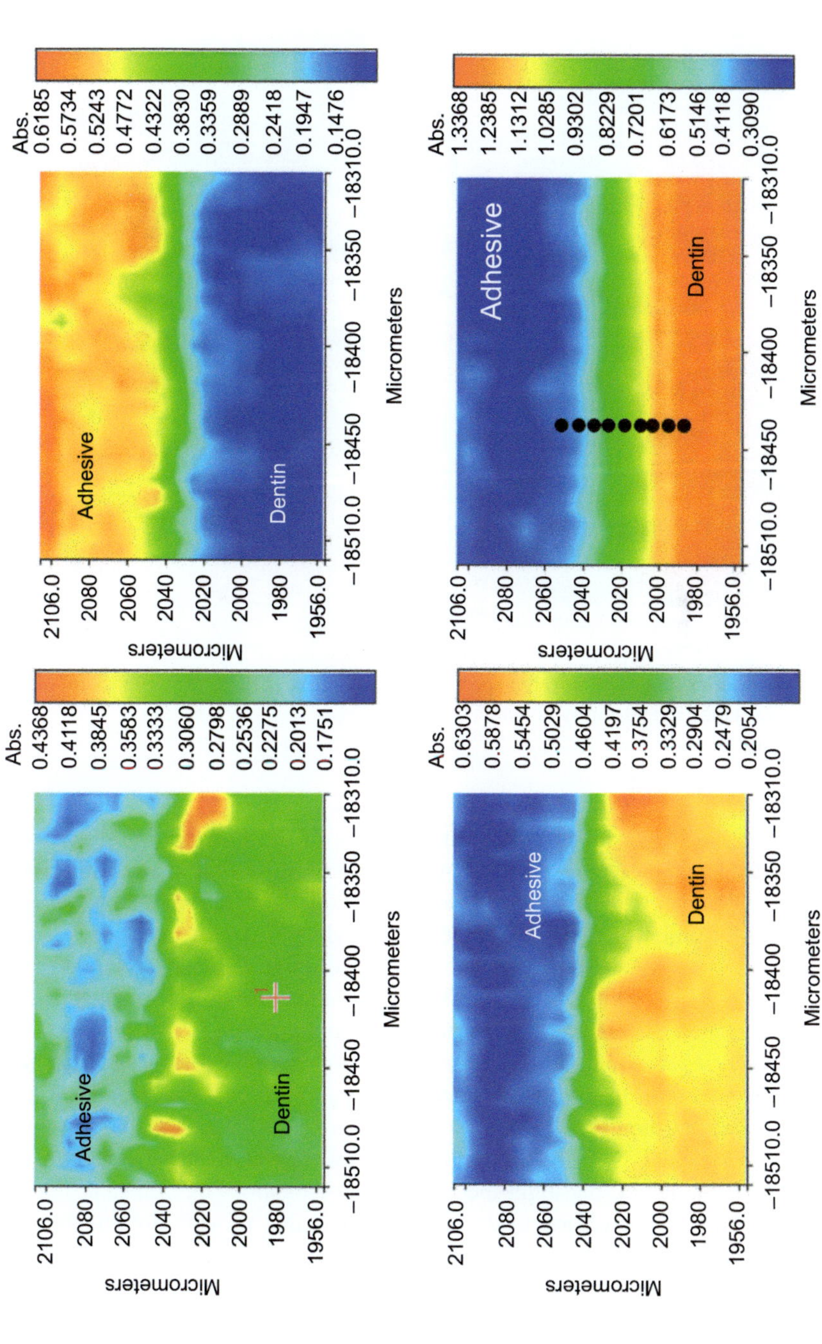

Figure 4.9 Fourier transform infrared spectroscopic image of the interfacial structure of the bond between adhesive and noncarious dentin.

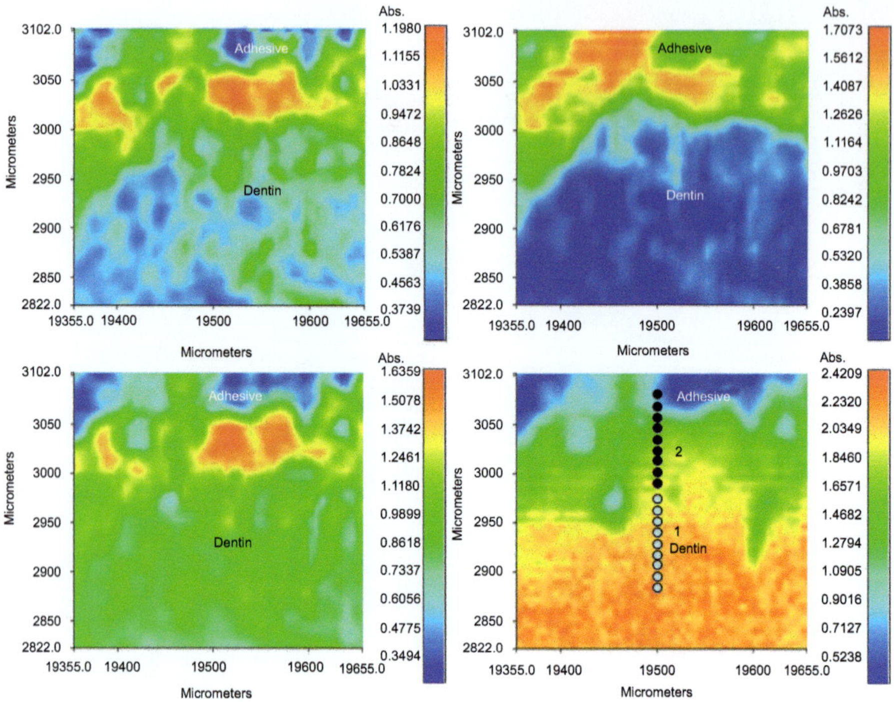

Figure 4.10 Fourier transform infrared spectroscopic image of the interfacial structure of the bond between adhesive and caries-affected dentin.
Ab, absorbance.

a result of adhesive phase separation, the majority of the intertubular adhesive/c-a dentin interface would be characterized by collagen fibrils with limited infiltration of the critical dimethacrylate component bisphenol A glycerolate dimethacrylate (Bis-GMA) (Spencer and Wang, 2002). The dimethacrylate BisGMA is the formulation component that contributes most to the cross-linked polymeric adhesive; the mono-methacrylate hydroxyethylmethacrylate (HEMA) cannot cross-link with itself and can only become part of a cross-linked system by copolymerizing with the BisGMA. Adhesive phase separation in combination with a (collagen) polymer-to-gel transition in the c-a dentin would translate to limited adhesive infiltration and poor bonding at the interface with c-a dentin.

These results, which describe distinct differences between bonding characteristics to healthy and c-a dentin, highlight the need for investigations on clinically relevant substrates as part of our efforts to develop materials that provide durable function under clinical conditions (Marangos et al., 2009). Our understanding of adhesive bonding to clinically relevant substrates such as c-a and sclerotic dentin is very limited. The factors and mechanisms involved in the very low bond strengths to c-a dentin remain unclear. The impact of c-a dentin on the distribution of stresses at the a/d interface is largely unknown.

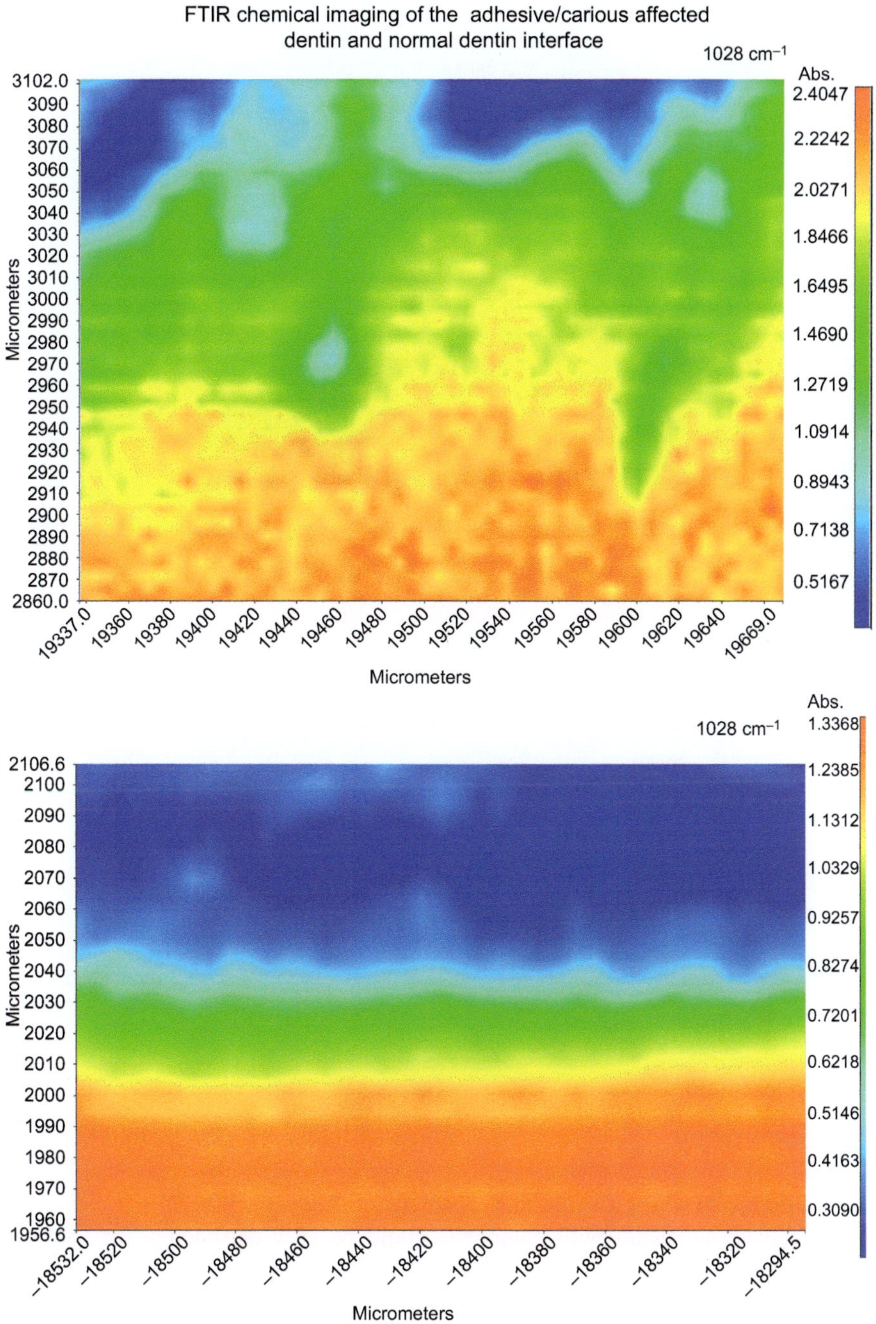

Figure 4.11 Fourier transform infrared (FTIR) spectroscopic image of the interfacial structure of the bond between adhesive and noncarious dentin compared with FTIR spectroscopic image of the adhesive/caries-affected dentin interface. The comparison illustrates the dramatic differences in the mineral/matrix ratio, crystallinity, and collagen organization at the interface between the adhesive and caries-affected dentin and noncarious dentin.

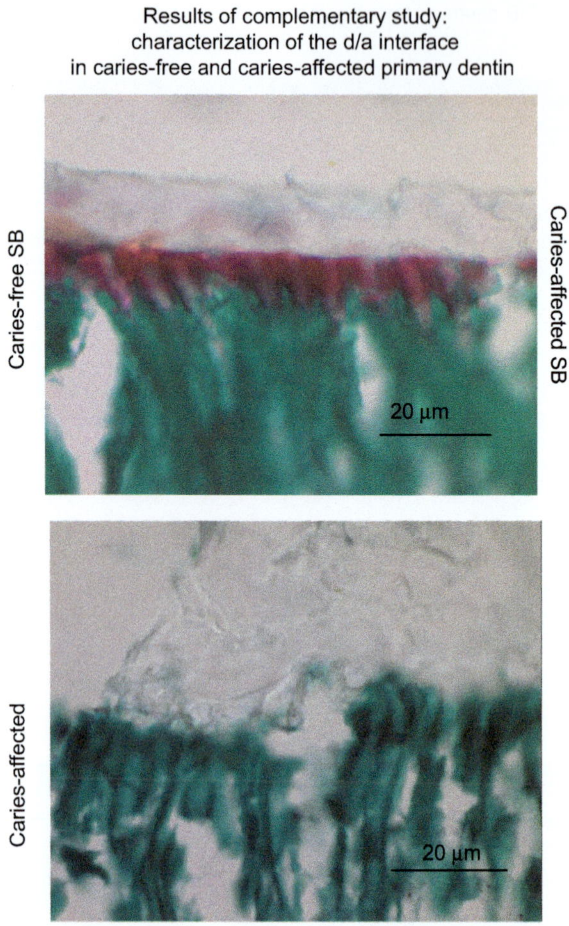

Figure 4.12 Goldner trichrome–stained section of the adhesive/caries-affected dentin interface. The dentin was recovered from an exfoliated primary molar. The Goldner trichrome image provides a clear illustration of the sporadic and irregular structure at the adhesive/caries-affected dentin interface.

4.8 Summary

With a failure rate nearly double that of amalgam (Ferracane, 2013) the increasing trend to replace amalgam with composite could be very detrimental for patients. Removal of these restorations leads to loss of sound tooth structure with concomitant weakening of the tooth and possible pulpal injury (Hunter et al., 1995). Over the lifetime of the patient, the repeated loss of sound tooth structure will translate into the need for more complex restorations and eventually total tooth loss. The higher failure rate and need for frequent replacement could translate to a significant reduction in the quality of life for nearly 32% of the US population with natural dentition who do not receive regular dental treatment (Health, 2007). Similarly, the higher total colony-forming units of *S. mutans* at the margins of composite when compared with that of comparable amalgam restorations could translate to an increase in untreated dental disease and a significant reduction in the quality of life for the 4 million US children who do not receive regular dental care (Census, 2013).

The a/d bond may be the first defense against substances that penetrate and ultimately undermine the composite restoration in vivo. The failure of the a/d bond, in concert with reports of increased levels of cariogenic bacteria at the perimeter of composite materials, points to an interesting interplay between microbiology and adhesive degradation as key elements in the premature failure of composite restorations. Adhesion of *S. mutans* to surfaces in the mouth creates an environment that supports the subsequent attachment and growth of other bacterial species, ultimately forming a microecosystem known as a biofilm. Although it is unlikely that dental plaque biofilm can be eliminated, it may be possible to reduce the pathogenic impact of the biofilm at the composite/tooth interface. One approach is novel resin matrices that are engineered to shift the microbial ecology at the composite/tooth interface from a disease-associated state to a "healthy" state (Spencer et al., 2014). Any change in the chemical structure of the resin will, however, likely alter other mechanical and physicochemical properties. The optimal adhesive will be produced by balancing the desired physical, chemical, and mechanical properties.

Natural material systems are inherently multifunctional and autonomic; these systems represent the ideal goal for advanced engineering applications. Robust interfaces within native constructs join widely disparate materials. These robust interfacial structures have long been an inspiration for synthetic materials. The rich hierarchical organization of complex composites, such as bone and teeth, is the genesis of extreme and unusual behavior, ie, high strength-to-weight ratios, damage tolerance, and adaptability, behavior that engineered materials cannot replicate.

Translating nature's principles to new materials demands a multiplicity of elements. For example, computational technologies must be merged with biological engineering approaches to systematically examine how nature's hierarchical structure–function relationships occur. In situ characterization must be integrated with multiscale modeling to provide a unified description of the structure and properties from molecular to macroscales. Although complementary analytical techniques can provide in situ detection of the interfacial molecular structure and micromechanical features, they do not provide complete constitutive behavior. Analytical techniques alone provide fragmented information that has to be interpreted and unified. In general, material constitutive behavior critically depends on the mechanisms that occur at scales smaller than the material scale. Thus, modeling methodologies that can account for these underlying mechanisms are required. The modeling in conjunction with multiscalar structure/property characterization can identify the weakest links at material/tissue interfaces. The combination of modeling and multiscale characterization can lead to the ability to predict behavior at interfacial structures.

The mouth is a particularly caustic environment. Synthetic and/or bioenabled materials that are used to repair damaged tissues in the mouth must resist a variety of physical, chemical, and mechanical challenges. These challenges are magnified at the material/tooth interface. Reactions at the atomic, molecular, and nanoscales initiate interfacial failure. Understanding the phenomena that underlie interfacial failure is confounded by several factors including the lack of techniques that allow in situ monitoring of the material/tissue bond. Much of our current understanding is based on techniques that view the material/tissue bond after failure. Unraveling the complexity of the material/tissue interface requires knowledge, experience, and expertise that crosses discipline boundaries. Solving the problems that are central to clinical failure requires clinicians, scientists, and engineers working collaboratively to develop novel materials with unique and extreme multifunctional capabilities.

Acknowledgments

The authors gratefully acknowledge support from the University of Missouri–Kansas City School of Dentistry, University of Missouri–Kansas City, University of Kansas and Department of Health and Human Services, and US Public Health Service R15 DE12252, R01 DE12487, S10 RR16710, NIH-NIDCR R01 DE014392, R01DE022054, and R01DE025476.

References

Armstrong SR, Boyer DB, Keller JC. Microtensile bond strength testing and failure analysis of two dentin adhesives. Dent Mater 1998;14:44–50.

Armstrong S, Geraldeli S, Maia R, Raposo LH, Soares CJ, Yamagawa J. Adhesion to tooth structure: a critical review of "micro" bond strength test methods. Dent Mater 2010;26(2):e50–62.

Balooch G, Marshall GW, Marshall SJ, Warren OL, Asif SA, Balooch M. Evaluation of a new modulus mapping technique to investigate microstructural features of human teeth. J Biomech 2004;37(8):1223–32.

Bohaty BS. (Ph.D. Dissertation). Kansas City: University of Missouri-Kansas City; 2010.

Bourbia M, Ma D, Cvitkovitch DG, Santerre JP, Finer Y. Cariogenic bacteria degrade dental resin composites and adhesives. J Dent Res 2013;92(11):989–94.

Brackett MG, Li N, Brackett WW, Sword RJ, Qi YP, Niu LN, et al. The critical barrier to progress in dentine bonding with the etch-and-rinse technique. J Dent 2011;39(3):238–48.

Bumrerraj S, Katz JL. Scanning acoustic microscopy study of human cortical and trabecular bone. Ann Biomed Eng 2001;29:1–9.

Census bureau targets unmet need. 2013;44(7).

Chai H, Lee JJ, Constantino PJ, Lucas PW, Lawn BR. Remarkable resilience of teeth. Proc Natl Acad Sci USA 2009;106(18):7289–93.

Chase B. A new generation of Raman instrumentation. Appl Spectrosc 1994;48:14A–8A.

Collins CJ, Bryant RW, Hodge KL. A clinical evaluation of posterior composite resin restorations: 8-year findings. J Dent 1998;26(4):311–7.

Delaviz Y, Finer Y, Santerre JP. Biodegradation of resin composites and adhesives by oral bacteria and saliva: a rationale for new material designs that consider the clinical environment and treatment challenges. Dent Mater 2014;30(1):16–32.

DeRouen TA, Martin MD, Leroux BG, Townes BD, Woods JS, Leitao J, et al. Neurobehavioral effects of dental amalgam in children: a randomized clinical trial. JAMA 2006;295(15):1784–92.

Dong XD, Ruse ND. Fatigue crack propagation path across the dentinoenamel junction complex in human teeth. J Biomed Mater Res A 2003;66(1):103–9.

Doukoudakis S, Kranias N, Spanou M, Stavridakis M. Morphologic characteristics of dentin at the dentinoenamel junction as viewed by scanning electron microscopy. J Esthet Dent 1997;9(2):94–9.

Drummond JL. Degradation, fatigue, and failure of resin dental composite materials. J Dent Res 2008;87(8):710–9.

Ferracane JL. Resin-based composite performance: are there some things we can't predict? Dent Mater 2013;29(1):51–8.

Finer Y, Santerre JP. Salivary esterase activity and its association with the biodegradation of dental composites. J Dent Res 2004;83:22–6.

Fong H, Sarikaya M, White SN, Snead ML. Nano-mechanical properties profiles across dentin-enamel junction of human incisor teeth. Mater Sci Eng 2000;C7:119–28.

Gallagher RR, Demos SG, Balooch M, Marshall Jr GW, Marshall SJ. Optical spectroscopy and imaging of the dentin-enamel junction in human third molars. J Biomed Mater Res A 2003;64(2):372–7.

Goldberg M, Septier D, Bourd K, Hall R, Jeanny JC, Jonet L, et al. The dentino-enamel junction revisited. Connect Tissue Res 2002;43(2–3):482–9.

Gordan VV, Garvan CW, Blaser PK, Mondragon E, Mjor IA. A long-term evaluation of alternative treatments to replacement of resin-based composite restorations: results of a seven-year study. J Am Dent Assoc 2009;140(12):1476–84.

Hayashi Y. High resolution electron microscopy in the dentino-enamel junction. J Electron Microsc 1992;41(5):387–91.

Health US. National center for health statistics. Health, United States, 2007 with chartbook on trends in the health of Americans. Hyattsville, MD. 2007.

Hunter GK, Wong KS, Kim JJ. Binding of calcium to glycosaminoglycans: an equilibrium dialysis study. Arch Biochem Biophys 1988;260(1):161–7.

Hunter AR, Treasue ET, Hunter AJ. Increases in cavity volume associated with the removal of class 2 amalgam and composite restorations. Oper Dent 1995;20(1):2–6.

Imbeni V, Kruzic JJ, Marshall GW, Marshall SJ, Ritchie RO. The dentin-enamel junction and the fracture of human teeth. Nat Mater 2005;4(3):229–32.

Katz JL, Meunier A. Scanning acoustic microscope studies of the elastic properties of osteons and osteon lamellae. J Biomechanical Eng 1993;115:543–8.

Katz JL, Yoon HS, Das PK, Meunier A. Scanning acoustic microscopy of bone-biomaterials interfaces. London: plastics and Rubber Institute; 1985. No. 19/1–4.

Katz JL, Bumrerraj S, Dreyfuss J, Wang Y, Spencer P. Micromechanics of the dentin/adhesive interface. J Biomed Mater Res 2001;58:366–71.

Katz JL, Spencer P, Wang Y, Wagh A, Nomura T, Bumrerraj S. Structural, chemical and mechanical characterization of the dentin/adhesive interface. In: Lewandrowski K, Wise D, Trantolo D, Gresser J, Yaszemski M, Altobelli D, editors. Tissue engineering and biodegradable equivalents: scientific and clinical applications. Marcel Decker; 2002. p. 775–93.

Katz JL, Spencer P, Nomura T, Wagh A, Wang Y. Micromechanical properties of demineralized dentin collagen with and without adhesive infiltration. J Biomed Mater Res 2003;66A:120–8.

Katz JL, Kinney JH, Spencer P, Wang Y, Fricke B, Walker MP, et al. Elastic anisotropy of bone and dentitional tissues. J Mater Sci Mater Med 2005a;16:803–6.

Katz JL, Wang Y, Bumrerraj S, Nomura T, Misra A, Eppell SJ, et al. Functional imaging of the hierarchical structure/property relationships in bone, dentin and the dentin/adhesive interface. In: Nalwa HS, editor. Handbook of nanostructured biomaterials and their applications. Stevenson Ranch, CA: American Scientific Publishers; 2005b.

Katz JL, Misra A, Spencer P, Wang Y, Bumrerraj S, Nomura T, et al. Multiscale mechanics of hierarchical structure/property relationships in calcified tissues and tissue/material interfaces. Mater Sci Eng A Struct Mater 2007;27(3):450–68.

Kingman A, Hyman J, Masten SA, Jayaram B, Smith C, Eichmiller F, et al. Bisphenol a and other compounds in human saliva and urine associated with the placement of composite restorations. J Am Dent Assoc 2012;143(12):1292–302.

Kodaka T, Kuroiwa M, Abe M. Fine structure of the inner enamel in human permanent teeth. Scanning Microsc 1990;4(4):975–85.

Kodaka T, Debari K, Kuroiwa M. Mineral content of the innermost enamel in erupted human teeth. J Electron Microsc 1991;40(1):19–23.

Laurence JS, Blanpain C, De Leener A, Parmentier M, LiWang PJ. Importance of basic residues and quaternary structure in the function of mip-1 beta: Ccr5 binding and cell surface sugar interactions. Biochemistry 2001;40(16):4990–9.

Leloup G, D'Hoore W, Bouter D, Degrange M, Vreven J. Meta-analytical review of factors involved in dentin adherence. J Dent Res 2001;80(7):1605–14.

Lemor RM, Kruger MB, Wieliczka DM, Swafford JR, Spencer P. Spectroscopic and morphologic characterization of the dentin/adhesive interface. J Biomed Opt 1999;4:22–7.

Li F, Chai ZG, Sun MN, Wang F, Ma S, Zhang L, et al. Anti-biofilm effect of dental adhesive with cationic monomer. J Dent Res 2009;88(4):372–6.

Li Y, Carrera C, Chen R, Li J, Lenton P, Rudney JD, et al. Degradation in the dentin-composite interface subjected to multi-species biofilm challenges. Acta Biomater 2014;10(1):375–83.

Lin CP, Douglas WH. Structure-property relations and crack resistance at the bovine dentin-enamel junction. J Dent Res 1994;73(5):1072–8.

Lin C, Douglas WH, Erlandsen SL. Scanning electron microscopy of type I collagen at the dentin-enamel junction of human teeth. J Histochem Cytochem 1993;41(3):381–8.

Lisy F, Hiltner A, Baer E, Katz JL, Meunier A. Application of scanning acoustic microscopy to polymeric materials. J Appl Polym Sci 1994;52:329–52.

Marangos O, Misra A, Spencer P, Bohaty B, Katz JL. Physico-mechanical properties determination using microscale homotopic measurements: application to sound and caries-affected primary tooth dentin. Acta Biomater 2009;5(4):1338–48.

Marangos O, Misra A, Spencer P, Katz JL. Scanning acoustic microscopy investigation of frequency-dependent reflectance of acid- etched human dentin using homotopic measurements. IEEE Trans Ultrason Ferroelectr Freq Control 2011;58(3):585–95.

Marshall Jr GW, Balooch M, Gallagher RR, Gansky SA, Marshall SJ. Mechanical properties of the dentinoenamel junction: AFM studies of nanohardness, elastic modulus, and fracture. J Biomed Mater Res 2001;54:87–95.

Marshall SJ, Balooch M, Habelitz S, Balooch G, Gallagher R, Marshall GW. The dentin-enamel junction – a natural, multilevel interface. J Eur Ceram Soc 2003;23(15):2897–904.

Meunier A, Katz JL, Christel P, Sedel L. A reflection scanning acoustic microscope for bone and bone-biomaterials interface studies. J Orthop Res 1988;6:770–5.

Misra A, Spencer P, Marangos O, Wang Y, Katz JL. Micromechanical analysis of dentin/adhesive interface by the finite element method. J Biomed Mater Res B Appl Biomater 2004;70(1):56–65.

Misra A, Marangos O, Parthasarathy R, Spencer P. Micro-scale analysis of compositional and mechanical properties of dentin using homotopic measurements. In: Biomedical Imaging and Computational Modeling in Biomechanics, Lecture Notes in Computational Vision and Biomechanics, vol. 4. 2013. pp. 131–141.

Montagner AF, Sarkis-Onofre R, Pereira-Cenci T, Cenci MS. Mmp inhibitors on dentin stability: a systematic review and meta-analysis. J Dent Res 2014;93(8):733–43.

Murray PE, Windsor LJ, Smyth TW, Hafez AA, Cox CF. Analysis of pulpal reactions to restorative procedures, materials, pulp capping, and future therapies. Crit Rev Oral Biol Med 2002;13(6):509–20.

NIH. Nidcr strategic plan 2009–13. Increasing the service life of dental resin composites. Rfa-de-10-005. 2009.

Opdam NJM, Bronkhorst EM, Loomans BAC, Huysmans M. 12-year survival of composite vs. amalgam restorations. J Dent Res 2010;89(10):1063–7.

Pashley DH, Tay FR, Yiu C, Hashimoto M, Breschi L, Carvalho RM, et al. Collagen degradation by host-derived enzymes during aging. J Dent Res 2004;83(3):216–21.

Rasmussen ST. Fracture properties of human teeth in proximity to the dentinoenamel junction. J Dent Res 1984;63(11):1279–83.

Roeder L, Pereira PN, Yamamoto T, Ilie N, Armstrong S, Ferracane J. Spotlight on bond strength testing–unraveling the complexities. Dent Mater 2011;27(12):1197–203.

Rudd TR, Guimond SE, Skidmore MA, Duchesne L, Guerrini M, Torri G, et al. Influence of substitution pattern and cation binding on conformation and activity in heparin derivatives. Glycobiology 2007;17(9):983–93.

Sano H, Takatsu T, Ciucchi B, Russell CM, Pashley DH. Tensile properties of resin-infiltrated demineralized human dentin. J Dent Res 1995;74(4):1093–102.

Schulze KA, Oliveira SSA, Marshall GW, Gansky SA, Marshall SJ. Technique sensitivity of a self-etching versus an acid etching system. J Dent Res 2002;81(Sp. Iss.):139.

Shimizu D, Macho GA. Functional significance of the microstructural detail of the primate dentino-enamel junction: a possible example of exaptation. J Hum Evol 2007;52(1):103–11.

Spencer P, Swafford JR. Unprotected protein at the dentin-adhesive interface. Quintessence Int 1999;30(7):501–7.

Spencer P, Wang Y. Adhesive phase separation at the dentin interface under wet bonding conditions. J Biomed Mater Res 2002;62(3):447–56.

Spencer P, Wang Y. Micro-Raman spectroscopy: principles and applications in dental research. Imperial College Press; 2007.

Spencer P, Wieliczka DM. A review of the chemical and morphological characterization of the dentin/adhesive interface. Recent Res Dev Appl Spectrosc 1999;2:183–93.

Spencer P, Wang Y, Walker MP, Wieliczka DM, Swafford JR. Interfacial chemistry of the dentin/adhesive bond. J Dent Res 2000;79:1458–63.

Spencer P, Wang Y, Walker MP, Swafford JR. Molecular structure of acid-etched dentin smear layers-in situ study. J Dent Res 2001;80:1802–7.

Spencer P, Katz JL, Tabib-Azar M, Wang Y, Wagh A, Nomura T. Hyperspectral analysis of collagen infused with bisGMA-based polymeric adhesive. In: Lewandrowski KU, Wise DL, Trantolo DJ, Hasirci V, Yaszemski M, Altobelli DE, editors. Tissue engineering and novel delivery systems. New York: Marcel Decker; 2003. p. 599–632.

Spencer P, Wang Y, Katz JL. Identification of collagen encapsulation at the dentin/adhesive interface. J Adhes Dent 2004;6:91–5.

Spencer P., Wang Y., Katz J.L., Misra A. Physicochemical interactions at the dentin/adhesive interface using FTIR chemical imaging. J Biomed Opt 2005;10(3):031104.

Spencer P, Wang Y, Bohaty B. Interfacial chemistry of moisture-aged class II composite restorations. J Biomed Mater Res B Appl Biomater 2006;77(2):234–40.

Spencer P, Ye Q, Park J, Topp EM, Misra A, Marangos O, et al. Adhesive/dentin interface: the weak link in the composite restoration. Ann Biomed Eng 2010;38(6):1989–2003.

Spencer P, Ye Q, Park J, Parthasarathy R, Marangos O, Misra A, et al. Dentin/adhesive interface in teeth. In: Thomopoulos S, Genin G, Birman V, editors. Structural interfaces and attachments in biology. New York: Springer; 2013. p. 133–51.

Spencer P, Ye Q, Misra A, Goncalves SEP, Laurence JS. Proteins, pathogens, and failure at the composite-tooth interface. J Dent Res 2014;93(12):1243–9.

Tanaka H, Arai T, Miyajima K, Shimabayashi S, Nakagaki M. Effect of adsorption of glycosaminoglycans on the dissolution properties of hydroxyapatite. Colloids Surfaces 1989;37:357–68.

Tay FR, Pashley DH. Water treeing–a potential mechanism for degradation of dentin adhesives. Am J Dent 2003;16(1):6–12.

Tay FR, Pashley DH. Guided tissue remineralisation of partially demineralised human dentine. Biomaterials 2008;29(8):1127–37.

Tay FR, Hashimoto M, Pashley DH, Peters MC, Lai SC, Yiu CK, et al. Aging affects two modes of nanoleakage expression in bonded dentin. J Dent Res 2003;82:537–41.

Tfayli A, Piot O, Draux F, Pitre F, Manfait M. Molecular characterization of reconstructed skin model by Raman microspectroscopy: comparison with excised human skin. Biopolymers 2007;87(4):261–74.

Tjaderhane L, Nascimento FD, Breschi L, Mazzoni A, Tersariol IL, Geraldeli S, et al. Strategies to prevent hydrolytic degradation of the hybrid layer-a review. Dent Mater 2013;29(10):999–1011.

Turner CH, Katz JL. Evaluating mechanical properties of bone using scanning acoustic microscopy. In: An YH, Draughn RA, editors. Mechanical testing of bone and the bone-implant interface. Boca Raton: CRC Press; 2000. p. 371–83.

Turrell G, Corset J. Raman microscopy-developments and applications. New York: Academic Press; 1996.

van de Sande FH, Opdam NJ, Rodolpho PA, Correa MB, Demarco FF, Cenci MS. Patient risk factors' influence on survival of posterior composites. J Dent Res 2013;92(Suppl. 7):78S–83S.

Varki A. Essentials of glycobiology. Cold Spring Harbor, NY: Cold Spring Harbor Laboratory Press; 2009.

Vidal CM, Tjaderhane L, Scaffa PM, Tersariol IL, Pashley D, Nader HB, et al. Abundance of MMPs and cysteine cathepsins in caries-affected dentin. J Dent Res 2014;93(3):269–74.

Wang Y, Spencer P. Analysis of acid-treated dentin smear debris and smear layers using confocal Raman microspectroscopy. J Biomed Mater Res 2002a;60:300–8.

Wang Y, Spencer P. Quantifying adhesive penetration in adhesive/dentin interface using confocal Raman microspectroscopy. J Biomed Mater Res 2002b;59:46–55.

Wang Y, Spencer P. Hybridization efficiency of the adhesive dentin interface with wet bonding. J Dent Res 2003;82:141–5.

Wang Y, Spencer P. Continuing etching of an all-in-one adhesive in wet dentin tubules. J Dent Res 2005a;84:350–4.

Wang Y, Spencer P. Evaluation of the interface between one-bottle adhesive systems and dentin by Goldner's trichrome stain. Am J Dent 2005b;18:66–72.

Wang Y, Spencer P. Interfacial chemistry of class II composite restoration: structure analysis. J Biomed Mat Res 2005c;75A:580–7.

Wang RR, Meyers E, Katz JL. Scanning acoustic microscopy study of titanium-ceramic interface of dental restorations. J Biomed Mater Res 1998;42(4):508–16.

Wang Y, Spencer P, Yao X, Brenda B. Effect of solvent content on resin hybridization in wet dentin bonding. J Biomed Mater Res A 2007;82:975–83.

White SN, Paine ML, Luo W, Sarikaya M, Fong H, Yu Z, et al. Dentino-enamel junction is a broad transitional zone uniting dissimilar bioceramic composites. J Am Ceram Soc 2000;83(1):238–40.

Whittaker DK. The enamel–dentine junction of human and *Macaca irus* teeth: a light and electron microscopic study. J Anat 1978;125(Pt 2):323–35.

Wieliczka DM, Spencer P, Kruger MB. Raman mapping of the dentin/adhesive interface. Appl Spectrosc 1996;50(12):1500–4.

Wieliczka DM, Kruger MB, Spencer P. Raman imaging of dental adhesive diffusion. Appl Spectrosc 1997;51:1593–6.

Yiu CK, King NM, Carrilho MR, Sauro S, Rueggeberg FA, Prati C, et al. Effect of resin hydrophilicity and temperature on water sorption of dental adhesive resins. Biomaterials 2006;27(9):1695–703.

Zaslansky P, Friesem AA, Weiner S. Structure and mechanical properties of the soft zone separating bulk dentin and enamel in crowns of human teeth: insight into tooth function. J Struct Biol 2006;153(2):188–99.

Understanding the mechanical behavior of the material–tissue and material–material interface in dental reconstructions

5

J.L. Ferracane[1], U. Lohbauer[2], W.M. Palin[3]
[1]Oregon Health & Science University, Portland, OR, United States; [2]Universitätsklinikum Erlangen, Friedrich-Alexander Universität Erlangen-Nürnberg, Erlangen, Germany; [3]University of Birmingham, Birmingham, United Kingdom

5.1 Introduction

The integrity of an interface is a function of the mechanical properties of the materials composing the interface, as well as the interaction between the two, ie, the adhesive forces. In dental and craniofacial sciences, frequently, the goal is to replace lost or damaged natural tissue with synthetic materials. For ideal function, these replacement materials must strongly bond to the existing tissue, but they must also form a hermetic seal that eliminates the passage of microorganisms and fluids, which would lead to further tissue destruction or weakening of the interface or the individual materials, compromising the final outcome. Therefore, the study of interfaces is crucial, and the manner in which they can be tested to predict the likelihood of success is of great interest to the field.

Because a variety of materials and material combinations are used for the repair or replacement of oral and craniofacial tissues, numerous types of material interfaces exist. A complete discussion of this important topic requires an examination of all of them. In this chapter, the three different types of interfaces are treated separately. First, the interface between the tooth tissue and restorative material is explored, specifically by considering resin-based materials such as dental adhesives and composites, and the manner in which they interact with dentin and enamel. Second, the interaction between these same resin-based materials and other structures, such as oxide ceramic dental crowns, are explored, because these tooth replacement materials are typically fixed to the remaining tooth structure through the use of resin-based adhesives and cements, or repaired intraorally with similar materials. Finally, the interface between different synthetic materials, such as metals and ceramics, with dental porcelain used as an esthetic veneering material is addressed.

Owing to the vast differences in the properties of the different materials that create these interfaces, the quality of the interface depend very much on the individual properties, as well as on the many factors that affect the adhesion between the two.

Material-Tissue Interfacial Phenomena. http://dx.doi.org/10.1016/B978-0-08-100330-5.00005-4

Describing the mechanical characteristics of this interfacial adhesion, and the manner in which it is accomplished, are the primary objectives of this chapter.

5.2 The material–tooth interface

5.2.1 The interface of resin and adhesive with dentin and enamel

Tooth structure is composed predominantly of hydroxyapatite, a calcium phosphate crystalline mineral (Fig. 5.1). The enamel is almost totally mineralized, incorporating only a very small amount of organic matrix, being mainly protein (3 vol%) and water (12 vol%) (Lussi, 2006). The crystals are arranged in long rods having a very well-defined radial anisotropy. Dentin is composed of approximately 47 vol% mineral; 33 vol% protein, mainly collagen with other noncollagenous proteins; and about 20 vol% water (Lussi, 2006). Dentin is arranged in a tubular structure, with a lower density of tubules near the dentin–enamel junction (DEJ), and a greater tubular density, and subsequently lower mineral density, near the dental pulp. Therefore, the properties of dentin vary based on location within the tooth.

Enamel, typical of many ceramics, is a very brittle material, possessing high elastic modulus (~70–110 GPa) but relatively low tensile strength (10–70 MPa) and fracture toughness (0.7–2.1 MPa $m^{1/2}$) (Arola et al., 2010). Dentin, in contrast, has a much lower elastic modulus (~20 GPa) than enamel, but has higher tensile strength (60–100 MPa) and is more fracture resistant (1.5–2.1 MPa $m^{1/2}$), all due to its higher organic content (Arola et al., 2010). Enamel is also about 56 times harder than dentin. The most important aspect of the enamel–dentin complex is the interface, or transition region (Fig. 5.2), between the two, called the DEJ, which is estimated to be anywhere from 10 to 100 μm thick (Bechtle et al., 2010), although Gallagher et al. (2010) used a combination of nanoindentation and Raman microspectroscopy to estimate the thickness as less than 10 μm.

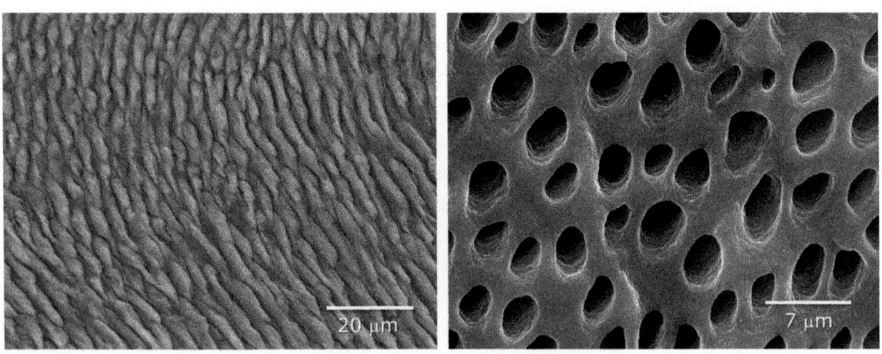

Figure 5.1 Microstructure of enamel (left) and dentin (right) revealed by acid treatment showing the dense structure of enamel, which is composed of rods of hydroxyapatite mineral, and the porous structure of dentin, which is composed of hydroxyapatite mineral with protein surrounding the tubules.

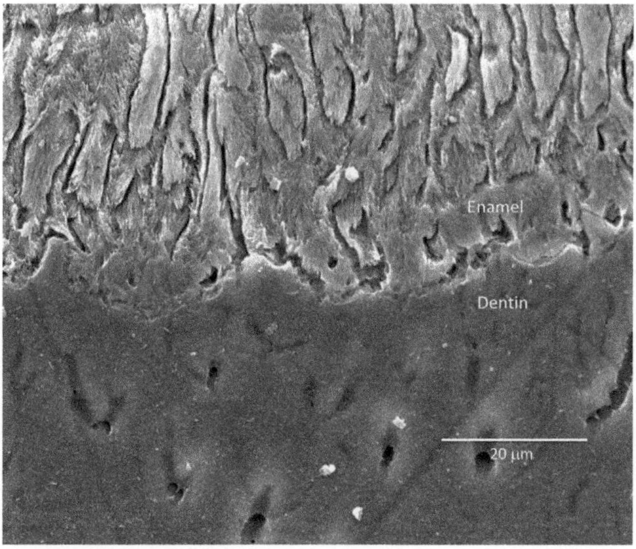

Figure 5.2 Microstructure of the enamel–dentin junction.

The tougher dentin provides significant toughening of the entire tooth complex by serving as a crack blunter at the DEJ. There are many views as to how this interface provides enhanced resistance to crack propagation. These include the mismatch in elastic modulus between the dentin and enamel that arrests cracks (Bechtle et al., 2010) and crack bridging and localized microcracking within the enamel as the junction is approached (Yahyazadehfar et al., 2014). The ultimate outcome is that there is significant energy dissipation at the interface, which often typically allows cracks to reach, but not breach, the dentin. In addition, there is strong adhesion between the enamel and dentin at the interface, with an apparent increase in fracture toughness as the DEJ is approached (Bechtle et al., 2010). Thus, the DEJ provides a dramatic advantage over the individual tooth components, which accounts for the fact that a very high proportion of teeth in humans have cracks, but they continue to function for many years, despite the fact that the outer enamel structure is compromised.

In modern dentistry, it is most typical to create bonded interfaces with enamel and dentin through resin-based adhesives and composites, both being composed of polymer matrices, and the latter especially being reinforced by inorganic particulates coupled to the polymer with a silane coupling molecule, thus securing that interface within the material. Resins are capable of flowing into micro- and macroscopic irregularities on the surface of the enamel or dentin and "locking" into the tooth structure once the resin becomes hardened. This curing process typically occurs through a light-activated initiation process that transforms dimethacrylate monomers into a highly cross-linked polymer network. The polymerization process is associated with a significant shrinkage that may be directed away from the interface, thus imposing stresses on the potential bond between the resin and the tooth material. This stress may compromise both the adhesiveness and the seal of the interface. This topic has resulted in a tremendous volume of work and the subject of numerous reviews (Carvalho et al., 1996; Braga and Ferracane, 2004; Lu et al., 2004; Stansbury et al., 2005; Ferracane, 2008; Mantri and Mantri, 2013). This work has focused on trying to quantitate the stress and quality of the interfacial seal, as well as quantitating the adhesive force. The adhesive force is predominantly a result of mechanical forces but also derives from secondary bonding, with a potential for chemical interactions for certain adhesive systems.

The literature varies widely in terms of the actual mechanical strength of the adhesive interface between dental resins and dentin. However, a comparison of several adhesive resins that have been tested in many studies over the years shows average adhesive strengths from approximately 22–54 MPa using the microtensile mode, with an actual range of 6–75 MPa, and an average of 12–26 MPa with the shear test method, with an actual range of 6–39 MPa (Ferracane et al., 2009). These data suggest that the adhesive strength of the interface may be approaching, or even exceeding, the tensile strengths of the dentin and enamel, respectively.

The multilayer interface that forms between the resin and dentin may be more appropriately termed an interphase. This region is composed of tooth structure and resin, and has been called the "hybrid" layer due to its dual composition. The layer is created by acid treatment of the dentin to demineralize and expose the collagen network, and subsequently impregnating the collagen with monomers that polymerize into a cross-linked polymer matrix surrounding the collagen fibrils. The layer may be fractions of a micrometer thick, as is typical with self-etching adhesives using milder organic acids, and up to several micrometers thick, as is more typical for etch-and-rinse type adhesives employing stronger acids, although the strength of the interface does not depend on the thickness (Fig. 5.3). This resin penetration process is usually incomplete, leaving porosities on the micro- and nanoscale within the hybrid layer that weaken it (Pinzon et al., 2013).

Studies have been conducted to evaluate the mechanical properties of the materials across this resin–dentin interface. Van Meerbeek et al. (1993) used nanoindentation of permanent teeth to study the hardness and elastic modulus and showed an expected transition from the dentin of higher modulus through the hybrid layer of

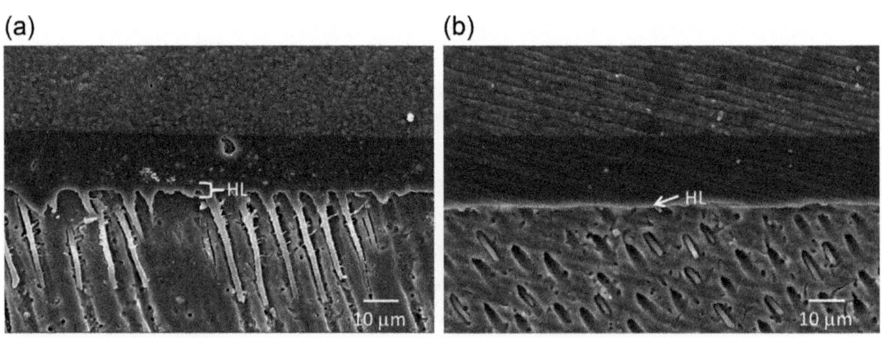

Figure 5.3 Microstructure of the interface between a resin adhesive and dentin treated with a strong acid showing a defined hybrid layer (HL) a few micrometers thick (a) and a milder acid in which the hybrid layer is very thin (b).

lower modulus to the unfilled resin adhesive of even lower modulus. Hardness followed a similar pattern. They suggested that this "elastic layer" may provide deformation that actually enhances the adhesive to remain bonded to the tooth structure during the polymerization shrinkage of the composite restorative, especially if the adhesive layer above the hybrid layer is thick. Hosoya and Marshall (2005) and Hosoya (2006) measured hardness across the interface of resin with sound and carious primary dentin with nanoindentation. They showed different results compared with permanent dentin in that the hardness and modulus were not significantly reduced within the interface when compared with sound dentin below the interface, and were possibly even higher when compared when carious dentin. Ryou et al. (2013) used nano–dynamic mechanical analysis to show that the storage modulus of the hybrid layer was heterogeneous due to the different properties of the resin tags and the resin-reinforced collagen areas that compose the interface. The resin–collagen interface had slightly higher modulus than the resin itself due to the greater stiffness of the collagen, but the properties of both components, as expected, depended highly on the hydration state. They also verified that this layer of resin-infiltrated collagen was extremely viscoelastic, and capable of significant time-dependent deformation. Thus, loading rate would have a significant effect on its properties, both during function and mechanical testing.

As the purpose of this chapter is to describe the mechanical aspects of this interface, the focus from here on will be directed at the methods used to test the adhesion between resin and tooth structure.

5.2.2 Interfacial testing methods

5.2.2.1 Tensile and shear

Historically, the predominant testing mode for tooth–resin interfaces has been the tensile or the shear-bond method, and the microtensile bond method (Fig. 5.4). It is likely that the purest method for testing the bond between the two materials is uniaxial

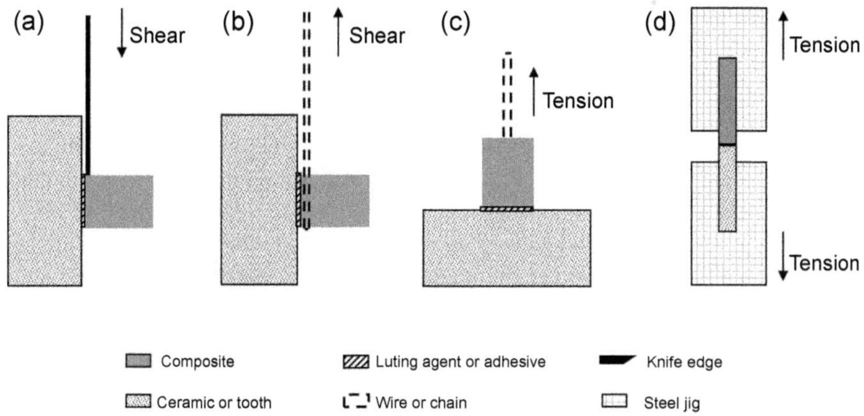

Figure 5.4 Test methods for bond strengths: (a) shear with a knife edge, (b) shear by pulling a wire loop in tension, (c) tension, and (d) microtensile.

tension of specimens of a size that is indicative of dental restorations. In this case, the material, in the form of a cylinder, is cured directly on a dentin or enamel surface, and then somehow gripped and pulled up off the surface. Failure stress is calculated as the force at fracture divided by the cross-sectional area, based on the assumption that the stresses are uniformly distributed within the joint area. Uniaxial tensile testing relies on critical alignment, gripping, and loading procedures that often are neglected or compromised, resulting in failures that do not provide an accurate indication of the true interfacial properties. For many, the shear test method provided a simpler approach. However, with either method, nonuniform stress distributions are typical at either the edges of the interface or in the center of the joint due to specimen production limitations and geometries, and these stress concentrations can significantly affect testing outcomes. It is common, and predictable, that failures originate from defects and critical flaws in the adhesive resin material near the interface, typically at the fillet formed during the joining/curing process, rather than directly at the interfacial joint (Van Noort et al., 1991).

Studies have also verified that cohesive failure of the components, typically the tooth structure, occurs due to these stress concentrations (Versluis et al., 1997). This is an interesting phenomenon that was not noticed when the adhesion strength between the polymer resin and dentin was of more limited magnitude. However, as described by Versluis et al. (1997), due to the more brittle nature of dentin and enamel, and the fact that in shear tests, the composite on which the load is applied is mostly in compression, whereas the tooth structure is predominantly in tension, failure via crack propagation directed within the tooth structure is more likely. If the two materials at the interface were more closely matched in terms of mechanical properties, cracking along the interface would be expected.

Using finite element (FE) analysis, Van Noort et al. (1989) examined these variables, as well as the manner in which the properties of the dental composite affects stress distributions. In shear test modes, they found that peak interfacial stresses could be 65% higher with composites of higher modulus. They concluded that although the actual adhesive strength of the interface might be the same, composites with greater modulus could show higher interfacial stress values simply due to the influence of their own mechanical properties, and the difference between the properties of the composite and the tooth. This outcome helped to explain a wide variability in the results of composite bond strength to tooth structure. Similarly, in tensile testing, the thickness of the materials on either side of the test joint influence stress distribution, with thinner sections causing greater stresses at the center of the joint as opposed to at the edges.

Another significant issue with shear stress tests is the location of the applied load to the actual tooth–resin interface. There are large stress concentrations in the material at the site of load application, the magnitude of which depends on the contact area between the loading device and the composite (DeHoff et al., 1995). Point source load applications understandably produce the highest stresses. In any case, the stresses are highest within the interface closest to the loading site, and diminish and become more uniform within the bulk of the joint. For this reason, some have suggested using a wire loop, as opposed to a knife edge, to engage more area of the composite cylinder during loading to minimize the stress concentrations. In either situation, tensile stresses become more prevalent than shear as the loading site moves further away from the interface (Braga et al., 2010). In any case, these analyses show that the method of calculating bond strength by dividing failure load by cross-sectional area severely underestimates the true failure stress in the bonded interface.

5.2.2.2 Microtensile

In an attempt to eliminate the failure of dentin during bond tests, and to be able to obtain multiple test specimens from various parts of a single tooth, the microtensile bond test was introduced by Sano et al. (1994). With this method, composite can be bonded either to a flat dentin or enamel surface, or within a cavity preparation in a whole tooth, and individual stick-shaped specimens, approximately 1 mm^2, are cut providing a bonded interface that can be tested in tension. The sticks are tested with a square cross section, or as originally designed, further shaped into a dumbbell to ensure failure at the interface. Typically, due to the smaller surface area being tested, bond strengths using the microtensile mode are higher than those obtained from macroscale tensile or shear tests, but the methods are highly correlated and tend to rank materials in the same order (Pinzon et al., 2013).

The quality and stability of the resin–dentin interface has been studied exhaustively. A clinical study has verified that the bond strength declines with time in the mouth (Hashimoto et al., 2000). The lack of stability of this interface is associated with the degradation of the exposed collagen and plasticizing of the polymer resin with time, leading to enhanced internal porosity and a weakened structure. This has been verified both in vivo (Hashimoto et al., 2001) and in vitro (Okuda et al., 2002).

The utility and appropriateness of interfacial strength testing using the microtensile test has been the subject of numerous articles (Pashley et al., 1999; Armstrong et al., 2010). Some have suggested that there is only very limited correlation of such tests with actual clinical performance of materials (Heintze et al., 2011). Recent reviews suggest that "simple" tests of interfacial bond strength via shear or microtensile methods, in general, are plagued by high levels of data scatter, in large part due to the fact that many failures are not truly interfacial, although they are considered as such in the data analysis (Scherrer et al., 2010). Often fractographic analysis of debonded interfaces is performed with optical microscopy with insufficient resolution to identify the true site of fracture, leading to the identification of the so-called mixed fractures in which the failure appears to have occurred within the substrates and also at the interface. Thus, the true bond strength cannot be determined. The use of scanning electron microscopy (SEM) for assessing the fracture surface offers better resolution and a more thorough analysis of the failure mode (Fig. 5.5).

The data from these studies showed that the change in geometry and properties as one crosses the interface between the tooth and the material make it impossible to achieve uniform interfacial stresses across the joint. These uncertainties cast considerable doubt upon the extent to which these tests then can actually predict the interfacial adhesion of the clinical situation, even if standardized test methods are employed. For these reasons, many have argued for adopting an alternative approach to bond strength testing involving fracture mechanics (Tam and Pilliar, 1993; DeHoff et al., 1995; Versluis et al., 1997; Tantbirojn et al., 2000; Far and Ruse, 2003; Soderholm, 2010).

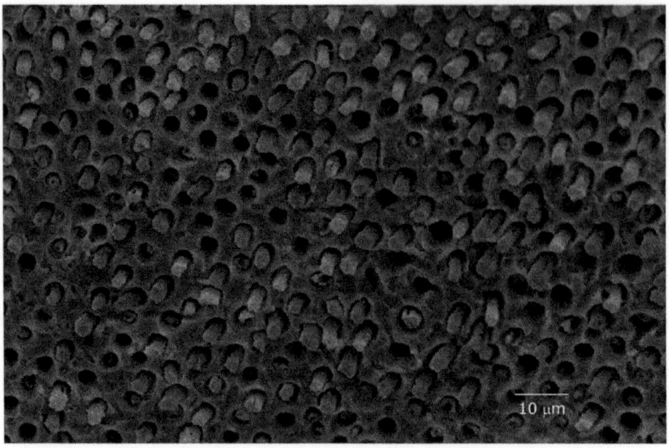

Figure 5.5 Scanning electron micrograph of a fractured interface between a resin adhesive and dentin, showing the failure at the bottom of the hybrid layer, and perhaps through the top layer of dentin. Note the resin tags that had penetrated the tubules, but offered no benefit to the bond because they do not bond to the dentin tubule walls.

5.2.2.3 *Fracture mechanics*

The first test of the fracture toughness of the interface between resin and tooth structure was conducted by De Groot et al. (1990) for dental enamel and composite using the single-edge notched beam method. They showed that the obtained value for the critical stress intensity, K_{Ic}, ranged from 0.84 to 1.02 MPa m$^{1/2}$ in the case of interfacial failure, being greater for the more heavily filled, stiffer composite. As noted earlier, higher bond strength values have been shown for stiffer composite using more conventional test methods. This work was followed by work by Tam and Pilliar (1993) using the chevron notch method for composite bonded to dentin. They reported fracture toughness values of 0.2–0.7 MPa m$^{1/2}$ depending on the type of adhesive. They also measured the value for the enamel interface as 1.11 MPa m$^{1/2}$, which is fairly consistent with the results of De Groot et al. (1990). Tam and Pilliar (1994) further assessed the microstructure of the fracture surfaces using SEM and X-ray microanalysis, which helped to explain the differences in toughness values for the different adhesives based on the extent of resin penetration and site of failure.

Many others have measured the fracture toughness of the interfacial bond (Armstrong et al., 1998, 2001; Walshaw et al., 2003). Armstrong et al. (2001) identified that the weakest interfaces in the joint were at the top of the hybrid layer and adhesive interface and at the bottom of the hybrid layer and dentin interface when tested with chevron-notched short bars. They also confirmed that when testing with the microtensile method, failures were typically within the substrates near the interface. A study by De Munck et al. (2013) compared the results of microtensile bond strength tests with the chevron notch beam (CNB) method for fracture toughness, and showed that although there was a reasonable correlation between the two methods for six dentin adhesives, there was significantly less scatter in the results for the CNB method.

Furthermore, most failures were interfacial for the CNB method, whereas most were not for the microtensile method. One may conclude that fracture toughness may serve as a more accurate and precise mode for testing the interfacial quality of the resin–tooth structure bond, although it may be more laborious in terms of specimen preparation and methodology, requiring a very sharp notch, or precrack, to be placed precisely at the bonded interface.

5.2.2.4 Fatigue

Dong and Ruse (2003) produced crack propagation across the DEJ through fatigue load cycling, and showed through SEM that the DEJ deflected cracks initiated in the enamel and running parallel to the plane of dentin tubules to a nearly perpendicular direction. They also measured fracture toughness using the notchless triangular prism geometry and recorded values for the complex of $1.5\,\mathrm{MPa\,m^{1/2}}$, which was consistent with other studies. Drummond et al. (1996) compared static shear tests with cyclic fatigue and shear punch bond tests and showed that the cyclic fatigue method provided a more conservative assessment of the true interfacial bond strength, being essentially one-half the value as that obtained in the other tests. They used a staircase approach where the cyclic stress level is increased or decreased by a defined level (ie, like a stair step) for each subsequent test based on the results (failure or survival of a given number of cycles) of the previous test.

Many others have used various types of fatigue tests, including bending, compression, rotary, and tensile, to study various aspects of the resin adhesive–tooth interface (Frankenberger et al., 2003; De Munck et al., 2005; Staninec et al., 2008; Belli et al., 2010; Mutluay et al., 2013; Yahyazadehfar et al., 2013). De Munck et al. (2005) and Belli et al. (2010) verified that the fatigue bond strength was approximately 25–70% of the static bond strength. Both showed evidence for microstructural damage accumulation during the fatigue testing that led to the reduced joint strength. This relationship of fatigue strength to static strength is similar to what is found for dental composites, where the fatigue strength is typically around 50% of the static strength (Turssi et al., 2006; Lohbauer et al., 2013). The studies by Mutluay et al. (2013) and Yahyazadehfar et al. (2013) introduced a novel method where the beam test specimen involves two similar bonded joints, one of which fails during the test to provide a value for the fatigue strength, and the other that allows microstructure analysis of the failure mechanisms. These studies verified that the dentin–composite joint had lower fatigue strength than the two joint materials, and that viscoelastic deformation during cyclic loading caused breakdown within the interface leading to failure, possibly through enhanced hydrolytic degradation. They also showed that for the joint with enamel, microfractures within the enamel itself led to failure of the joint.

The results of these studies suggest that tests involving the static evaluation of the adhesive–tooth bond are likely to overestimate the true durability of the adhesive interface. It is apparent that methods incorporating fracture toughness testing or fatigue loading are likely to be more appropriate for truly testing the interfacial integrity, and possibly for correlating with clinical performance of various materials.

5.3 The resin–ceramic interface—cementation

Resin-based cements are commonly used for permanent fixation of dental ceramics and have become the material of choice in modern adhesive dentistry providing enhanced clinical longevity compared with more traditional luting methods. Similar to the progression of resin composite restorative adhesive systems, developments in materials science have provided the dental practitioner with a variety of resin-based cement materials. However, dissimilar surface chemistries, variations in surface preparation, and the degradative effects of the oral environment may significantly affect the mechanical performance of the prosthesis, specifically at the adhesive interface. This section aims to review the effect of ceramic surface preparation and modification, materials chemistry, and mechanical testing modality on the interfacial mechanical properties and adhesion of dental ceramics, including those based on silica with a significant glassy phase and those that are almost exclusively crystalline, such as zirconia, with modern dental resin cements.

5.3.1 Resin strengthening of predominantly glassy ceramics

For several decades the use of traditional luting agents such as zinc phosphate cements were considered the gold standard for cementation purposes, and have been so successful that they are still used today. However, such materials simply act as a sealant between the tooth and restoration offering only weak micromechanical retention with no chemical adhesive potential. Although the introduction of zinc polycarboxylate and glass ionomer cements improved the chemical affinity between tooth and restoration, the low initial acidity of the mixed cement is known to extend the inherent defect population at the ceramic surface and reduce the mechanical reliability of the ceramic–lute interface (Fleming and Narayan, 2003). For over 15 years, it has been known that the clinical longevity of traditional, predominantly glassy ceramic prostheses can be significantly improved by interfacial adhesion of the ceramic restoration to tooth structure using resin-based cements (Krämer et al., 2008; Malament and Socransky, 1999a,b). The surface of silica-based glassy ceramics is amenable to modification by hydrofluoric acid, which increases the surface area and energy, as well as the wettability of the cement system. Subsequent surface priming using amphiphilic silane chemistry provides efficient coupling of the inorganic glass and organic moiety of the resin cement.

There has been much research concerned with the effect of surface conditioning of predominantly glassy ceramics having a silica-based glassy matrix with crystalline inclusions on the mechanical properties and performance of all-ceramic restorations. Ever since the introduction of the porcelain jacket crown and porcelain veneer in the early 20th century, it is known that the predominant failure mode of traditional dental ceramics initiates from the tensile surface, or internal fit surface of the restoration. Ultimately, failure occurs from the extension of a critical flaw within a preexisting defect population (Kelly, 1999; Quinn et al., 2005; Scherrer et al., 2006). If the flaw population can be modified at the ceramic surface, the probability of extending a critical defect can be significantly reduced. Consequently, precementation surface preparation is important not only to increase the surface energy and provide a greater surface area for resin penetration but also to modify the defect population to improve mechanical properties of the entire system.

Previous studies have proposed various mechanisms for improving the mechanical properties of the resin–ceramic interface. Marquis (1992) suggested that resin penetration within existing surface microporosities effectively decreased the crack length and blunted the crack tip thus reducing the stress intensity factor and improving toughness. Nathanson (1993) further postulated that shrinkage of the resin cement provided a residual compressive stress state within the defect population and thereby reduced the probability of crack extension. Moreover, resin cement strengthening has been suggested to occur by modifying the entire defect population through the creation of a hybrid layer of resin and ceramic consisting of an interpenetrating phase of ceramic surface porosity and infiltrated resin cement (Addison et al., 2007a; Fleming and Addison, 2009). Thus, the microstructure of this interface has similarities to that between resin and tooth.

The extent of resin–ceramic strengthening also depends on the thickness of the resin cement (Wang et al., 1995) and its intrinsic mechanical properties (Addison et al., 2007a). A positive linear correlation was observed between flexural modulus of the resin cement and ceramic strengthening (Addison et al., 2007b), and it has been previously suggested that resin cements with higher stiffness may result in increased clinical performance of glassy ceramic restorations (Addison et al., 2007b; Fleming et al., 2006). However, for stiffer cements that are manufactured with increased filler content (or higher molecular weight base resins), the initial increased viscosity is likely to reduce intimate contact with the ceramic surface preparation and lessen the strengthening effect (Belli et al., 2014a; Fleming et al., 2012).

5.3.2 Resin cementation of zirconia polycrystalline ceramics

Unlike ceramics that contain a silica glass phase that is readily modifiable by acid etching (Fig. 5.6), high-density polycrystalline ceramics such as zirconia are much less easily prepared. Furthermore, direct chemical adhesion of a conventional silane primer layer is more problematic as the surface of a polycrystalline ceramic is more stable and comparatively nonpolar, which eliminates the possibility of forming silanol groups as the surface is not readily hydrolyzed (Thompson et al., 2011). Consequently, either tribomechanical or chemical modification or the use of an appropriate coupling agent at the ceramic surface is required.

The literature is awash with various surface pretreatment protocols, development of primer and adhesive chemistry, and characterization of their adhesive potential between resin cements for luting purposes or resin composite restorative materials for intraoral repair. Mechanical alteration of the ceramic surface tribology can involve various methods.

Airborne particle abrasion, or "grit blasting" using various particle types, sizes, and application (Derand et al., 2005; Kern et al., 2009; Foxton et al., 2011) to increase roughness and surface energy and create micromechanical retentive features. Owing to the superior hardness of polycrystalline ceramic materials, it is difficult to roughen

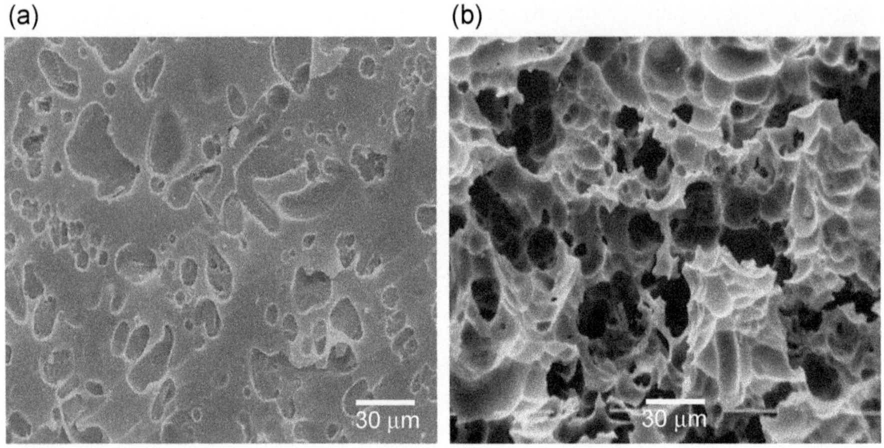

Figure 5.6 The two-phase structure of a typical glassy ceramic, before (a) and after the application of hydrofluoric acid (b), which readily etches the glass phase to provide a micromechanical key for infiltration of the resin cement.

the surface to a degree similar to that of traditional glassy ceramics. However, previous reports suggest that adhesion to grit blasted polycrystalline surfaces is improved, presumably by surface decontamination, increased roughness (albeit to a limited extent), and improved wettability of the resin cement material (Kern and Wenger, 1998; Amaral et al., 2008).

Laboratory findings also suggest that grit blasting can increase load-to-failure strengths under biaxial flexure (Sato et al., 2008; Kosmac et al., 1999) or fatigue strengthening (Scherrer et al., 2011) as a result of the well-known phase transformation within the metastable crystal lattice, and subsequent volume change that may induce an increased compressive strength at the ceramic surface. On the other hand, previous researchers have suggested that surface abrasion may induce critical surface flaws that reduce mechanical properties and potentially affect the longevity of zirconia crowns (Casucci et al., 2009). Such effects are largely dictated by numerous abrasion factors, such as particle size/type (Valandro et al., 2008; Ozcan et al., 2013a), nozzle distance/orientation, duration (Ozcan et al., 2013b), and application pressure (Souza et al., 2013). Even if phase transformation provides an immediate strengthening effect, the presence of microcracks under cyclic loading is known to substantially reduce fatigue strength and potentially the clinical lifetime of the ceramic restoration (Zhang et al., 2006; Mitov et al., 2011).

Microstructural variations within different commercial zirconia ceramic formulations are likely to significantly affect the extent and depth of phase transformation at the ceramic surface (known as the "transformed zone depth") following grit blasting. That, coupled with extensive variability in surface grit blasting protocols, provides a complex recipe for optimization of mechanical properties and longevity at the resin–ceramic interface. Although there are vast amounts of laboratory evidence for improved interfacial adhesion to zirconia, little clinical evidence of durable bonding using rather complex and time-consuming procedures currently exists, and that which

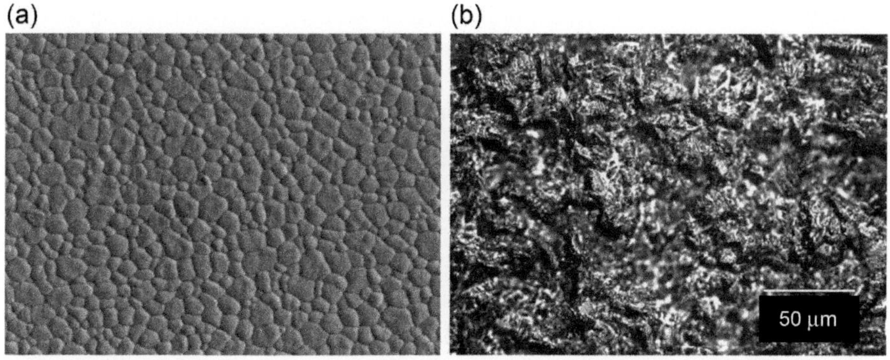

Figure 5.7 The predominantly single-phase microstructure of a typical polycrystalline zirconia dental ceramic before (a) and after air abrasion (b). Grit blasting provides increased roughness (albeit to a lesser extent than acid etching of a glassy ceramic) for micromechanical retention and increased surface area of hydroxyl groups important for adhesion of zirconate-coupling agents.

does, suggests that moderate-pressure grit blasting and appropriate (phosphate-based) resin cements (see later) provide good clinical longevity (Kern, 2015).

Modern techniques for bonding to dental zirconia ceramics often include zirconate-coupling agents, which contain phosphate groups that readily bind to metal oxides and a photopolymerizable organic group with methacrylate functionality that provides immediate adhesive stability to the resin cement. Zirconia dental restorations with cements that include phosphate-based monomers such as 10-methacryloyloxydecyl dihydrogen phosphate are strongly recommended due to the recognized superior clinical durability (Kern and Sasse, 2011; Sasse et al., 2012), evidenced by long-term hydrolytically stable adhesion between the phosphate moieties of the cement and surface hydroxyl groups of the ceramic (Thompson et al., 2011). Even if the potential for increasing surface roughness is somewhat limited by the high hardness of zirconia, grit blasting remains a critical step, not only to increase roughness for micromechanical retention (Fig. 5.7) but also to increase the number of hydroxyl groups available at the surface (Amaral et al., 2014; Tsuo et al., 2006).

The extent to which a zirconia ceramic surface should be roughened remains controversial. As previously mentioned, although grit blasting has been reported to provide enhanced strength characteristics (Guazzato et al., 2005; Wolfhart et al., 2007; Song et al., 2013; Erdem et al., 2014), others have suggested a strength-limiting effect (Zhang et al., 2006; Guazzato et al., 2004). In 2015, a review article presented strong clinical evidence for long-term durability of zirconia ceramic restorations using grit blasting with moderate air pressure and phosphate-based cement systems (Kern, 2015). The same review also quoted a previous clinical study, which identified the risk associated with the use of resin cements on unprepared (non grit blasted) zirconia restorations. A failure rate of 13.3% over 53 months was reported (Sailer and Hämmerle, 2014), which would otherwise support precementation grit blasting of the ceramic surface. Even assessment of modern self-adhesive or "universal" resin cements still advocates mechanical modification of the ceramic surface by grit blasting rather than relying on the self-adhesive quality of the cement alone (Pereira et al., 2015; Amaral et al., 2014).

Tribochemical modification is a popular technique to improve adhesive potential using airborne particle abrasion techniques. These methods typically employ silica-modified alumina particles to silicatize the ceramic surface to allow subsequent adhesion of a silane molecule (Thompson et al., 2011). Most in vitro studies report improved bond strengths to modified, silica-coated surfaces (Bottino et al., 2014; Erdem et al., 2014; May et al., 2012; Aboushelib et al., 2008b), although some show no significant difference with or without tribochemical treatment using the same resin cement (Ernst et al., 2005) and decreased strengthening effects (Attia et al., 2011; Chai et al., 2010) or even report evidence of ineffective penetration of the silica-coated layer (Matinlinna et al., 2006).

Born from the catastrophic failures of zirconia hip joint arthroplasties in the early 2000s, concerns exist over the effects of particle abrasion (whether that be from tribochemical or surface roughening treatments) on damage accumulation and low-temperature degradation of dental ceramics that may significantly affect their long-term clinical performance (Kim et al., 2010; Kohorst et al., 2012; Inokoshi et al., 2015). To eliminate the use of airborne particle abrasion techniques in an attempt to reduce the potential of long-term degradation, other (additive) surface treatments have been suggested such as a simple feldspathic surface glaze (Derand et al., 2005; Cattell et al., 2009; Everson et al., 2012; Şanlı et al., 2015), which provides a surface layer that is amenable to etching and subsequently infiltrated with the resin cement system. A further technique known as "selective infiltration etching" (Aboushelib et al., 2007) introduces a glass melt at relatively a low temperature (750°C), which effectively thermally etches the surface, providing microretentive features (without mechanical stress) for infiltration of the cement system. The authors report superior-aged bond strength compared with grit blasting. Other alternative surface modification techniques include fluorination pretreatments (Piascik et al., 2011), vapor deposition of silicalike "seed-layers" (Piascik et al., 2009), and in situ silica nanoparticle deposition (Oliveira-Ogliari et al., 2015).

5.3.3 Adhesion test methods for the resin cement–ceramic interface

As with adhesion testing for other interfaces discussed in this chapter, interrogation of the mechanical properties and bond strength at the resin–ceramic interface is fraught with problems. The wide variation in strength data has been discussed previously, but generally relates to in vitro tests that barely relate to the clinical situation, inappropriate test method designs that do not effectively test the adhesive joint, and other variables that are commonly not controlled.

The test methods in use at present for assessing the bond strength of resin cement to glassy and polycrystalline dental ceramics are very similar to those used for the material–tooth interface described previously (Fig. 5.4). Generally, macroshear and tensile tests are most popular for adhesion testing of the resin and glassy ceramic interface, although macroshear remains the predominant testing modality for studying the adhesion of resin cements to zirconia (Ozcan and Bernasoni, 2015; Inokoshi et al., 2014), likely due to the ease of specimen preparation without the need for cutting fully sintered zirconia into rectangular- or hourglass-shaped specimens. However, shear tests have long been criticized for their inability to accurately forecast clinical outcomes (Van Noort et al., 1989; Sudsangiam and van Noort, 1999; Heintze, 2013), as well as for unpredictable stress distributions, which lead to failure initiation away from the adhesive interface with the inevitable misinterpretation of the meaning of the bond strength data (Della Bona and van Noort, 1995). Although shear bond strength tests are the most used for resin cement–zirconia adhesion, they are reported as providing generally the lowest bond strength values and are the least discriminative when compared with microshear and macro- and microtensile tests (Inokoshi et al., 2014).

Alternative, less common, approaches include tensile bond strength by flexural testing (Şanlı et al., 2015; Mirmohammadi et al., 2010; Staninec et al., 2008). Here, the bonded surface is placed centrally under three- or four-point loading, the latter method requiring less accuracy in the alignment of the adhesive joint directly beneath the central load (Fig. 5.7). Nonetheless, for either method, obtaining a pure state of tension through the adhesive interface is difficult. The perceived advantages of interrogating the adhesive interface using a four-point flexure over direct tension tests are the ease of specimen preparation and better fixation and alignment. Polycrystalline ceramic blocks can be machined in their presintered state into oversized bar-shaped specimens that allow for shrinkage following full densification (Fig. 5.8). The test configuration should allow a span width to specimen depth ratio of greater than 10 to prevent shear stresses within the adhesive joint (Şanlı et al., 2015; Mirmohammadi et al., 2010). Previous researchers have used specimen dimensions of 25 mm length, 2 mm width, 2 mm depth (Mirmohammadi et al., 2010), or 5 mm width according to American Society for Testing Materials (ASTM) C164-11 (Şanlı et al., 2015; ASTM C1674-11, 2011). It has been suggested that the maximum tensile load at the convex surface of the four-point bend specimen and subsequent gradient stress field along the load axis is more clinically relevant than either direct tension or shear tests (Şanlı et al., 2015).

5.4 Sintered and soldered joints–bilayer interfaces in dentistry

A definition of interface in dentistry in not only assigned to adhesive dentistry but also includes sintered and soldered joints. Those interfaces are commonly found in prosthetic dentistry and mainly represent the application of veneers in fixed partial dentures (FPDs), the purpose of which is to enhance the overall esthetic quality of the final prosthesis. Especially, issues related to metal–ceramic and ceramic–ceramic interfaces are repeatedly addressed and updated in dental research.

The veneering process itself actually long precedes any dental application. Ceramic glaze and enamel technology has been invented in ancient Japan and was applied on earthenware or metals either for esthetic reasons or simply to seal and make them

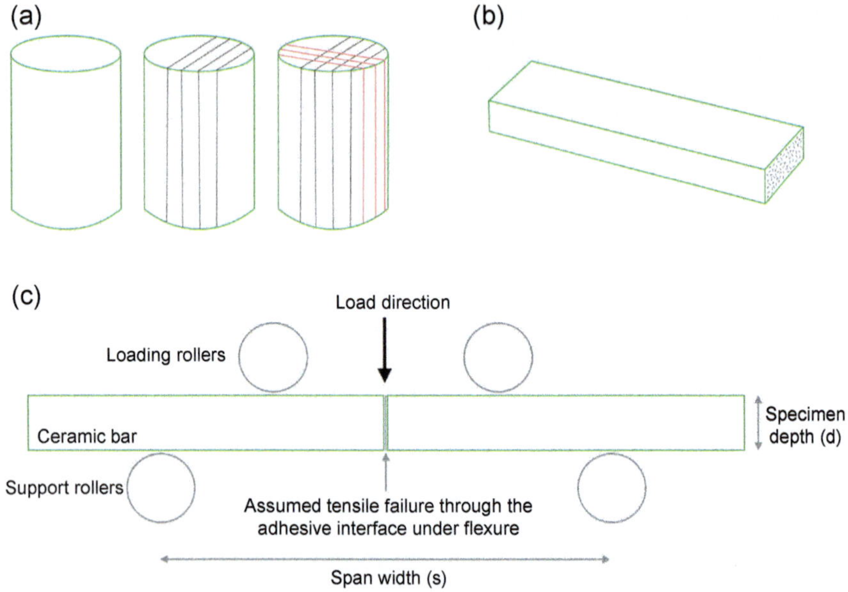

Figure 5.8 The adhesive joint between resin cements can be investigated using four-point flexural strength testing. Oversized polycrystalline ceramic *bar-shaped* specimens are cut from presintered blocks (a) to allow for full densification shrinkage prior to testing. The adhesive surface is prepared (grit blasted, silica coated, surface glazed, etc.) (b) and rejoined using a suitable resin cement material. The interface is positioned centrally under the load within a four-point bend apparatus and tested under flexure with failure assumed to initiate through the adhesive under tensile stress (c). To reduce the effect of shear deformation under flexure a span-width-to-specimen-depth ratio of at least 10 should be used (Şanlı et al., 2015; Mirmohammadi et al., 2010).

waterproof and chemically stable. Today, still applied mainly on whitewares, this thin coating layer is well researched. Much is known from early research into glazes and enamels, eg, most delamination problems related to a mismatch in the thermal expansion of the substrate and the veneer (Taylor and Bull, 1986).

In contrast to technical coatings, the unique characteristic in dentistry is that the veneer layer is applied in largely varying thicknesses and curvatures that are unique to each single FPD (Fig. 5.9). Veneers thereby serve many purposes. First, the esthetic appearance of glassy feldspathic ceramics is very natural, and second, with the use of fine-grained, reinforced glass ceramics, the hardness and thus the potential abrasivity of a restoration surface have been adjusted to better mimic those of the natural, human enamel (Oh et al., 2002).

5.4.1 Internal residual stresses

Dental veneering in the majority of cases is a sintering process based on a slurry technique, commonly conducted in repeated cycles by building up layer-by-layer. In recent years however, the method of soldering or even cementing computer-aided design/

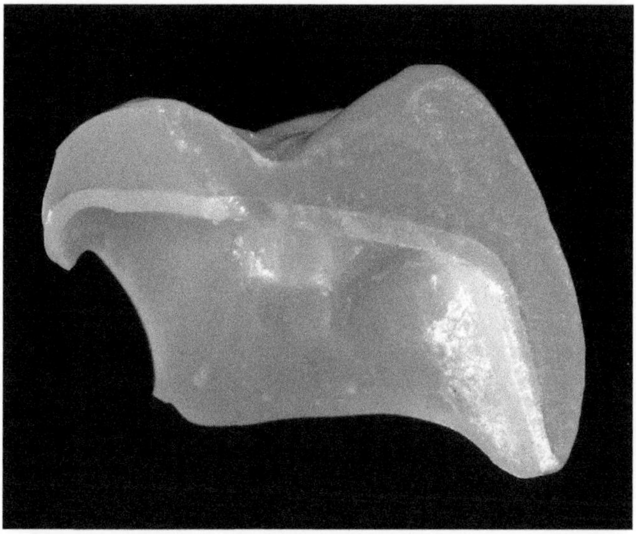

Figure 5.9 Cross-section through a veneered all-ceramic molar restoration showing the varying thickness and curvature of the veneer layer.

computer-aided manufacturing (CAD/CAM) veneers onto a framework substrate has become relatively popular (Kurbad, 2011). This alternative manufacturing protocol intended to minimize internal stresses at the core–veneer interface. This development was intrinsically related to the rapid improvement in CAD/CAM technology, which provided a perfect fit between both layers.

The key requirement for sintering veneers onto either metal or ceramic substrates is an optimal, mechanically stable adhesive joint (Borba et al., 2011). Several factors contribute to this adhesion. Chemical forces are mainly responsible, although they are assisted by microretentive interlocking via surface roughness of the substrate (Wataha, 2002; Lenz and Kessel, 1998). Metal alloys suitable for the veneering process contain certain metals that preferably oxidize at the interface during sintering (such as iron, chrome, tin, indium) and thus form a primary chemical bonding to the silica of the veneering ceramics. On the other hand, a (micro-) rough substrate surface, achieved by, eg, sandblasting techniques, is known to increase the interfacial adhesion (Lenz and Kessel, 1998; Taskonak et al., 2008; Schneider and Swain, 2015). On a macroscopic level, the contraction forces that build up during cooling from sintering temperatures is reported to further increase the interfacial adhesion (Baldassarri et al., 2012; Benetti et al., 2013; DeHoff and Anusavice, 1992; Taskonak et al., 2005; Benetti et al., 2010; Aboushelib et al., 2008a). A common ceramic slurry shrinks between 20% and 30% during sintering. Part of the contraction occurs due to densification as the solvent evaporates and the particles begin to fuse. In addition, there is a solid-state contraction defined by the thermal coefficient of expansion (CTE) α as the material cools below its glass-transition temperature T_g (DeHoff and Anusavice, 1992; Anusavice et al., 1989).

The shrinkage behavior of the veneer and the core materials would ideally be slightly mismatched to produce a buildup of internal stresses at the surface (Isgro

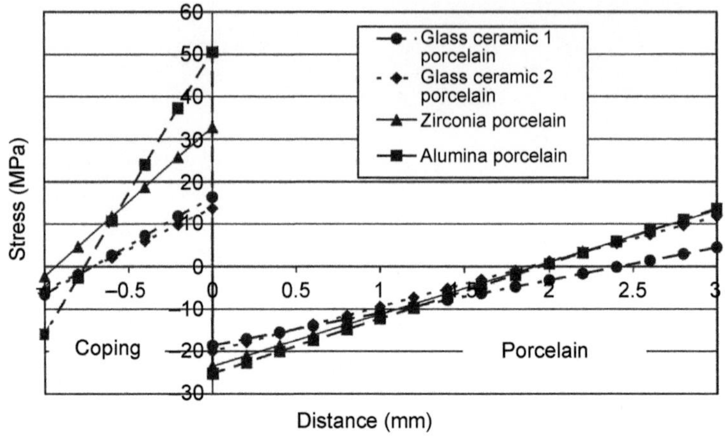

Figure 5.10 Calculation of internal stresses in the core and veneer layers according to Swain (2009).

et al., 2005; Belli et al., 2013; Fischer et al., 2007). The CTE of the veneering material has traditionally been selected to be slightly lower when compared with the substrate CTE (within a range of maximum 10% mismatch) (Anusavice and DeHoff, 1989). Fig. 5.10 shows the result of the calculation of expected stresses in a 3-mm-thick veneer layer due to a CTE mismatch of 10%. The theory explains this by the introduction of reinforcing, compressive stresses in the weak and brittle veneering ceramic (Benetti et al., 2013; DeHoff and Anusavice, 1992; Taskonak et al., 2005; Swain, 2009). However, individual dental restorations show a large variation in veneering thickness and curvature. Alternating concave and convex curvatures combined with, eg, thick cusps and thin fissures accounts for a multiaxial stress state in the veneering ceramic (Taskonak et al., 2008; Al-Amleh et al., 2014). Beneficial compressive stresses thus need to be compensated by deleterious tensile or shear stresses (Swain, 2009). As a consequence, the current technical advice for the veneer CTE should be to match the substrate CTE as close as possible to minimize internal residual stresses (Tholey et al., 2011; Benetti et al., 2014).

5.4.2 The zirconia–veneer interface

The adhesion between feldspathic veneers and zirconia, however, is not completely understood. Early research on the zirconia interface to borosilicate glasses proved a certain solubility of zirconia in the glass at elevated temperatures of 815 to 1200°C (King and Andrews, 1941). It has also been shown that zirconia enters the glass network as a six- or eight-coordinated network modifier (Takahashi et al., 1977). Durand analyzed the interface between veneer and zirconia using Raman spectroscopy and detected an interdiffusion zone of about 2 μm (Durand et al., 2012). Other work has shown that zirconia acts as nucleating element for glass crystallization and is able to enhance crystal growth (Ramos and Gandais, 1990). Fig. 5.11 shows a cross-section of the interface under transmission electron microscope. No voids, thus complete wetting and sealing is shown, even on rather rough sandblasted zirconia surfaces

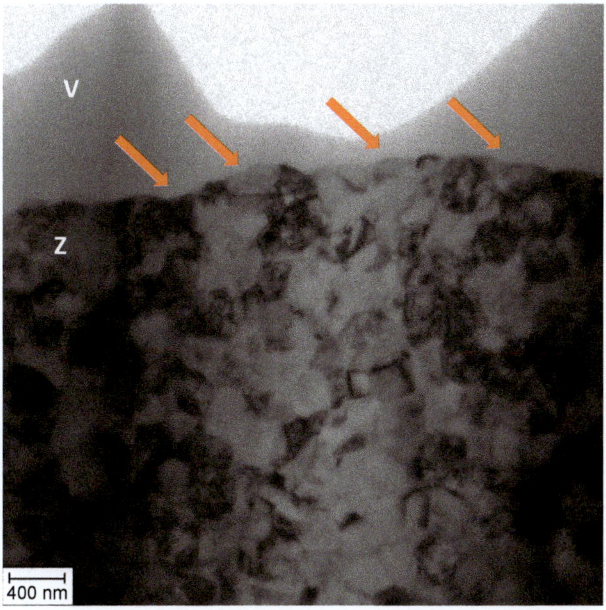

Figure 5.11 Cross-section of a sandblasted zirconia (z)–veneer (v) interface through a transmission electron microscope showing perfect wetting and interlocking (*arrows*) (Grigore et al., 2013).

(Grigore et al., 2013; Tholey et al., 2009). However, some disintegrated zirconia particles become solved in the glass matrix, most likely due to the preceding sandblasting procedure. Tholey et al. (2009) further suggested that tetragonal to monoclinic phase transformation could be triggered by the veneering process via local low-temperature degradation induced by the veneering liquid.

5.4.3 Mechanical properties of bilayer interfaces

The quantification of the interfacial adhesion and assessment of internal stresses is of central interest to the practical use of veneered restorations. Several techniques and protocols have been developed in the past to measure the bonding potential. Mainly of an indirect nature, the procedures descriptively monitor and test crack initiation, either due to mechanical or dynamic thermal loading. The most common tests reported in the literature are based on the so-called crunch-the-crown principles (Fischer et al., 2007). Those tests, however, due to the complexity of a veneered restoration, are not very sensitive and discriminatory, and provide only little information on the underlying principles and mechanisms (Kelly et al., 2012). Furthermore, the load-to-failure data from those tests far exceeds the maximum masticatory forces in vivo and are thus lacking clinical relevance. More standardized research has been developed into (uni- or bi-) axial strength testing of veneered and flat specimens (DeHoff and Anusavice, 1992). Based on those tests, variations in layer thickness and orientation, crack initiation, and crack path development can be investigated. The most prevalent procedure, however, has been adopted as a International Organization for

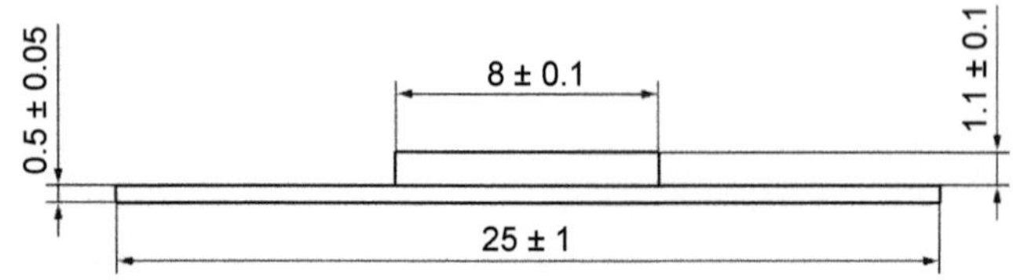

Figure 5.12 Sample preparation for the crack initiation test according to ISO 9693-1.

Standardization (ISO) procedure (ISO 9693-1, 2012; ISO/DIS 9693-2, 2014). The test was originally developed to determine the interfacial resistance of metal–ceramic bilayers against crack initiation or debonding in three-point flexure (Lenz and Kessel, 1998; Faihurst et al., 1981). Basically, the test specimens are made of a thin substrate and a short veneer layer (Fig. 5.12), which is loaded under bending conditions until initial cracks are formed at the interface between both layers. The veneered side of the specimens is thereby placed under tension. The procedure will soon be extended to ceramic–ceramic systems (ISO/DIS 9693-2) and will also include a test procedure for dynamic and cyclic thermal shock stress testing to prove the thermal compatibility of material combinations.

The ISO procedure is designed first for practical use and is easy to perform by dental technicians (to control the veneering procedure), but it provides limited insight into the underlying mechanisms. Because it is conducted on flat specimens, the interpretation of the data and its relevance to the clinical situation is limited. For example, the orientation of the veneer layer on the tensile side of the bending setup does not realistically reflect the clinical scenario. Interestingly, ISO 9693-1 provides a numerical solution for interfacial shear strength calculations. This approach uses the elastic modulus, thickness, and failure load as input variables, but only of the substrate, not of the veneering material. Furthermore, mismatch in CTE remains unaddressed. However, Schneider and Swain (2015) applied a linear elastic approach to the ISO test setup by calculating strain energies and proposed to extend the ISO procedure by the calculation of an intrinsic fracture toughness.

5.4.4 Clinical findings on veneered zirconia restorations

In recent years, with the success of zirconia as a framework material, the clinical experience revealed some serious concerns related to the veneering procedure. In contrast with restorations on metal substrates, the chipping rate for zirconia-veneered restorations was found in early studies to be significantly increased. Failure rates up to 25% after 2.5 years (Raigrodski et al., 2006), 36% in 5 years (Molin and Karlsson, 2008), or 32% after a period of 10 years (Sax et al., 2011) were reported, with more severe clinical consequences often leading to a complete restoration replacement (Heintze and Rousson, 2010; Christensen, 2009; Sailer et al., 2015). Fig. 5.13 shows an example of a zirconia-veneered five-unit bridge with a severe chipping of the buccal wall of the most distal abutment tooth. However, more recent clinical reports on the success of veneered zirconia restorations have shown a more promising performance compared

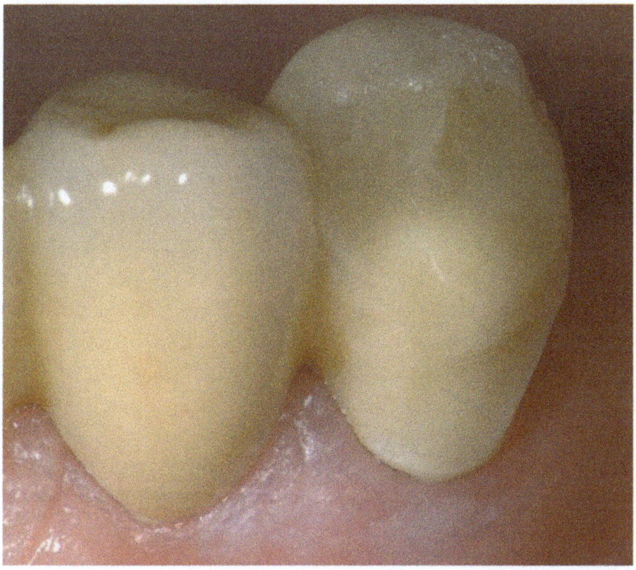

Figure 5.13 Veneer chipping of a zirconia-veneered five-unit bridge after 2.6 years in situ (Belli et al., 2014b).

with the earlier studies and a comparable success rate as with metal-based FPDs (Raigrodski et al., 2012; Al-Amleh et al., 2010).

5.4.5 Measurement of residual stresses

Inspired by the chipping issue, intensive research has been carried out to acquire more insight into the stress state of a sintered all-ceramic core-veneer interface. Pioneering work has been published by Swain (2009), in which he first discussed the specific features of Y-TZP zirconia and identified how its low thermal diffusivity ($D = 0.74 \times 10^{-6}\, m^2/s$) compared with metals ($D = 1.1 \times 10^{-4}\, m^2/s$) significantly contributed to the buildup of internal residual stresses within the veneer layer. The influence of a low thermal diffusivity is of practical importance during cooling a restoration from the veneering temperature (DeHoff and Anusavice, 1992; Tholey et al., 2011; Benetti et al., 2014; Asaoka et al., 1992; Zhang et al., 2013; Gostemeyer et al., 2010). Fast cooling is thereby identified as a major contributor to the internal stress buildup and has been implicated in the increased chipping rates on zirconia (Swain, 2009; Kim et al., 2008). As a consequence, current practical recommendations to dental technicians include a slow cooling protocol in the final step of the veneering procedure (Swain, 2009; Belli et al., 2012). The dental industry has adapted this recommendation to their sintering furnaces, which today include slow cooling programs or retarded door opening times.

Consequently, the role of residual stresses in bilayer structures and their measurement has been intensively addressed in dental research. The majority of experiments in the past decade have focused on the measurement of dimensional changes in the veneer layer because of variation of processing variables such as veneer thickness, substrate curvature, firing conditions, and CTE mismatch (Aboushelib et al., 2008a; Isgro et al., 2005; Al-Amleh et al., 2014; Jakubowicz-Kohen et al., 2014; DeHoff and Anusavice, 1989; Costa et al., 2014). More recently, it has become possible to investigate and quantify the amount of residual stresses in clinically relevant model structures and to relate them to their effect on bilayer integrity and strength. The precision of these techniques strongly relates to the resolution of the deformation control. Optical and profilometric techniques, as well as surface evaluation via strain gauges, have been investigated. The method of hole drilling into the veneer layer perpendicular to the core–veneer interface also provides an opportunity to measure the dimensional changes within the veneer layer (Mainjot et al., 2011). The drilling procedure induces a release of local stresses and thus generates a microrelaxation in the veneer layer depending on the residual stress state. Circular strain gages attached to the surface sensitively measure the dimensional changes. Problems, however, arise due to an extreme local heating during drilling, which might significantly change the local stress state, and even result in microcracking (Chang et al., 2011). Furthermore, this approach provides only global surface information on residual stresses in a plane-strain configuration parallel to the interface. The method consequently involves an invasive removal of incremental surface layers.

Another interesting approach focuses on transmittance of polarized light through thin, transparent, or translucent slices utilizing the birefringence effect (Tholey et al., 2011; Belli et al., 2012). Double refraction (birefringence) is measured based on the photoelasticity of materials and results from the retardation of polarized light through a translucent material with heterogeneous density. Stress-free glasses and ceramics, which are optically isotropic, become anisotropic when exposed to internal residual stresses or external mechanical actions (Marshall and Lawn, 1978; Katte, 2009). Fig. 5.14 shows an example of the photoelastic effect in thin crown slices, where a two-dimensional mapping of stress distribution in tension and compression becomes possible. The advantage is the ability to investigate the stress state in different planes, eg, perpendicular to the interface. Still the method presents an invasive approach due to the cutting process and an expected strain release, thus requiring a careful, slow cutting procedure under sustained water cooling.

To better understand crack development and crack path profiles, indentation crack measurements present an interesting complement to the aforementioned techniques (Marshall and Lawn, 1977; Zeng and Rowcliffe, 1994; Anunmana et al., 2009; Choi et al., 2011; Fischer and Marx, 2002; Anstis et al., 1981; Peitl et al., 2010). Basically, a surface indentation (eg, using Vickers indenters) initiates and drives cracks into a plain ceramic surface thereby allowing analysis of the length, nature, and orientation of the respective crack paths (Nishide et al., 2011). Crack deviations close to the interface, especially in a residual stress field, became a matter of interest (Kvam, 1992). Indenter modifications using Knoop or Berkovich indenters allow for targeted orientation of the crack initiation process (Nishide et al., 2011). Indentation analysis can be easily performed on individual plane orientations (Wendler et al., 2015). With the use of nanoindentation techniques, this kind of analysis can be performed close to the core–veneer interface.

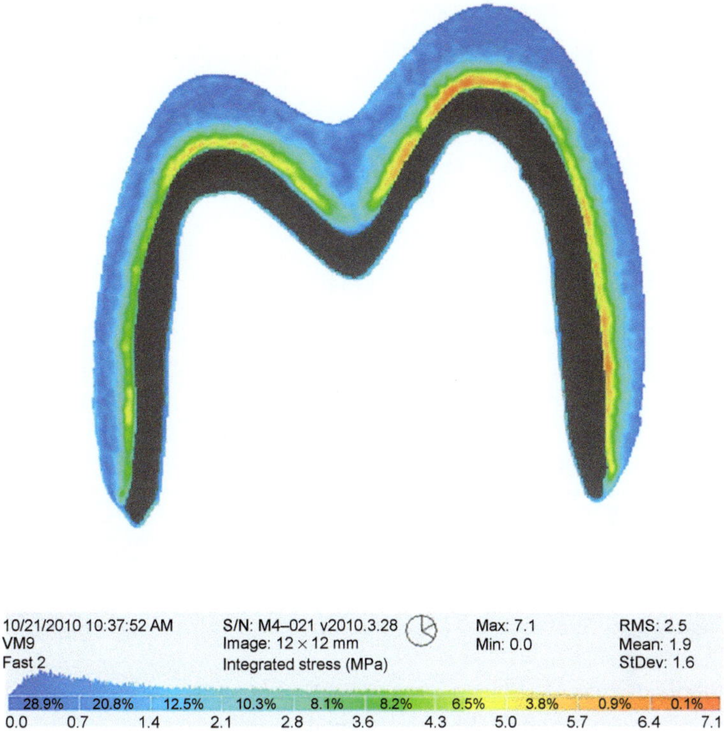

Figure 5.14 Residual stress map of a veneered cross-section under polarized light (birefringence), highlighting the development of internal stresses on different cooling protocols (Belli et al., 2012).

Residual stresses in a surface or subsurface layer can also be determined using X-ray diffraction (Sindel, 1998). The microstructural lattice space of a crystalline material changes due to internal residual stresses. Based on Bragg's law, X-ray diffraction presents a precise measure of the lattice parameters to quantitatively describe a residual stress state via lattice strain measurements (Mastelaro and Zanotto, 1996). This technique provides high resolution and precise outcomes. The penetration depth of X-rays, however, is limited to a few micrometers from the surface and thus involves an invasive removal of incremental surface layers.

An efficient tool for analyzing the residual stress state in bilayer structures and complementary to all experimental approaches is the numeric approximation of the problem using finite element (FE) models (Zhang et al., 2013; Costa et al., 2014; Bonfante et al., 2012; Hu et al., 2013; Anami et al., 2015; Meira et al., 2013). The major advantage of this tool is the simulation of dynamic thermal or mechanical processes as they occur during sintering or intraoral mastication (Costa et al., 2014; Anami et al., 2015). Also unique to this method is its application to individual geometries, allowing the research findings on planar structures to potentially be extrapolated to curved and thus more clinically realistic geometries (Hu et al., 2013). A common difficulty with

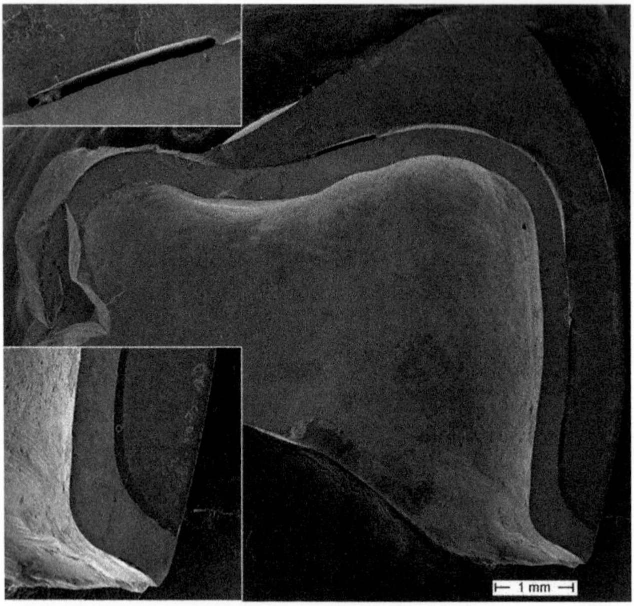

Figure 5.15 SEM image of a veneer soldered onto a zirconia framework.

FE modeling is that the significance is extremely limited to step-by-step verification and confirmation of the model with experimental results.

5.4.6 Future perspectives

The recent developments from industry have aimed to overcome the problems regarding internal residual stress buildup. The idea behind the new approaches involves a simultaneous CAD/CAM manufacturing of both parts followed by a separate bonding step (Kurbad, 2011). Two different concepts are currently marketed. The "Cad-On" technique (Ivoclar Vivadent, Schaan, Liechtenstein) includes a heating procedure and soldering a CAD/CAM produced veneer via a fusion glass ceramic onto a zirconia framework, while the "Rapid Layering Technique" (Vita Zahnfabrik, Bad Säckingen, Germany) favors an adhesive cementation of both layers. However, to date, little is known about the clinical success, manufacturing quality, process complications, and basic research for the two concepts. Fig. 5.15 shows a soldered interface between the veneer and zirconia framework foretelling some of the possible complications and deficiencies of these techniques. The image is taken from a clinically failed three-unit bridge after the 18 months in situ.

Acknowledgments

The authors would like to thank Dr. Carolina Bosso André for providing the scanning electron micrographs of the dentin-resin interface and the fracture surface.

References

Aboushelib MN, Kleverlaan CJ, Feilzer AJ. Selective infiltration-etching technique for a strong and durable bond of resin cements to zirconia-based materials. J Prosthet Dent 2007;98(5):379–88.

Aboushelib MN, Matinlinna JP, Salameh Z, Ounsi H. Innovations in bonding to zirconia-based materials: part I. Dent Mater 2008a;24(9):1268–72.

Aboushelib M, Feilzer A, De Jager N, Kleverlaan C. Prestresses in bilayered all-ceramic restorations. J Biomed Mater Res B Appl Biomater 2008b;87(1):139–45.

Addison O, Marquis PM, Fleming GJP. Resin strengthening of dental ceramics – the impact of surface texture and silane. J Dent 2007a;35(5):416–24.

Addison O, Marquis PM, Fleming GJP. Resin elasticity and the strengthening of all-ceramic restorations. J Dent Res 2007b;86(6):519–23.

Al-Amleh B, Neil Waddell J, Lyons K, Swain MV. Influence of veneering porcelain thickness and cooling rate on residual stresses in zirconia molar crowns. Dent Mater 2014;30(3):271–80.

Al-Amleh B, Lyons K, Swain M. Clinical trials in zirconia: a systematic review. J Oral Rehabil 2010;37(8):641–52.

Amaral R, Özcan M, Valandro LF, Balducci I, Bottino MA. Effect of conditioning methods on the microtensile bond strength of phosphate monomer-based cement on zirconia ceramic in dry and aged conditions. J Biomed Mater Res B Appl Biomater 2008;85(1):1–9.

Amaral M, Belli R, Cesar P, Valandro L, Petschelt A, Lohbauer U. The potential of novel primers and universal adhesives to bond to zirconia. J Dent 2014;42(1):90–8.

Anami LC, Lima JM, Corazza PH, Yamamoto ET, Bottino MA, Borges AL. Finite element analysis of the influence of geometry and design of zirconia crowns on stress distribution. J Prosthodont 2015;24(2):146–51.

Anstis G, Chantikul P, Lawn B, Marshall D. A critical evaluation of indentation techniques for measuring fracture toughness: I, direct crack measurements. J Am Ceram Soc 1981;64(9):533–8.

Anunmana C, Anusavice KJ, Mecholsky Jr JJ. Residual stress in glass: indentation crack and fractography approaches. Dent Mater 2009;25:1453–8.

Anusavice KJ, DeHoff PH, Hojjatie B, Gray A. Influence of tempering and contraction mismatch on crack development in ceramic surfaces. J Dent Res 1989;68(7):1182–7.

Armstrong SR, Boyer DB, Keller JC, Park JB. Effect of hybrid layer on fracture toughness of adhesively bonded dentin-resin composite joint. Dent Mater 1998;14(2):91–8.

Armstrong SR, Keller JC, Boyer DB. Mode of failure in the dentin-adhesive resin-resin composite bonded joint as determined by strength-based (muTBS) and fracture-based (CNSB) mechanical testing. Dent Mater 2001;17(3):201–10.

Armstrong S, Geraldeli S, Maia R, Raposo LH, Soares CJ, Yamagawa J. Adhesion to tooth structure: a critical review of "micro" bond strength test methods. Dent Mater 2010;26(2):e50–62.

Arola D, Bajaj D, Ivancik J, Majd H, Zhang D. Fatigue of biomaterials: hard tissues. Int J Fatigue 2010;32(9):1400–12.

Asaoka K, Kuwayama N, Tesk JA. Influence of tempering method on residual stress in dental porcelain. J Dent Res 1992;71(9):1623–7.

ASTM International Designation: C1674-11. Standard test method for flexural strength of advanced ceramics with engineered porosity (Honeycomb Cellular Channels) at ambient temperatures. West Conshohocken, PA, USA: ASTM International; 2011.

Attia A, Lehmann F, Kern M. Influence of surface conditioning and cleaning methods on resin bonding to zirconia ceramic. Dent Mater 2011;27(3):207–13.

Baldassarri M, Stappert C, Wolff M, Thompson V, Zhang Y. Residual stresses in porcelain-veneered zirconia prostheses. Dent Mater 2012;28(8):873–9.

Bechtle S, Fett T, Rizzi G, Habelitz S, Klocke A, Schneider GA. Crack arrest within teeth at the dentinoenamel junction caused by elastic modulus mismatch. Biomaterials 2010;31(14):4238–47.

Belli R, Baratieri LN, Braem M, Petschelt A, Lohbauer U. Tensile and bending fatigue of the adhesive interface to dentin. Dent Mater 2010;26(12):1157–65.

Belli R, Monteiro Jr S, Baratieri L, Katte H, Petschelt A, Lohbauer U. A photoelastic assessment of residual stresses in zirconia- veneer crowns. J Dent Res 2012;91(3):316–20.

Belli R, Frankenberger R, Appelt A, Schmitt J, Baratieri L, Greil P, et al. Thermal-induced residual stresses affect the lifetime of zirconia-veneer crowns. Dent Mater 2013;29(2):181–90.

Belli R, Kreppel S, Petschelt A, Hornberger H, Boccaccini AR, Lohbauer U. Strengthening of dental adhesives via particle reinforcement. J Mech Behav Biomed Mater 2014a;37:100–8.

Belli R, Scherrer SS, Reich S, Petschelt A, Lohbauer U. In vivo shell-like fractures of veneered-ZrO_2 fixed dental prostheses. Case Stud Eng Failure Anal 2014b;2(2):91–9.

Benetti P, Della Bona A, Kelly JR. Evaluation of thermal compatibility between core and veneer dental ceramics using shear bond strength test and contact angle measurement. Dent Mater 2010;26(8):743–50.

Benetti P, Kelly JR, Della Bona A. Analysis of thermal distributions in veneered zirconia and metal restorations during firing. Dent Mater 2013;29(11):1166–72.

Benetti P, Kelly JR, Sanchez M, Della Bona A. Influence of thermal gradients on stress state of veneered restorations. Dent Mater 2014;30(5):554–63.

Bonfante EA, Rafferty BT, Silva NRFA, Hanan JC, Rekow ED, Thompson VP, et al. Residual thermal stress simulation in three-dimensional molar crown systems: a finite element analysis. J Prosthodont 2012;21(7):529–34.

Borba M, De Araujo MD, De Lima E, Yoshimura HN, Cesar PF, Griggs JA, et al. Flexural strength and failure modes of layered ceramic structures. Dent Mater 2011;27(12):1259–66.

Bottino MA, Bergoli C, Lima EG, Marocho SM, Souza RO, Valandro LF. Bonding of Y-TZP to dentin: effects of Y-TZP surface conditioning, resin cement type, and aging. Oper Dent May–June 2014;39(3):291–300.

Braga RR, Ferracane JL. Alternatives in polymerization contraction stress management. Crit Rev Oral Biol Med 2004;15(3):176–84.

Braga RR, Meira JB, Boaro LC, Xavier TA. Adhesion to tooth structure: a critical review of "macro" test methods. Dent Mater 2010;26(2):e38–49.

Carvalho RM, Pereira JC, Yoshiyama M, Pashley DH. A review of polymerization contraction: the influence of stress development versus stress relief. Oper Dent 1996;21(1):17–24.

Casucci A, Osorio E, Osorio R, Monticelli F, Toledano M, Mazzitelli C, et al. Influence of different surface treatments on surface zirconia frameworks. J Dent 2009;37(11):891–7.

Cattell MJ, Chadwick TC, Knowles JC, Clarke RL. The development and testing of glaze materials for application to the fit surface of dental ceramic restorations. Dent Mater 2009;25(4):431–41.

Chai J, Chu FC, Chow TW. Effect of surface treatment on shear bond strength of zirconia to human dentin. J Prosthodont 2010;20(3):173–9.

Chang CW, Waddell JN, Lyons KM, Swain MV. Cracking of porcelain surfaces arising from abrasive grinding with a dental air turbine. J Prosthodont 2011;20(8):613–20.

Choi JE, Waddell JN, Swain MV. Pressed ceramics onto zirconia. Part 2: indentation fracture and influence of cooling rate on residual stresses. Dent Mater 2011;27(11):1111–8.

Christensen GJ. Porcelain-fused-to-metal versus zirconia-based ceramic restorations, 2009. J Am Dent Assoc 2009;140(8):1036–9.

Costa AK, Borges AL, Fleming GJ, Addison O. The strength of sintered and adhesively bonded zirconia/veneer-ceramic bilayers. J Dent 2014;42(10):1269–76.
De Groot R, Van Elst HC, Peters MC. Fracture-mechanics parameters of the composite-enamel bond. J Dent Res 1990;69(1):31–5.
De Munck J, Braem M, Wevers M, Yoshida Y, Inoue S, Suzuki K, et al. Micro-rotary fatigue of tooth-biomaterial interfaces. Biomaterials 2005;26(10):1145–53.
De Munck J, Luehrs AK, Poitevin A, Van Ende A, Van Meerbeek B. Fracture toughness versus micro-tensile bond strength testing of adhesive-dentin interfaces. Dent Mater 2013;29(6):635–44.
DeHoff PH, Anusavice KJ. Tempering stresses in feldspathic porcelain. J Dent Res 1989;68(2):134–8.
DeHoff PH, Anusavice KJ. Analysis of tempering stresses in bilayered porcelain discs. J Dent Res 1992;71(5):1139–44.
DeHoff PH, Anusavice KJ, Wang Z. Three-dimensional finite element analysis of the shear bond test. Dent Mater 1995;11(2):126–31.
Della Bona A, Van Noort R. Shear vs. tensile bond strength of resin composite bonded to ceramic. J Dent Res 1995;74(9):1591–6.
Derand T, Molin M, Kvam K. Bond strength of composite luting cement to zirconia ceramic surfaces. Dent Mater 2005;21(12):1158–62.
Dong XD, Ruse ND. Fatigue crack propagation path across the dentinoenamel junction complex in human teeth. J Biomed Mater Res A 2003;66(1):103–9.
Drummond JL, Sakaguchi RL, Racean DC, Wozny J, Steinberg AD. Testing mode and surface treatment effects on dentin bonding. J Biomed Mater Res 1996;32(4):533–41.
Durand JC, Jacquot B, Salehi H, Fages M, Margerit J, Cuisinier FJG. Confocal Raman microscopic analysis of the zirconia/feldspathic ceramic interface. Dent Mater 2012;28(6):661–71.
Erdem A, Akar G, Erdem A, Kose T. Effects of different surface treatments on bond strength between resin cements and zirconia ceramics. Oper Dent May–June 2014;39(3):E118–27.
Ernst CP, Cohnen U, Stender E, Willershausen B. In vitro retentive strength of zirconium oxide ceramic crowns using different luting agents. J Prosthet Dent 2005;93(6):551–8.
Everson P, Addison O, Palin WM, Burke FJ. Improved bonding of zirconia substructures to resin using a "glaze-on" technique. J Dent April 2012;40(4):347–51.
Fairhurst CW, Anusavice KJ, Ringle RD, Twiggs SW. Porcelain-metal thermal compatibility. J Dent Res 1981;60(4):815–9.
Far C, Ruse ND. Effect of bleaching on fracture toughness of composite-dentin bonds. J Adhes Dent 2003;5(3):175–82.
Ferracane JL, Dossett JM, Pelogia F, Macedo MRP, Hilton TJ. Navigating the dentin bond strength testing highway: lessons and recommendations. In: Adhesion aspects in dentistry. Leiden: Koninklijke Brill NV; 2009. p. 245–60.
Ferracane JL. Buonocore Lecture. Placing dental composites – a stressful experience. Oper Dent 2008;33(3):247–57.
Fischer H, Marx R. Fracture toughness of dental ceramics: comparison of bending and indentation method. Dent Mater 2002;18(1):12–9.
Fischer J, Stawarczyk B, Tomic M, Strub JR, Hammerle CH. Effect of thermal misfit between different veneering ceramics and zirconia frameworks on in vitro fracture load of single crowns. Dent Mater J 2007;26(6):766–72.
Fleming GJP, Addison O. Adhesive cementation and the strengthening of all-ceramic dental restorations. J Adhes Sci Technol 2009;23:945–59.
Fleming GJP, Narayan O. The effect of cement type and mixing on the bi-axial fracture strength of cemented aluminous core porcelain discs. Dent Mater 2003;19(1):69–76.

Fleming GJ, Maguire FR, Bhamra G, Burke FM, Marquis PM. The strengthening mechanism of resin cements on porcelain surfaces. J Dent Res 2006;85(3):272–6.

Fleming GJ, Hooi P, Addison O. The influence of resin flexural modulus on the magnitude of ceramic strengthening. Dent Mater 2012;28(7):769–76.

Foxton RM, Cavalcanti AN, Nakajima M, Pilecki P, Sherriff M, Melo L, et al. Durability of resin cement bond to aluminium oxide and zirconia ceramics after air abrasion and laser treatment. J Prosthodont 2011;20(2):84–92.

Frankenberger R, Strobel WO, Krämer N, Lohbauer U, Winterscheidt J, Winterscheidt B, et al. Evaluation of the fatigue behavior of the resin-dentin bond with the use of different methods. J Biomed Mater Res B Appl Biomater 2003;67(2):712–21.

Gallagher RR, Balooch M, Balooch G, Wilson RS, Marshall SJ, Marshall GW. Coupled nanomechanical and Raman microspectroscopic investigation of human third molar DEJ. J Dent Biomech 2010:1–7.

Gostemeyer G, Jendras M, Dittmer MP, Bach FW, Stiesch M, Kohorst P. Influence of cooling rate on zirconia/veneer interfacial adhesion. Acta Biomater 2010;6(12):4532–8.

Grigore A, Spallek S, Petschelt A, Butz B, Spiecker E, Lohbauer U. Microstructure of veneered zirconia after surface treatments: a TEM study. Dent Mater 2013;29(11):1098–107.

Guazzato M, Albakry M, Quach L, Swain MV. Influence of grinding, sandblasting, polishing and heat treatment on the flexural strength of a glass-infiltrated alumina-reinforced dental ceramic. Biomaterials 2004;25(11):2153–60.

Guazzato M, Quach L, Albakry M, Swain MV. Influence of surface and heat treatments on the flexural strength of Y-TZP dental ceramic. J Dent 2005;33(1):9–18.

Hashimoto M, Ohno H, Kaga M, Endo K, Sano H, Oguchi H. In vivo degradation of resin-dentin bonds in humans over 1 to 3 years. J Dent Res 2000;79(6):1385–91.

Hashimoto M, Ohno H, Kaga M, Endo K, Sano H, Oguchi H. Resin-tooth adhesive interfaces after long-term function. Am J Dent 2001;14(4):211–5.

Heintze SD, Rousson V. Survival of zirconia- and metal-supported fixed dental prostheses: a systematic review. Int J Prosthodont 2010;23(6):493–502.

Heintze SD, Thunpithayakul C, Armstrong SR, Rousson V. Correlation between microtensile bond strength data and clinical outcome of Class V restorations. Dent Mater 2011;27(2):114–25.

Heintze SD. Clinical relevance of tests on bond strength, microleakage and marginal adaptation. Dent Mater 2013;29(1):59–84.

Hosoya Y, Marshall GW. The nano-hardness and elastic modulus of sound deciduous canine dentin and young premolar dentin – preliminary study. J Mater Sci Mater Med 2005;16(1):1–8.

Hosoya Y. Hardness and elasticity of bonded carious and sound primary tooth dentin. J Dent 2006;34(2):164–71.

Hu J, Dai N, Bao Y, Gu W, Ma J, Zhang F. Effect of different coping designs on all-ceramic crown stress distribution: a finite element analysis. Dent Mater 2013;29(11):e291–298.

Inokoshi M, De Munck J, Minakuchi S, Van Meerbeek B. Meta-analysis of bonding effectiveness to zirconia ceramics. J Dent Res April 2014;93(4):329–34.

Inokoshi M, Vanmeensel K, Zhang F, De Munck J, Eliades G, Minakuchi S, et al. Aging resistance of surface-treated dental zirconia. Dent Mater February 2015;31(2):182–94.

Isgro G, Wang H, Kleverlaan CJ, Feilzer AJ. The effects of thermal mismatch and fabrication procedures on the deflection of layered all-ceramic discs. Dent Mater 2005;21(7):649–55.

ISO 9693-1. Dentistry: compatibility testing – part 1: metal-ceramic systems. 2012.

ISO/DIS 9693-2. Dentistry: compatibility testing – part 2: ceramic-ceramic systems. 2014.

Jakubowicz-Kohen BD, Sadoun MJ, Douillard T, Mainjot AK. Influence of firing time and framework thickness on veneered Y-TZP discs curvature. Dent Mater 2014;30(2):242–8.
Katte H. Imaging measurements of stress birefringence in optical materials and components. Photonik Int 2009;1:39–41.
Kelly JR, Benetti P, Rungruanganunt P, Bona AD. The slippery slope: critical perspectives on in vitro research methodologies. Dent Mater 2012;28(1):41–51.
Kelly JR. Clinically relevant approach to failure testing of all-ceramic restorations. J Prosthet Dent 1999;81(8):652–61.
Kern M, Sasse M. Ten-year survival of anterior all-ceramic resin-bonded fixed dental prostheses. J Adhes Dent 2011;13:407–10.
Kern M, Wegner SM. Bonding to zirconia ceramic: adhesion methods and their durability. Dent Mater 1998;14(1):64–71.
Kern M, Barloi A, Yang B. Surface conditioning influences zirconia ceramic bonding. J Dent Res 2009;88(9):817–22.
Kern M. Bonding to oxide ceramics – laboratory versus clinical outcome. Dent Mater 2015;31(1):8–14.
Kim JW, Covel NS, Guess PC, Rekow ED, Zhang Y. Concerns of hydrothermal degradation in CAD/CAM zirconia. J Dent Res 2010;89(1):91–5.
Kim JW, Kim JH, Janal MN, Zhang Y. Damage maps of veneered zirconia under simulated mastication. J Dent Res 2008;87(12):1127–32.
King Jr BW, Andrews AI. Solubility of zirconia in soda-borosilicate glasses. J Am Ceram Soc 1941;24(11):367–72.
Kohorst P, Borchers L, Strempel J, Stiesch M, Hassel T, Bach FW, et al. Low-temperature degradation of different zirconia ceramics for dental applications. Acta Biomater 2012;8(3):1213–20.
Kosmac T, Oblak C, Jevnikar P, Funduk N, Marion L. The effect of surface grinding and sandblasting on flexural strength and reliability of Y TZP zirconia ceramic. Dent Mater November 1999;15(6):426–33.
Krämer N, Taschner M, Lohbauer U, Petschelt A, Frankenberger R. Totally bonded ceramic inlays and onlays after eight years. J Adhes Dent 2008;10(4):307–14.
Kurbad A. Digital veneering – manufacturing computer-generated veneers with the CAD-on technique. Int J Comput Dent 2011;14(3):255–71.
Kvam K. Fracture toughness determination of ceramic and resin-based dental composites. Biomaterials 1992;13(2):101–4.
Lenz J, Kessel S. Thermal stresses in metal-ceramic-specimens for the ISO crack initiation test (three-point flexure bond test). Dent Mater 1998;14(4):277–80.
Lohbauer U, Belli R, Ferracane JL. Factors involved in mechanical fatigue degradation of dental resin composites. J Dent Res 2013;92(7):584–91.
Lu H, Stansbury JW, Bowman CN. Towards the elucidation of shrinkage stress development and relaxation in dental composites. Dent Mater 2004;20(10):979–86.
Lussi A. Dental erosion – from diagnosis to therapy. 1st ed. Basel: Karger; 2006.
Mainjot AK, Schajer GS, Vanheusden AJ, Sadoun MJ. Residual stress measurements in veneering ceramic by hole-drilling. Dent Mater 2011;27(5):439–44.
Malament KA, Socransky SS. Survival of Dicor glass-ceramic dental restoratives over 14 years. Part I. Survival of Dicor complete coverage restorations and effect of internal surface acid etching, tooth position, gender and age. J Prosthet Dent 1999a;81(1):23–32.
Malament KA, Socransky SS. Survival of Dicor glass-ceramic dental restoratives over 14 years. Part II. Effect of thickness of Dicor material and design on tooth preparation. J Prosthet Dent 1999b;81(6):662–7.

Mantri SP, Mantri SS. Management of shrinkage stresses in direct restorative light-cured composites: a review. J Esthet Restor Dent 2013;25(5):305–13.

Marquis PM. The influence of cements on the mechanical performance of dental ceramics. Bioceramics 1992;5:317–24.

Marshall DB, Lawn BR. An indentation technique for measuring stresses in tempered glass surfaces. J Am Ceram Soc 1977;60(1–2):86–7.

Marshall DB, Lawn BR. Measurement of nonuniform distribution of residual stress in tempered glass. Glass Technol 1978;19(3):57–8.

Mastelaro VR, Zanotto ED. Residual stresses in a soda-lime-silica glass-ceramic. J Non-Cryst Solids 1996;194(3):297–304.

Matinlinna JP, Heikkinen T, Ozcan M, Lassila LV, Vallittu PK. Evaluation of resin adhesion to zirconia ceramic using some organosilanes. Dent Mater 2006;22(9):824–83.

May LG, Kelly JR, Bottino MA, Hill T. Effects of cement thickness and bonding on the failure loads of CAD/CAM ceramic crowns: multi-physics FEA modeling and monotonic testing. Dent Mater 2012;28(8):e99–109.

Meira JB, Reis BR, Tanaka CB, Ballester RJ, Cesar PF, Versluis A, et al. Residual stresses in Y-TZP crowns due to change in the thermal contraction coefficient of veneers. Dent Mater 2013;29(5):594–601.

Mirmohammadi H, Aboushelib MN, Kleverlaan CJ, Ager N, Feilzer AJ. The influence of rotating fatigue on the bond strength of zirconia-composite interfaces. Dent Mater 2010;26(7):627–33.

Mitov G, Gessner J, Lohbauer U, Woll K, Muecklich F, Pospiech P. Subcritical crack growth behavior and life data analysis of two types of dental Y-TZP ceramics. Dent Mater July 2011;27(7):684–91.

Molin MK, Karlsson SL. Five-year clinical prospective evaluation of zirconia-based Denzir 3-unit FPDs. Int J Prosthodont 2008;21(3):223–7.

Mutluay MM, Yahyazadehfar M, Ryou H, Majd H, Do D, Arola D. Fatigue of the resin-dentin interface: a new approach for evaluating the durability of dentin bonds. Dent Mater 2013;29(4):437–49.

Nathanson D. In: Gaber DA, Goldstein RE, editors. Porcelain and composite inlays and onlays: esthetic posterior restorations. Chicago, IL, USA: Quintessence; 1993. p. 23–32.

Nishide A, Yamamoto T, Momoi Y, Swain MV. Cracks formed by Vickers indentation adjacent to the interface in bonded dental ceramics with various marginal angles. Dent Mater J 2011;30(3):308–14.

Oh WS, Delong R, Anusavice KJ. Factors affecting enamel and ceramic wear: a literature review. J Prosthet Dent 2002;87(4):451–9.

Okuda M, Pereira PN, Nakajima M, Tagami J, Pashley DH. Long-term durability of resin dentin interface: nanoleakage vs. microtensile bond strength. Oper Dent 2002;27(3):289–96.

Oliveira-Ogliari A, Collares FM, Feitosa VP, Sauro S, Ogliari FA, Moraes RR. Methacrylate bonding to zirconia by in situ silica nanoparticle surface deposition. Dent Mater January 2015;31(1):68–76.

Ozcan M, Bernasconi M. Adhesion to zirconia used for dental restorations: a systematic review and meta-analysis. J Adhes Dent 2015;17(1):7–26.

Ozcan M, Melo RM, Souza RO, Machado JP, Felipe Valandro L, Botttino MA. Effect of air-particle abrasion protocols on the biaxial flexural strength, surface characteristics and phase transformation of zirconia after cyclic loading. J Mech Behav Biomed Mater April 2013a;20:19–28.

Ozcan M, Raadschelders J, Vallittu P, Lassilla L. Effect of particle deposition parameters on silica coating of zirconia using a chairside air-abrasion device. J Adhes Dent June 2013b;15(3):211–4.

Pashley DH, Carvalho RM, Sano H, Nakajima M, Yoshiyama M, Shono Y, et al. The microtensile bond test: a review. J Adhes Dent 1999;1(4):299–309.

Peitl O, Serbena FC, Mastelaro VR, Zanotto ED. Internal residual stress measurements in a bioactive glass-ceramic using Vickers indentation. J Am Ceram Soc 2010;93(8):2359–68.

Pereira Lde L, Campos F, Dal Piva AM, Gondim LD, Souza RO, Özcan M. Can application of universal primers alone be a substitute for airborne-particle abrasion to improve adhesion of resin cement to zirconia? J Adhes Dent April 2015;17(2):169–74.

Piascik JR, Swift EJ, Thompson JY, Grego S, Stoner BR. Surface modification for enhanced silanation of zirconia ceramics. Dent Mater 2009;25(9):1116–21.

Piascik JR, Wolter SD, Stoner BR. Development of a novel surface modification for improved bonding to zirconia. Dent Mater 2011;27(5):e99–105.

Pinzon LM, Watanabe LG, Reis AF, Powers JM, Marshall SJ, Marshall GW. Analysis of interfacial structure and bond strength of self-etch adhesives. Am J Dent 2013;26(6):335–40.

Quinn JB, Quinn GD, Kelly JR, Scherrer SS. Fractographic analyses of three ceramic whole crown restoration failures. Dent Mater 2005;21(10):920–9.

Raigrodski AJ, Chiche GJ, Potiket N, Hochstedler JL, Mohamed SE, Billiot S, et al. The efficacy of posterior three-unit zirconium-oxide-based ceramic fixed partial dental prostheses: a prospective clinical pilot study. J Prosthet Dent 2006;96(4):237–44.

Raigrodski AJ, Hillstead MB, Meng GK, Chung KH. Survival and complications of zirconia-based fixed dental prostheses: a systematic review. J Prosthet Dent 2012;107(3):170–7.

Ramos A, Gandais M. Earliest stages of crystal growth in a silicate glass containing titanium and zirconium as nucleating elements – HRTEM and XAS study. J Cryst Growth 1990;100(3):471–80.

Ryou H, Pashley DH, Tay FR, Arola D. A characterization of the mechanical behavior of resin-infiltrated dentin using nanoscopic Dynamic Mechanical Analysis. Dent Mater 2013;29(7):719–28.

Sailer I, Hämmerle CH. Zirconia ceramic single-retainer resin-bonded fixed dental prostheses (RBFDPs) after 4 years of clinical service: a retrospective clinical and volumetric study. Int J Periodontics Rest Dent 2014;34(3):333–43.

Sailer I, Makarov NA, Thoma DS, Zwahlen M, Pjetursson BE. All-ceramic or metal-ceramic tooth-supported fixed dental prostheses (FDPs)? A systematic review of the survival and complication rates. Part I: single crowns (SCs). Dent Mater 2015;31(6):603–23.

Şanli S, Çömlekoğlu MD, Çömlekoğlu E, Sonugelen M, Pamir T, Darvell BW. Influence of surface treatment on the resin-bonding of zirconia. Dent Mater June 2015;31(6):657–68.

Sano H, Shono T, Sonoda H, Takatsu T, Ciucchi B, Carvalho R, et al. Relationship between surface area for adhesion and tensile bond strength – evaluation of a micro-tensile bond test. Dent Mater 1994;10(4):236–40.

Sasse M, Eschbach S, Kern M. Randomized clinical trial on single retainer all-ceramic resin-bonded fixed partial dentures: influence of the bonding system after up to 55 months. J Dent 2012;40(9):783–6.

Sato H, Yamada K, Pezzotti G, Nawa M, Ban S. Mechanical properties of dental zirconia ceramics changed with sandblasting and heat treatment. Dent Mater 2008;27(3):408–14.

Sax C, Hammerle CH, Sailer I. 10-year clinical outcomes of fixed dental prostheses with zirconia frameworks. Int J Comput Dent 2011;14(3):183–202.

Scherrer SS, Quinn JB, Quinn GD, Kelly JR. Failure analysis of ceramic clinical cases using qualitative fractography. Int J Prosthodont 2006;19(2):185–92.

Scherrer SS, Cesar PF, Swain MV. Direct comparison of the bond strength results of the different test methods: a critical literature review. Dent Mater 2010;26(2):e78–93.

Scherrer SS, Cattani-Lorente M, Vittecoq E, De Mestral F, Griggs JA, Wiskott HW. Fatigue behavior in water of Y-TZP zirconia ceramics after abrasion with 30 μm silica-coated alumina particles. Dent Mater February 2011;27(2):e28–42.

Schneider GA, Swain MV. The Schwickerath adhesion test: a fracture mechanics analysis. Dent Mater 2015;31(8):986–91.

Sindel J. Randzonenschädigung von CAD/CAM-bearbeiteten Dentalkeramiken. [Dissertation]. Germany: University of Erlangen; 1998. ISBN: 3000031073.

Soderholm KJ. Review of the fracture toughness approach. Dent Mater 2010;26(2):e63–77.

Song JY, Park SW, Lee K, Yun KD, Lim HP. Fracture strength and microstructure of Y-TZP zirconia after different surface treatments. J Prosthet Dent October 2013;110(4):274–80.

Souza RO, Valandro LF, Melo RM, Machado JP, Bottino MA, Ozcan M. Air-particle abrasion on zirconia ceramic using different protocols: effects on biaxial flexural strength after cyclic loading, phase transformation and surface topography. J Mech Behav Biomed Mater October 2013;26:155–63.

Staninec M, Kim P, Marshall GW, Ritchie RO, Marshall SJ. Fatigue of dentin-composite interfaces with four-point bend. Dent Mater 2008;24(6):799–803.

Stansbury JW, Trujillo-Lemon M, Lu H, Ding X, Lin Y, Ge J. Conversion-dependent shrinkage stress and strain in dental resins and composites. Dent Mater 2005;21(1):56–67.

Sudsangiam S, Van Noort R. Do dentin bond strength tests serve a useful purpose? J Adhes Dent 1999;1(1):57–67.

Swain M. Unstable cracking (chipping) of veneering porcelain on all-ceramic dental crowns and fixed partial dentures. Acta Biomater 2009;5(5):1668–77.

Takahashi K, Mochida N, Yoshida Y. Properties and structure of silicate glasses containing tetravalent cations. J Ceram Soc Japan 1977;85(7):26–36.

Tam LE, Pilliar RM. Fracture toughness of dentin/resin-composite adhesive interfaces. J Dent Res 1993;72(5):953–9.

Tam LE, Pilliar RM. Fracture surface characterization of dentin-bonded interfacial fracture toughness specimens. J Dent Res 1994;73(3):607–19.

Tantbirojn D, Cheng YS, Versluis A, Hodges JS, Douglas WH. Nominal shear or fracture mechanics in the assessment of composite-dentin adhesion? J Dent Res 2000;79(1):41–8.

Taskonak B, Mecholsky Jr JJ, Anusavice KJ. Residual stresses in bilayer dental ceramics. Biomaterials 2005;26(16):3235–41.

Taskonak B, Borges G, Mecholsky Jr JJ, Anusavice K, Moore B, Yan J. The effects of viscoelastic parameters on residual stress development in a zirconia/glass bilayer dental ceramic. Dent Mater 2008;24(9):1149–55.

Taylor JR, Bull AC. Ceramic glaze technology. Oxford: Pergamon Press; 1986.

Tholey MJ, Swain MV, Thiel N. SEM observations of porcelain Y-TZP interface. Dent Mater 2009;25(7):857–62.

Tholey MJ, Swain MV, Thiel N. Thermal gradients and residual stresses in veneered Y-TZP frameworks. Dent Mater 2011;27(11):1102–10.

Thompson JY, Stoner BR, Piascik JR, Smith R. Adhesion/cementation to zirconia and other non-silicate ceramics: where are we now? Dent Mater 2011;27(1):71–82.

Tsuo Y, Yoshida K, Atsuta M. Effects of alumina-blasting and adhesive primers on bonding between resin luting agent and zirconia ceramics. Dent Mater 2006;25(4):669–74.

Turssi CP, Ferracane JL, Ferracane LL. Wear and fatigue behavior of nano-structured dental resin composites. J Biomed Mater Res B Appl Biomater 2006;78(1):196–203.

Valandro LF, Özcan M, Amaral R, Vanderlei A, Bottino MA. Effect of testing methods on the bond strength of resin to zirconia-alumina ceramic: microtensile versus shear test. Dent Mater 2008;27(6):849–55.

Van Meerbeek B, Willems G, Celis JP, Roos JR, Braem M, Lambrechts P, et al. Assessment by nano-indentation of the hardness and elasticity of the resin-dentin bonding area. J Dent Res 1993;72(10):1434–42.
Van Noort R, Noroozi S, Howard IC, Cardew G. A critique of bond strength measurements. J Dent 1989;17(2):61–7.
Van Noort R, Cardew GE, Howard IC, Noroozi S. The effect of local interfacial geometry on the measurement of the tensile bond strength to dentin. J Dent Res 1991;70(5):889–93.
Versluis A, Tantbirojn D, Douglas WH. Why do shear bond tests pull out dentin? J Dent Res 1997;76(6):1298–307.
Walshaw PR, Tam LE, Mccomb D. Bond failure at dentin-composite interfaces with 'single-bottle' adhesives. J Dent 2003;31(2):117–25.
Wang FH, Hand RJ, Ellis B, Seddon AB. Glass strengthening using epoxy coatings. Phys Chem Glass 1995;36:201–5.
Wataha JC. Alloys for prosthodontics restorations. J Prosthet Dent 2002;87(4):351–63.
Wendler M, Belli R, Petschelt A, Lohbauer U. Characterization of residual stresses in zirconia veneered bilayers assessed via sharp and blunt indentation. Dent Mater 2015;31(8):948–57.
Wolfart M, Lehmann F, Wolfart S, Kern M. Durability of the resin bond strength to zirconia ceramic after using different surface conditioning methods. Dent Mater 2007;23(1):45–50.
Yahyazadehfar M, Mutluay MM, Majd H, Ryou H, Arola D. Fatigue of the resin-enamel bonded interface and the mechanisms of failure. J Mech Behav Biomed Mater 2013;21:121–32.
Yahyazadehfar M, Ivancik J, Majd H, An B, Zhang D, Arola D. On the mechanics of fatigue and fracture in teeth. Appl Mech Rev 2014;66(3):0308031–3080319.
Zeng K, Rowcliffe D. Experimental measurement of residual stress field around sharp indentation in glass. J Am Ceram Soc 1994;77(2):524–30.
Zhang Y, Lawn BR, Malament K, Thompson VP, Rekow ED. Damage accumulation and fatigue life of particle-abraded ceramics. Int J Prosthodont 2006;19(5):442–8.
Zhang Z, Guazzato M, Sornsuwan T, Scherrer S, Rungsiyakull C, Li W, et al. Thermally induced fracture for core-veneered dental ceramic structures. Acta Biomater 2013;9(9):8394–402.

Understanding the chemistry and improving the durability of dental resin–dentin bonded interface

6

F. Li[1,2], *L. Zhang*[1,2], *M.D. Weir*[2], *L. Cheng*[2,3], *K. Zhang*[2,4], *H.H.K. Xu*[2]
[1]Fourth Military Medical University, Xian, China; [2]University of Maryland, Baltimore, MD, United States; [3]Sichuan University, Chengdu, China; [4]Capital Medical University, Beijing, China

6.1 Introduction

Resin composites and adhesives are increasingly used in dental restorations due to their esthetics and direct-filling capabilities (Ferracane, 2011; Peumans et al., 2005; Sakaguchi, 2005). The restoration–tooth structure bond, or the resin–tooth interface, is the weak link whose failure is the main reason for the failure of the restoration. Replacing the failed dental restorations accounts for 50–70% of all operative work. Therefore, a stronger and durable adhesion to tooth structure, especially to dentin, is a key factor of restoration longevity (Breschi et al., 2008; Spencer et al., 2010). It is important to understand the mechanism of dentin–resin bonding and the limitation for bond durability, and further to know the strategies for improving the stability of dentin–resin bonded interface.

6.2 Mechanisms of dentin–resin bonding

To produce a dentin surface suitable for bonding to resin, the dentin surface needs to be prepared to remove the carious-infected or stained tissues. After tooth cavity preparation, the dentin surface is covered with a 0.5- to 2-μm-thick "smear layer" of residual organic and inorganic debris (Eick, 1992). According to the different treatments with smear layer, current dental adhesives are classified into two major types:

1. Etch-and-rinse (or total-etch) adhesives: Etch-and-rinse adhesives are characterized by an initial etching step, followed by a compulsory rinsing procedure, which is responsible for the complete removal of the smear layer and smear plugs. In the bonding step, the adhesive resin is applied on the prepared surface, leading to the penetration of hydrophobic monomers not only into the interfibrilar spaces of the collagen network but also into the dentine tubules. After infiltration, these adhesive monomers are polymerized to form the hybrid layer (HL), which in combination with the presence of resin tags inside dentine tubules provides micromechanical retention to the composite restoration. According to

Material-Tissue Interfacial Phenomena. http://dx.doi.org/10.1016/B978-0-08-100330-5.00006-6

the bonding procedure, the etch-and-rinse adhesive can be classified into two subtypes: three-step etch-and-rinse adhesives (acid + primer + bonding) and; two-step etch-and-rinse adhesives (acid + primer and bonding).

2. Self-etch adhesives: They include an acidic monomer that simultaneously demineralizes and penetrates into the dentin surface, making the smear layer permeable without removing it completely. Different from their etch-and-rinse counterparts, self-etch adhesives do not require a separate etching step. The self-etch adhesives can be classified into two subtypes: two-step self-etch adhesives (acidic primer + bonding) and one-step self-etch adhesives (all in one).

After partial removal of the mineral phase from the dentin substrate using an etching agent or an acidic monomer, the adhesive monomers penetrate into the spaces in the demineralized dentin substrate and form a zone after polymerization of the adhesive. This zone is called "hybrid layer" or "resin-infiltrated layer" (Perdigao, 2010). The penetrating ability of adhesive resin, the permeability of dentin substrate, as well as the resin polymerization properties affect the HL and thus the resin–dentin bonding (Perdigao, 2010; Spencer et al., 2010). The resin monomers infiltrate into the dentin tubules to form resin tags. The thickness of the HL and the length of resin tags depend on the aggressiveness of the etching agent or the acidic monomer (Eliades et al., 2005; McCabe and Walls, 2008; Nakabayashi and Pashley, 1998). The HL for total-etch adhesives is about 5 μm thick, whereas for mild or moderate self-etch adhesives, it is approximately 0.5–1.5 μm thick and the resin tags are shorter. However, the thickness of the HL and the length of resin tags have no effect on the resin–dentin bonding strength (Nakabayashi and Pashley, 1998). In addition to the HL, chemical bonding between the adhesive and the mineral and protein components in dentin also contributes to the adhesive–dentin bond (Stangel et al., 2007). Organic compounds that can bond to the ions in apatite of dentin include (1) phosphate-based adhesives, (2) amino acid– or amino alcohol–based adhesives, and (3) adhesives based on dicarboxylates. Monomers that contain hydroxyl, carboxyl, amino, and amido groups can potentially react with the bonding sites inherent to collagen. These reactions involved transesterification, secondary amide formation, or possibly hydrogen bonding. Therefore, several mechanisms of adhesion including HL and chemical bond formation can operate simultaneously and synergistically in forming the bonds to dentin.

6.3 Factors that compromise the durability of dentin–resin bond

As the most common alternative to dental amalgam, composites are increasingly being used because of their esthetics and improved performance (Ferracane, 2011; Peumans et al., 2005; Sakaguchi, 2005). However, secondary (recurrent) caries at the tooth–restoration margins is a frequent reason for the failure of composite restorations (Spencer et al., 2014). According to the minimally invasive treatment concept (Mount and Ngo, 2000), more dentin tissues are recommended to be preserved, which is accompanied by a certain amount of caries-infected and caries-affected dentin with residual bacteria in the prepared cavity. Compared with other restorative materials such as amalgams and ceramics, composites tend to accumulate more biofilms/plaques (Beyth et al., 2007). Poor marginal adaptation, marginal discoloration, and loss of retention of composite restorations were reported when the resin—dentin interface is exposed to the oral environment and under the challenge of chemical and mechanical stresses (Spencer et al., 2010, 2014). The loss of marginal seal leads to microleakage along the bonded interface, which can provide pathways for the invading bacteria from the oral environment (Delaviz et al., 2014; Fruits et al., 2006). Bacterial growth and biofilm formation can produce acids to destroy the resin–dentin interfaces and result in failure of the bonded restorations.

Current adhesive materials and techniques have been improved yielding good immediate and short-term bonding effectiveness (Inoue et al., 2001). However, the long-term durability and stability of the resin–dentin bond still remain questionable (Carvalho et al., 2012; Liu et al., 2011c; Spencer et al., 2010). In fact, a 2005 review highlighted that the immediate dentin bond strength values did not correlate with long-term bond stability (De Munck et al., 2005). The degradation of the adhesive interface may occur in a relatively short time, even in the absence of detectable gaps and bacteria on the bonded interfaces (Breschi et al., 2008). For almost all of the contemporary adhesives, including both etch-and-rinse and self-etch adhesive systems, substantial degradation of the resin-dentin bond over time was detected (Breschi et al., 2008; Carvalho et al., 2012; De Munck et al., 2005; Liu et al., 2011c). In the etch-and-rinse strategy, after the preliminary etching to dentin, bonding monomers impregnated the porous etched substrate (Nakabayashi and Pashley, 1998). Thus stable bonds could be achieved if the etched substrate was fully infiltrated by the adhesive to avoid different degrees of incomplete impregnation. However, discrepancies between the depth of dentin demineralization and adhesive infiltration were reported with an unprotected demineralized zone or "defection zone" at the bottom of the HL (Pashley et al., 2011). In the self-etch strategy, adhesive stability was related to the effective coupling of the comonomers with the infiltrated substrate since acidic comonomers simultaneously demineralize and infiltrate dentin. For strong self-etch adhesives with a pH of around 1, the interfaces were similar to etch-and-rinse systems with incompletely infiltrated defection zone at the bottom of the HL. For mild self-etch adhesives, high percentages of hydrophilic monomers were used to facilitate infiltration and thus to increase the degree of permeability of adhesive. This resulted in nanoleakage expression and impaired the quality and stability of the HL (Van Meerbeek et al., 2011). Generally, the more simple an adhesive is, the less stable the adhesive–dentin interface. Overall, the bond durability of contemporary dentin adhesives is listed here in decreasing order: two-step self-etch (mild and moderately aggressive) > three-step etch-and-rinse > two-step self-etch (aggressive) > two-step etch-and-rinse > one-step self-etch (Van Meerbeek et al., 2010). The better durability of the mild two-step self-etch adhesives may be attributed to the use of a separate, relatively more hydrophobic resin layer on top of the hydrophilic self-etch primer, which renders the interface less susceptible to water sorption. Moreover, the mild self-etch primer can only partially dissolve the apatite minerals and the hydroxyapatite crystallites on collagen fibers can protect collagen against degradation.

HL is the hybridization of collagen matrix, residual hydroxyapatite crystallites, and resin. HL degradation has been attributed to several factors. These include the heterogeneity of the structure and composition of dentin, the dentin surface characteristics after bur cutting and chemical treatments, the bond strategy and physicochemical properties of the adhesives, and other variables (Breschi et al., 2008; Pashley et al., 2011; Van Meerbeek et al., 2011). Both physical and biochemical factors, including the occlusal forces, the repetitive expansion, and contraction stresses from temperature changes, dentinal fluids, saliva, acidic attacks from food and cariogenic bacteria, and proteases, continuously challenge the HL and accelerate the degradation of HL. Indeed, it is now accepted that hydrolytic degradation of adhesive resin by water sorption, as well as collagenolysis by endogenous matrix metalloproteinases (MMPs) and cysteine cathepsins, are the main factors that degrade the stability and durability of the HL and the resin–dentin bond (Breschi et al., 2008; Carvalho et al., 2012; De Munck et al., 2005; Liu et al., 2011c; Pashley et al., 2011; Van Meerbeek et al., 2011).

Hydrolytic degradation of adhesive resin involves hydrolysis and leaching of the adhesive that has infiltrated the collagen matrix. The incomplete removal of water from the demineralized dentin or hydrophilic bonding agent results in the trapping of water within the adhesive, which affects the polymerization. Incomplete polymerization of the adhesive resin is the main reason for the elution of resin monomer. The elusion can be facilitated by water ingress into the loosely cross-linked or hydrophilic domains of the adhesive (Parthasarathy et al., 2012). Hydrolysis is a chemical process that breaks the covalent bonds between the polymers by the addition of water to the ester bonds. To facilitate the adhesive infiltration, after acid etching, water-wet bonding technique was applied to keep the collagen loose and expanded (Kanca, 1992). The contents of hydrophilic and ionic monomers were accordingly increased to improve the wetting ability and compatibility of adhesives to the moist, acid-etched dentin surfaces (Van Landuyt et al., 2007); 2-hydroxyethyl methacrylate (HEMA) was incorporated into many dentin adhesives to improve their hydrophilicity and reduce phase separation of these monomers (Spencer and Wang, 2002; Van Landuyt et al., 2007). However, these hydrophilic monomers could hamper water evaporation from the adhesive and increase the water permeability of the HL (Liu et al., 2011c). This could then accelerate the hydrolysis of methacrylate ester bonds. It was demonstrated that the hydrolysis of adhesive resin was promoted by the increase in acidity of the monomer components (Aida et al., 2009) or by the esterase activity from saliva and from oral bacteria (Shokati et al., 2010).

The ideal HL should be an adhesive–dentin interface with the etched substrate being fully infused and reinforced by the polymer. However, deficient resin infiltration, nanoleakeage due to residual water within polymerized adhesive resin, and degradation of adhesive during aging were all detected in adhesive–dentin interfaces. As a result, collagen was exposed in the HL (Breschi et al., 2008; Carvalho et al., 2012; De Munck et al., 2005; Liu et al., 2011c; Pashley et al., 2011; Van Meerbeek et al., 2011). Unprotected and denuded collagen fibrils could be degraded by the host-derived proteases, which would produce voids in the HL and promote the degradation of the adhesive–dentin bond. MMPs and cysteine cathepsins are the major endogenous proteases that were reported to play an important role in collagen degradation. MMPs are a family of Ca/Zn-dependent endopeptidases that degrade a variety of extracellular matrices. MMP-1 and MMP-8 (collagenases), MMP-2 and MMP-9 (gelatinases), as well as MMP-3 (matrilysin) and MMP-20 have already been detected in human sound dentin (Boukpessi et al., 2008; Mazzoni et al., 2007; Sulkala et al., 2007; Van Strijp et al., 2003). These MMPs are secreted by odontoblasts during dentinogenesis and enwrapped in mineralized dentin in an inactive and latent form. Dentinal MMP-2, MMP-8, MMP-9, and MMP-20 (van Strijp et al., 2003) were reported to participate in the degradation of resin–dentin bonds both in vivo and in vitro (Boukpessi et al., 2008; Sulkala et al., 2007). MMPs may be exposed by dentin etching and then activated by the low-pH environment, thermal changes, and mechanical stresses during bonding application and aging process (Chaussain-Miller et al., 2006; Mazzoni et al., 2006). Among these possible factors that may activate the latent form of MMPs (pro-MMPs), the mechanism of low-pH environment was studied the most. The acidic resin monomers incorporated into either etch-and-rinse or self-etch adhesives were shown to increase the collagenolytic and gelatinolytic activities of completely or partially demineralized collagen matrices (Mazzoni et al., 2006, 2013; 2015). These acidic resins produced a low-pH environment and activated latent forms of MMPs (pro-MMPs) via the cysteine-switch mechanism, which exposed the catalytic domains of these enzymes that were blocked by propeptides (Mazzoni et al., 2013). Mildly acidic resin monomers could also activate MMPs by inhibiting tissue inhibitor of metalloproteinases-1 (TIMP-1) (Ishiguro et al., 1994) in TIMP–MMP complexes, therefore producing active MMPs (Sulkala et al., 2001). In addition, the acidic monomer in self-etch adhesive was shown to increase MMP-2 expression in human dentin–pulp complex (Lehmann et al., 2009), possibly increasing MMP-2 penetration into the HL via dentinal fluid. Cysteine cathepsins were the other important proteases that were expressed by mature human odontoblasts and were present in intact dentin (Tersariol et al., 2010). The low-pH environment induced by adhesives also provided excellent conditions for the activation of dentin cysteine cathepsins. Acid activation of dentin-bound cathepsins may further result in activation of matrix-bound MMPs (Cox et al., 2006). Therefore, during the application of acidic monomers, not only MMPs but also cysteine cathepsins were activated and were likely involved in the degradation of HL over time (Tersariol et al., 2010). Therefore, to ensure the longevity of the tooth cavity restoration, the dentin–resin bond durability needs to be improved.

6.4 Strategies to improve the dentin–resin bond durability

6.4.1 Modification of hybrid layer with antibacterial bonding system

Bacterial invasion and the consequent caries development are the microbial factors for dentin–resin bond failure. To deal with this issue, the modification of HL with antibacterial bonding system has been extensively studied. Half of all dental restorations fail within 10 years, with secondary caries as a primary reason (Mjor and Toffenetti, 2000; Sakaguchi, 2005). Composites are bonded in cavities via adhesives (Ferracane et al., 2010; Pashley et al., 2011; Spencer et al., 2010). Residual bacteria could exist in the prepared cavity, and microleakage could allow new bacteria to invade the tooth–restoration interfaces. To address these challenges, attempts were made to render the primer and adhesive antibacterial; this approach was intended to inhibit bacteria and the associated demineralization that occurred as a result of acid produced by the bacteria (Cheng et al., 2012b; Imazato et al., 1998a, 2003; Li et al., 2009b). Since quaternary ammonium methacrylates (QAMs) can be covalently bonded with the polymer matrix, QAMs have been introduced to develop antibacterial dental adhesive systems. Extensive studies reported the incorporation of methacryloyloxydodecyl pyridinium bromide (MDPB) in dental adhesive systems with long-lasting antibacterial activity, without releasing the antibacterial agent or compromising the bonding efficiency (Imazato et al., 2003b, 2004; 2007).

Quaternary ammonium compounds (QACs) are a group of cationic antimicrobials widely used for numerous industrial and pharmaceutical purposes (Buffet-Bataillon et al., 2012). In 1994, to develop antibacterial dental resin without agent release, Imazato et al. combined alkylpyridinium, a QAC, with a methacrylate group, and successfully synthesized MDPB (Imazato et al., 1994). The QAC group is responsible for the antibacterial activity of MDPB, whereas the methacrylate group allows for copolymerization with other conventional dental monomers to provide antibacterial effect without leaching out or being lost over time (Imazato et al., 1994).

Besides MDPB, several other QAMs were also developed for use in resinous dental materials. Methacryloxylethyl cetyl dimethyl ammonium chloride (DMAE-CB) was synthesized by Chen et al., providing a commercial etch-and-rinse adhesive with stable antibacterial activities that did not damage the bonding capacity (Li et al., 2009a,b). QAMs with two methacrylate groups [2-methacryloxylethyl dodecyl methyl ammonium bromide (MAE-DB) and quaternary ammonium dimethacrylate (QADM)] were synthesized to enhance the polymerization capacity (Cheng et al., 2012b; Huang et al., 2011, 2012). Recently, a series of QAMs were synthesized with different side chain lengths (CLs) for antibacterial modifications of dentin adhesives and composites (Cheng et al., 2012b; Li et al., 2013c, 2014b). Antibacterial resins greatly reduced biofilm growth and acid production, potentially exerting a protection on the restoration and the margins against recurrent caries (Cheng et al., 2012b; Li et al., 2013c, 2014b). Indeed, the dentin bond strength of a commercial bonding agent was decreased by about one-third after water-aging for 6 months, whereas the new antibacterial bonding agents yielded dentin bond strengths at 6 months that were nearly the same as those at 1 d (Fig. 6.1(a)) (Zhang et al., 2013a).

6.4.1.1 Antibacterial effects

Antibacterial bonding agents were first prepared by incorporating MDPB into the primer of commercial self-etching adhesive Liner Bond 2 (Imazato et al., 1997). Since then, the antibacterial activity of this prototype was confirmed by a number of in vitro studies (Imazato et al., 1997, 2001). Based on these studies, Clearfil Protect Bond, employing a 5% MDPB-containing primer was developed and commercialized, which was sold as Clearfil SE Protect in the United States and Clearfil Mega Bond FA in Japan (Imazato et al., 2014).

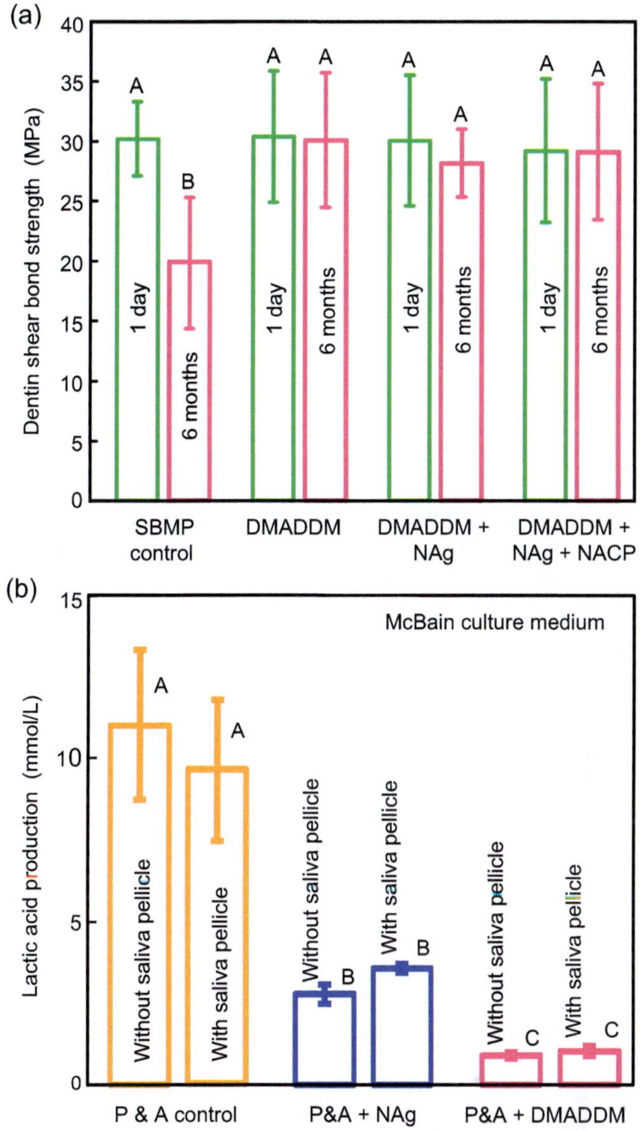

Figure 6.1 Development of antibacterial bonding agents. (a) Dentin shear bond strengths [mean ± standard deviation (SD); $n = 10$]. There was a 35% loss in bond strength for commercial bonding agent in 6 months' water-aging. There was no strength loss for new antibacterial bonding agents incorporating dimethylaminododecyl methacrylate (DMADDM), nanoparticles of silver (NAg), and nanoparticles of amorphous calcium phosphate. (b) Lactic acid production by biofilm on resin disks cultured in McBain artificial saliva medium, which produced a salivary coating on the resin surfaces (mean ± SD; $n = 6$). SBMP is a commercial bonding agent from 3 M. P is SBMP primer. A is SBMP adhesive. The incorporation of NAg or DMADDM greatly decreased acid production of biofilms. In each plot, values with dissimilar letters are significantly different from each other ($p < .05$).
Adapted from Zhang K, Cheng L, Wu EJ, Weir MD, Bai Y, Xu HH. Effect of water-ageing on dentine bond strength and anti-biofilm activity of bonding agent containing new monomer dimethylaminododecyl methacrylate. J Dent 2013a;41(6):504–13 and Li F, Weir MD, Fouad AF, Xu HH. Effect of salivary pellicle on antibacterial activity of novel antibacterial dental adhesives using a dental plaque microcosm biofilm model. Dent Mater 2014c;30(2):182–91, with permission.

The MDPB-containing primer before curing can kill bacteria rapidly because of the bactericidal activity of the unpolymerized MDPB, thereby acting as a cavity disinfectant (Imazato et al., 1997, 2001; 2006). It is noteworthy that the QAM-containing primer was able to penetrate into dentin tubules and eradicate caries-related species inside the dentin (Cheng et al., 2013b; Imazato et al., 2002; Schmalz et al., 2004). In vivo studies using beagle dogs found that the MDPB-containing primer could also inactivate *Streptococcus mutans* in the cavity (Imazato et al., 2004). Since residual bacteria are one of the primary causes of secondary caries, the cavity-disinfecting effect of QAM-containing primer may improve the outcomes of restorative treatments of caries lesions.

The human oral cavity supports a diverse microbial consortium composed of hundreds of bacterial species (Moore and Moore, 1994; Paster et al., 2001). A 2013 study (Li et al., 2013b) tested the antibacterial effect of QAMs against eight important oral bacteria species: *streptococci* (*S. mutans* and *Streptococcus sanguinis*), *Lactobacillus*, *Actinomyces*, *Porphyromonas*, *Prevotella*, *Staphylococcus aureus*, and *Enterococcus faecalis*. The results showed that *E. faecalis* was less susceptibility to QAMs, whereas *S. sanguinis* was the easiest to kill. Dimethylaminododecyl methacrylate (DMADDM), a monomer with an alkyl chain of 12 carbons, showed strong bactericidal activity against all bacteria with a minimum inhibitory concentration (MIC) of 1.2–9.8 μg/mL (Li et al., 2013b). DMADDM exhibited rapid killing effects against all eight oral bacterial species at the concentration of eightfold MIC (Li et al., 2013b).

After photocuring, QAMs such as MDPB were copolymerized with dental monomers to form antibacterial polymer matrices to reduce bacterial growth (Imazato et al., 1998a,b). Adhesives containing MDPB substantially reduced the growth of *S. mutans*. Adhesives containing QAMs such as QADM and DMAE-CB reduced biofilm growth and inhibited biofilm accumulation on resin surface via selectively downregulating *gtf* gene expression of *S. mutans* (Li et al., 2009a, 2013a). These polymerizable cationic monomers were covalently bonded within the polymer matrix and could exert antibacterial or antibiofilm effects upon contact without releasing compounds that might be toxic to mammalian cells.

Saliva in oral cavity can be absorbed onto dental restoration surfaces to provide anchor points for bacteria (Lendenmann et al., 2000) and may block certain functional groups on the resin surfaces. The contact-killing/inhibiting mechanism of QAM-containing resin would imply that when a salivary protein pellicle separates the antibacterial resin surface from the overlaying biofilm, the antibacterial effect of the resin could decrease. Several studies suggested that proteins adsorbed from physiological fluids, such as saliva-derived protein films, were able to attenuate the antibacterial properties of the underlying surfaces (Ebi et al., 2001; Imazato et al., 2003a; Muller et al., 2009). MDPB-immobilized fillers, which contained MDPB at a concentration of 15.8%, could greatly inhibit bacterial growth; however, saliva pretreatment of the surface reduced its antibacterial potency (Imazato et al., 2003a). The reduction in the antibacterial effect by the adsorption of proteins on the resin surfaces was a drawback of contact-killing dental materials. Similar results were reported with QADM, indicating that precoating the resin with salivary pellicles or the use of saliva-mimicking culture media such as the McBain medium are needed to avoid overestimating the antibacterial efficacy of a dental resin (Li et al., 2014c). Nonetheless, even with saliva coating of the resin surface, strong antibacterial resins were able to greatly reduce oral biofilm growth and lactic acid production, compared with counterparts without a QAM (Fig. 6.1(b)) (Li et al., 2014c).

6.4.1.2 The antibacterial mechanism of quaternary ammonium methacrylates

QAMs possess bacteriolysis effects, because their positively charged quaternary amine N^+ can attract the negatively charged cell membrane of bacteria, which can disrupt the cell membrane and cause cytoplasmic leakage (Beyth et al., 2006; Namba et al., 2009). Fluorescent indicators for membrane integrity in conjunction with confocal laser scanning microscopy were adopted to illustrate the detrimental effects of immobilized cationic moieties on bacterial membranes (Li et al., 2009b).

For short-chain QACs, the antimicrobial activity relies solely on the positively charged ammonium group coupling with the negatively charged bacterial membrane to disrupt membrane functions, alter the balance of essential ions (i.e., K^+, Na^+, Ca^{2+}, and Mg^{2+}), interrupt protein activity, and damage bacterial DNA (Simoncic and Tomcis, 2010). Long-chain QACs have double-killing effects, namely, (1) the positive charges and (2) the additional antimicrobial activity by inserting into bacterial membrane, resulting in physical disruption (Simoncic and Tomcis, 2010).

Quaternary amine charge density is important because when the negatively charged bacteria contact the positive quaternary amine charge, the electrical balance is disturbed and the bacterium could be disrupted. A 2014 study (Li et al., 2014b) investigated the effects of quaternary amine charge density of bonding agent on its antibacterial efficiency. QAM monomer was incorporated into a bonding system at a series of mass fractions to obtain resins with varied charge density, and the results demonstrated that increasing the charge density increased the antibacterial efficacy, as shown in Fig. 6.2 (Li et al., 2014b).

The alkyl CL is another important factor in the antibacterial efficacy of QAMs. Another study (Li et al., 2013c) developed dental bonding agents containing new QAMs with various CLs. The results showed monotonically increasing antibacterial potency with increasing CL from 3 to 16. However, when CL was further increased to 18, the antibacterial efficacy decreased. The reason might be that when the alkyl chain was too long, it might bend/curl and hence cover the positively charged quaternary ammonium groups, thereby blocking the electrostatic interactions with the bacteria and diminishing the antibacterial potency. A CL of 16 may be the critical point for the alkyl chain to extend without burying the quaternary ammonium sites. Dental resin containing new QAM with a CL of 16 appeared to be the optimum for inhibiting biofilm growth, as shown in Fig. 6.3(a) (Li et al., 2013c). Furthermore, adding QAMs with different CLs into the bonding agent did not adversely affect the dentin microtensile bond strength (Fig. 6.3(b)) (Li et al., 2013c). Therefore, the new QAM is promising for use in primer and adhesive to kill the residual bacteria inside tooth cavity and inhibit the invading bacteria at the tooth–composite margins to protect the bonded interface.

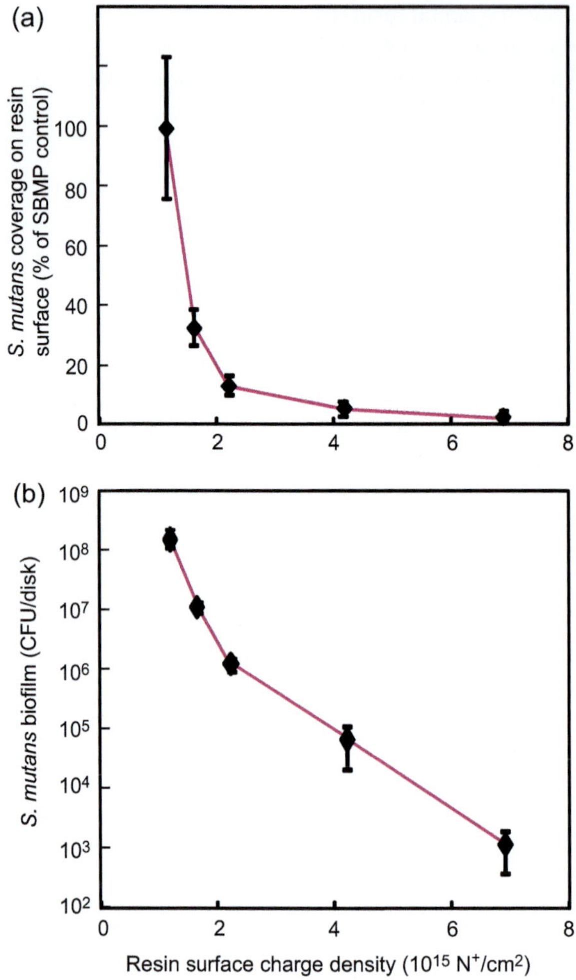

Figure 6.2 Development of antibacterial bonding agent as a function of quaternary amine surface charge density. (a) Bacterial early attachment to resin at 4h. (b) Mature biofilm colony-forming unit (CFU) counts after culturing for 2 days (mean ± SD; $n = 6$). Bonding agent charge density was strongly and inversely proportional to bacterial early attachment and biofilm CFU.
Adapted from Li F, Weir M.D, Chen J, Xu HH. Effect of charge density of bonding agent containing a new quaternary ammonium methacrylate on antibacterial and bonding properties. Dent Mater 2014b;30(4):433–41, with permission.

6.4.1.3 Cytotoxicity of quaternary ammonium methacrylates

New bonding materials need to be compatible with the dentin–pulp complex. It is important to investigate the influence of antibacterial monomers on pulpal healing after cavity restoration. MDPB exhibited a low level of toxicity to human pulpal cells, similar to triethyleneglycol dimethacrylate (Imazato et al., 1999). The incorporation of

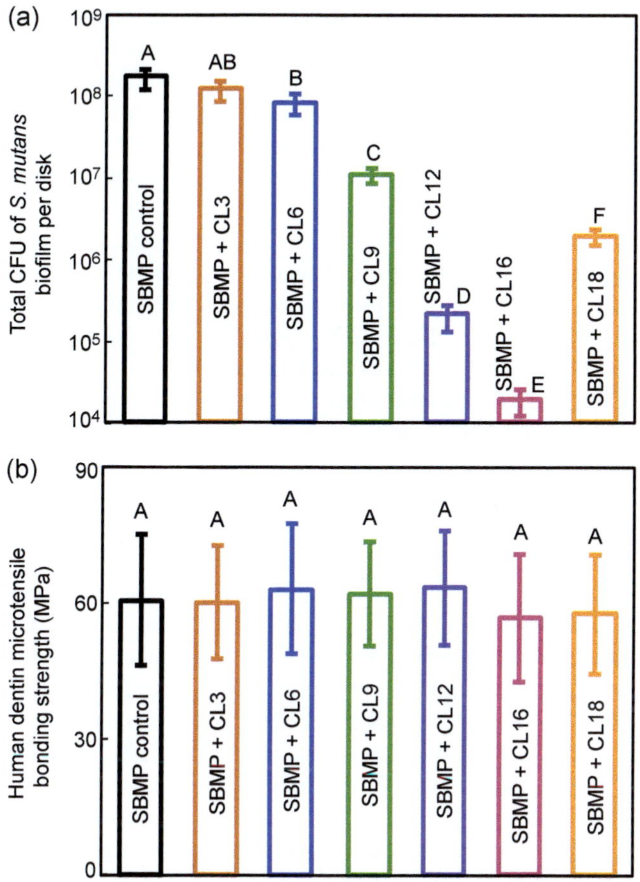

Figure 6.3 Development of antibacterial dental monomers with different chain lengths (CLs). (a) Colony-forming units (CFU) of biofilms at 2 days on resin surfaces (mean ± SD; $n=6$). (b) Human dentin microtensile bond strength (mean ± SD; $n=40$). Antibacterial efficacy increased with CL from 3 to 16 and then decreased at CL = 18. Biofilm CFU for SBMP with quaternary ammonium methacrylate at CL = 16 was reduced by four orders of magnitude, compared with SBMP control ($p<.05$). For dentin bond test, 8 teeth were used for each group. Five microtensile beams were obtained from each tooth, yielding 40 beams/group. In each plot, values with dissimilar letters are significantly different from each other ($p<.05$). Adapted from Li F, Weir MD, Xu HH. Effects of quaternary ammonium chain length on antibacterial bonding agents. J Dent Res 2013c;92(10):932–8, with permission.

MDPB into a primer did not increase the toxicity on pulpal cells (Imazato et al., 2000). The inhibitory effects of MDPB on the proliferation and mineralization of odontoblastlike MDPC-23 mouse cells were lower than those of bisphenol A glycidyl methacrylate (BisGMA), indicating that MDPB had better biocompatibility than BisGMA (Nishida et al., 2010). A 2013 study on a series of monomers with varied CLs revealed that increasing the CL increased the cytotoxicity; however, all the tested antibacterial monomers had less cytotoxicity than BisGMA (Li et al., 2013c).

A rat molar model was used to investigate the influence of antibacterial QAM-containing adhesives and composites on the dentin–pulp complex in vivo (Li et al., 2014a). Rat molars were considered to be anatomically, biologically, and physiologically similar to human molars (Dammaschke, 2010). An occlusal cavity was prepared in rat molars with remaining dentin thickness of approximately 200 μm. The DMADDM-containing composite and adhesive generated pulp response similar to that of the control group without DMADDM, exhibiting mild inflammatory reaction at 8 d and virtually no inflammatory reaction at 30 d (Li et al., 2014a). Furthermore, the restorations containing DMADDM and nanoparticles of amorphous calcium phosphate (NACP) generated much more tertiary dentin thickness than the control in vivo at 30 days (Fig. 6.4) (Li et al., 2014a). Therefore, although QAMs are promising in protecting the bonded tooth–restoration interfaces and inhibiting recurrent caries, they have better biocompatibility than the widely used dental monomers, such as BisGMA, and could be used in adhesive modification without adversely influencing the pulp healing ability.

6.4.1.4 Nanoparticles for antibacterial activity

Silver, both as a metal and in ionic form, exhibits strong antibacterial activity against a broad range of microorganisms (Peng et al., 2012; Shahverdi et al., 2007). The effective biocidal concentration of silver nanoparticles is at the nanomolar level in contrast to the micromolar level of silver ions (Kong and Jang, 2008). Due to the strong antibacterial activity, nanoparticles of silver (NAg) were incorporated in resins for antibacterial activity (Cheng et al., 2011; Shahverdi et al., 2007). Recent studies prepared NAg by dissolving Ag salt in 2-(tert-butylamino)ethyl methacrylate monomer, which was then mixed with the resin and photopolymerized, thus forming the NAg in situ (Cheng et al., 2011). This yielded well-dispersed NAg in the resin without agglomeration (Cheng et al., 2011). The small particle size of NAg, about 2.7 nm in diameter, yielded a high specific surface area, allowing the use of a low filler level of NAg in the adhesive to achieve antibacterial efficacy. The incorporation of NAg at a low concentration of 0.03% also provided a strong antibacterial activity (Cheng et al., 2011). Bonding agent containing NAg and QAM could flow into dentinal tubules and kill the bacteria inside dentin blocks to protect the dentin and the interface (Fig. 6.5) (Cheng et al., 2013b).

It is generally accepted that the mode of antibacterial action of NAg involves Ag ion release (Pallavicini et al., 2010). Ag ions could target the thiol groups (–SH) of proteins exposed to the extracellular portion of the bacterial membrane (Feng et al., 2000; Gupta et al., 1999; Morones et al., 2005) and inactivate the vital enzymes of bacteria, thus causing DNA in the bacteria to lose its replication ability, which leads to cell death (Rai et al., 2009). The Ag ion release could not only influence the *S. mutans* biofilm in direct contact with material surface but also exerted a long-distance antibacterial effect against planktonic bacteria. Therefore, QAM and NAg could show complementary behavior for inhibiting bacteria. Experimental adhesives containing QAM + NAg exhibited significantly stronger antibacterial potency, than those using one agent alone (Cheng et al., 2012b, 2013a,b; Li et al., 2013a; Zhang et al., 2012, 2013b).

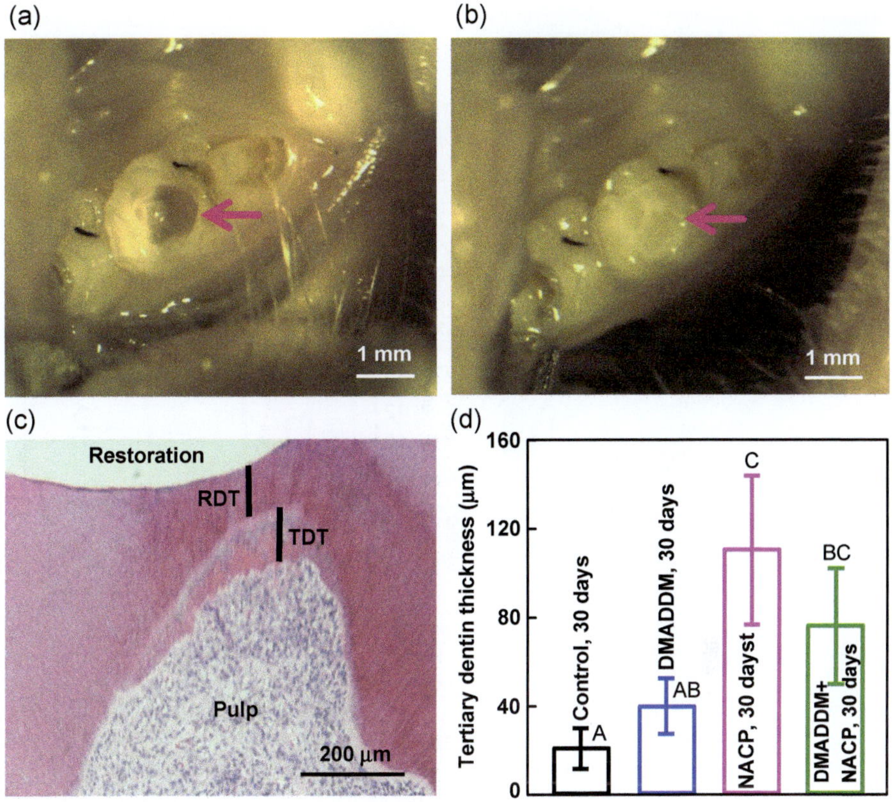

Figure 6.4 Rat tooth cavity model. (a) Rat right and left molar teeth were used. (b) Cavity was restored with bonding agent and composite and light-cured. (c) Example of histological image showing the remaining dentin thickness, as well as new tertiary dentin thickness (TDT) after 30 days in vivo in the rats. (d) TDT measured from hematoxylin and eosin histological images (mean ± SD; $n=6$). The arrows indicate the prepared molar cavity. Values with different letters are significantly different from each other ($p<.05$). There was no significant difference between the control and dimethylaminododecyl methacrylate (DMADDM) ($p>.1$). There was no difference between nanoparticles of amorphous calcium phosphate (NACP) and DMADDM + NACP ($p>.1$). NACP and DMADDM + NACP had TDT that were five- to sixfold that of control. Adapted from Li F, Wang P, Weir MD, Fouad AF, Xu HH. Evaluation of antibacterial and remineralizing nanocomposite and adhesive in rat tooth cavity model. Acta Biomater 2014a;10(6):2804–13, with permission.

This ion-releasing antibacterial action mode of NAg might raise concerns about the persistence of its bioactivity. Previous studies showed that Ag-containing resins could inhibit *S. mutans* growth for more than 6 months (Yoshida et al., 1999), which could be sufficient in killing residual bacteria inside dentinal tubules with NAg in the primer and adhesive.

Another approach to combat caries is to use nanoparticles of CaP to impart remineralizing capability (Dickens et al., 2003; Katoh et al., 2010; Langhorst et al., 2009;

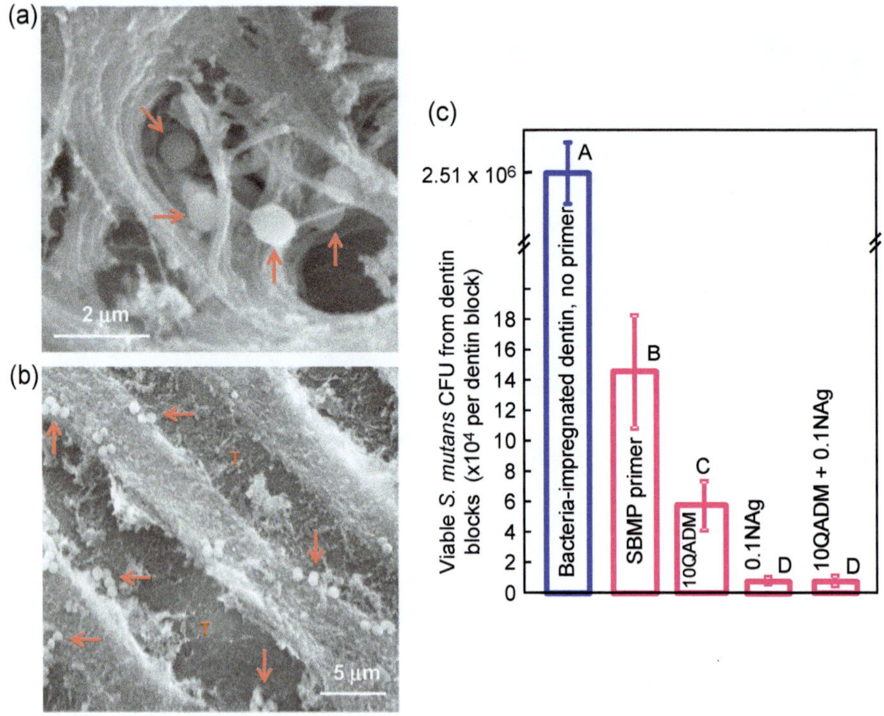

Figure 6.5 Killing *Streptococcus mutans* impregnated into dentin blocks. (a) Scanning electron microscopic image of *S. mutans* impregnation into tubules, viewed on the external surface of dentin with the tubules perpendicular to the surface. (b) *S. mutans* in tubules, in the cross-section of dentin by opening the dentin block after bacterial impregnation. *Arrows* indicate *S. mutans* in tubules. (c) *S. mutans* colony-forming unit (CFU) harvested from dentin blocks (mean ± SD; $n = 6$). The CFU of the bacterial-impregnated dentin without primer was 2.51×10^6 (CFU/dentin block). The other groups had the units of 10^4 CFU/dentin block. CFU of dentin treated with primer 10QADM + 0.1NAg was 3 log less than the CFU of control dentin without primer. Therefore, the novel antibacterial primer killed bacteria in the dentinal tubules. *NAg*, nanoparticles of silver.
Adapted from Cheng L, Zhang K, Weir MD, Liu H, Zhou X, Xu HH. Effects of antibacterial primers with quaternary ammonium and nano-silver on Streptococcus mutans impregnated in human dentin blocks. Dent Mater 2013b;29(4):462–72,with permission.

Weir et al., 2012; Xu et al., 2006, 2010, 2011). Previous studies incorporated CaP particles of about 1–55 μm in size into resins (Dickens et al., 2003; Langhorst et al., 2009). These traditional CaP composites released calcium (Ca) and phosphate (P) ions and remineralized tooth lesions in vitro (Dickens et al., 2003; Langhorst et al., 2009). Dental resins containing NACP with a high surface area released high levels of Ca and P ions, while possessing mechanical properties nearly twofold those of traditional CaP composites (Xu et al., 2006, 2010). Recent studies combined NACP with QAM or NAg and achieved a novel dental bonding agent with remineralization capacity and long-lasting antibacterial activity (Cheng et al., 2012a; Melo et al., 2013a,b). Due to their small particle sizes, the NACP and NAg readily flowed into the dentinal tubules

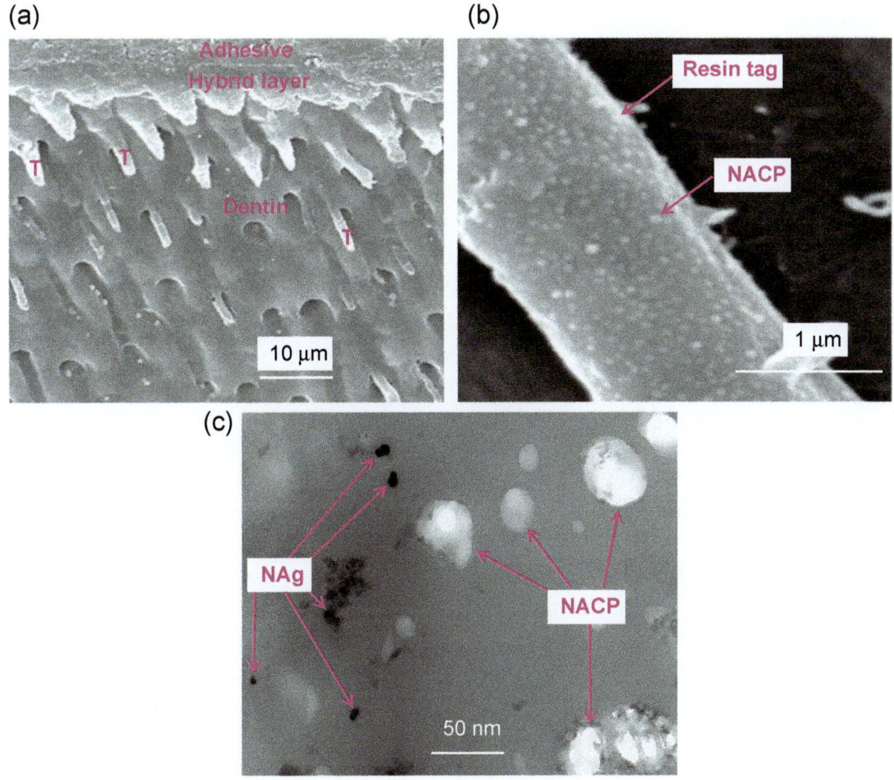

Figure 6.6 Scanning and transmission electron microscopic examination of the dentin–adhesive interface. (a, b) Representative SEM images at low and high magnification, and (c) TEM image. "T" in (a) indicates resin tags. The example in (a) is for group DMADDM + NAg + NACP; other groups had similar features. (b) Higher magnification for DMADDM + NAg + NACP shows NACP inside a resin tag. (c) At an even higher magnification in TEM, both NACP and NAg are visible inside resin tags. Therefore, both NACP and NAg were successfully flowed into the dentinal tubules. *DMADDM*, dimethylaminododecyl methacrylate; *NACP*, nanoparticles of amorphous calcium phosphate; *NAg*, nanoparticles of silver.
Adapted from Zhang K, Cheng L, Wu EJ, Weir MD, Bai Y, Xu HH. Effect of water-ageing on dentine bond strength and anti-biofilm activity of bonding agent containing new monomer dimethylaminododecyl methacrylate. J Dent 2013a;41(6):504–13, with permission.

with the bonding agent (Fig. 6.6) (Zhang et al., 2013a). Such new materials having both remineralization and antibacterial properties may be of great benefit to preserve the bonded interface durability and combat secondary caries, which requires further study.

6.4.2 Improvement of esterase resistance and infiltration of adhesive

Hydrolysis, inadequate monomer conversion, and incomplete infiltration of the adhesive are the main material factors for dentin–resin bond failure. To address this challenge, the modification of the adhesive with water-compatible and esterase-resistant properties has been extensively studied (Park et al., 2008, 2009). In addition, ethanol-wet bonding technique has been examined to improve resin infiltration.

6.4.2.1 Development of water-compatible, esterase-resistant adhesives

Spencer's group attempted to reduce the hydrolytic degradation of methacrylate adhesives and promote bonding to wet dentin by molecular design (Spencer et al., 2010). Methacrylate side chains were selectively modified to be both water compatible and esterase resistant. This was accomplished by using bulky and/or branched functional groups that were poor esterase substrates but sufficiently hydrophilic to be water compatible (Park et al., 2008, 2009). For example, a new trimethacrylate monomer with urethane-linked groups [1,1,1-tri-[4-(methacryloxyethylamino-carbonyloxy)-phenyl] ethane (MPE)] was synthesized and used as a comonomer to improve the esterase resistance of dentin adhesives (Park et al., 2009). Moreover, the adhesive modified with MPE showed a degree of double bond conversion comparable to the control, good penetration into the dentin surface, and a uniform adhesive/dentin interface, as shown in Fig. 6.7 (Park et al., 2009).

Another strategy involved increasing the matrix hydrophobicity following initial monomer penetration into the dentin layer (Spencer et al., 2010). Secondary cross-linking of polar functional groups on methacrylate side chains could be employed to achieve this goal. In addition, water-compatible photoinitiators were developed to promote polymer conversion, thereby reducing the susceptibility to esterase hydrolysis by reducing the number of unreacted pendant groups (Guo et al., 2008, 2009; Park et al., 2010; Ye et al., 2009). These efforts are expected to contribute to preserving the tooth–resin bond and increasing the restoration longevity.

6.4.2.2 Ethanol-wet bonding technique

Ethanol-wet bonding technique has always been advocated to be used with hydrophobic adhesive (Hosaka et al., 2009; Pashley et al., 2007; Sadek et al., 2008, 2010b; Tay et al., 2007), which aims to both provide superior sealing of collagen and absorb little water to avoid the degradation of collagen peptides. In the ethanol-wet bonding technique, ethanol instead of water is used to support the demineralized dentin collagen matrix (Pashley et al., 2007; Sadek et al., 2008; Tay et al., 2007). The voids between the microfibrils are filled with ethanol, which is a much better solvent for resin monomers and may promote the intimate coating of adhesive on collagen.

In addition to providing better solubility of adhesive resin, ethanol is also capable of collapsing the proteoglycan hydrogel, which is claimed to stuff the collagen matrix (Oyarzun et al., 2000; Pereira et al., 2007) and interfere with resin infiltration (Scott and Thomlinson, 1998). Therefore, adhesive resin could penetrate in ethanol-wet collagen matrix more easily. Moreover, ethanol has been demonstrated to shrink the diameter of collagen fibrils (Hosaka et al., 2009; Tay et al., 2007) more than it shrinks the volume of the matrix, thereby enlarging the interfibrillar spaces and allowing for more resin infiltration. Accordingly, ethanol-wet bonding technique may guarantee an intimate association between collagen fibers and resin to provide better resin sealing

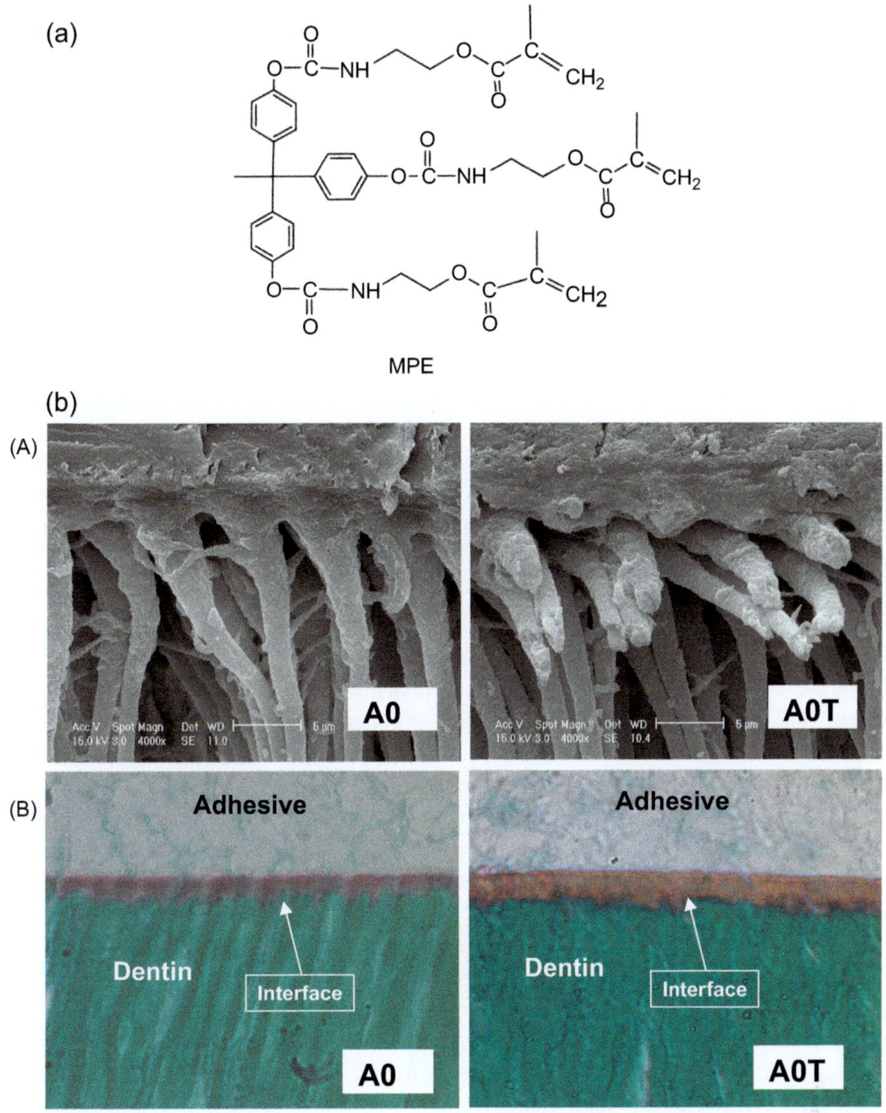

Figure 6.7 (a) Structure of 1,1,1-tri-[4-(methacryloxyethylamino-carbonyloxy)-phenyl] ethane (MPE). (b) Representative scanning electron micrographs (A) and staining/light microscopy (B) of dentin/adhesive interface for control (C0) and experimental (MPE0) resins. The scanning electron microscopic images indicated good resin penetration into the prepared dentin surface for both adhesive formulations. The color of the interface zone is dark red when treated with control adhesive and the width is about 2.4 μm, whereas the experimental adhesive is orange/red and 3.5 μm in width. The difference in color represents the extent of exposed collagen at the interface. The red color represents exposed collagen at the interface that is available for reaction with stains. The orange color indicates that the resin-infiltrated layer where exposed collagen was slightly more encapsulated with adhesive. Adhesive resin composition: (C0: HEMA/BisGMA = 45/55 w/w ratio + 40 wt% EtOH; MPE0: HEMA/BisGMA/MPE = 45/30/25 w/w ratio + 40 wt% EtOH). *BisGMA*, bisphenol A glycidyl methacrylate; *EtOH*, ethyl alcohol; *HEMA*, 2-hydroxyethyl methacrylate.
Adapted from Park JG, Ye Q, Topp EM, Spencer P. Enzyme-catalyzed hydrolysis of dentin adhesives containing a new urethane-based trimethacrylate monomer. J Biomed Mater Res B Appl Biomater 2009;91(2):562–71, with permission.

of the collagen matrix (Shin et al., 2009). This may reduce the permeability of the resin–dentin bonding interface (Cadenaro et al., 2009), thereby minimizing harmful endogenous collagenolytic activities.

6.4.3 Endogenous protease inhibition and collagen biomineralization

6.4.3.1 Inhibition of endogenous proteases

The degradation of the mineral depleted, resin-sparse, water-rich collagen fibrils along the bonded interface is the biological factor contributing to dentin–resin bond failure. To solve this problem, three main strategies have been proposed: the inhibition of endogenous proteases, the biomineralization of denuded collagen fibrils, and the biomodification of collagen. The collagen fibrils are exposed by dentin demineralization with acids or acidic resin monomers from self-etch adhesive systems (Liu et al., 2011c). Resin penetration and entanglement of exposed collagen fibrils in the partially or completely demineralized dentin provide micromechanical retention for the dentin–resin bond. However, it is impossible for resin monomers to completely displace water within the extrafibrillar and intrafibrillar compartments of a demineralized collagen matrix, and to infiltrate the collagen network completely (Breschi et al., 2008; Carvalho et al., 2012; Sauro et al., 2009). The mineral-depleted, resin-sparse, water-rich collagen fibrils along the bonded interface (Breschi et al., 2008; Carvalho et al., 2012) are the weak link in the dentin–resin bond. It is susceptible to degradation under the combined challenges of enzymes, temperature, and functional stresses, resulting in damage of the interfacial integrity, reduction in bond strength, and ultimately, the failure of dentin–resin bonds.

Dentin bonding not only is a physicochemical process of the dissolution of hydroxyapatite and the penetration of adhesive resin but also has biological characteristics. MMPs, a group of zinc- and calcium-dependent host-derived proteases, and cysteine cathepsins, have been confirmed to be deeply involved in this process (Pashley et al., 2004; Tersariol et al., 2010). MMP-2, MMP-8, MMP-9, and MMP-20, which exist in mineralized dentin (Sulkala et al., 2007), can be exposed and activated by the acid etchants used in adhesive bonding systems (Mazzoni et al., 2006). They can also be activated by the mildly acidic adhesive resin components of self-etching adhesive system (Nishitani et al., 2006), and by the lactic acid released by oral pathogenic bacteria (Tjaderhane et al., 1998). The activated collagen-bound MMPs and/or non–collagen-bound MMPs may progressively degrade the uncovered collagen fibrils in the bonded dentin. The breakdown of collagen may increase the water content, causing further collagen degradation, and inducing deterioration of the durability of the dentin–resin bond (Manuja et al., 2012; Spencer and Wang, 2002).

To protect the integrity of dentin collagen in HL and improve the bond durability, chlorhexidine (CHX), a biguanide antimicrobial agent with the ability to inhibit the activities of MMP-2, MMP-8, and MMP-9 (Gendron et al., 1999), was used as a nonspecific MMP inhibitor in the dentin-bonding process (Carrilho et al., 2007a; De Munck et al., 2009; Hebling et al., 2005; Pashley et al., 2004). For etch-and-rinse adhesives, CHX was applied to the demineralized dentin directly or incorporated into an acid conditioner prior to the application of adhesives, which was shown to be effective for reducing degradation of resin–dentin bonds after in vivo aging (Brackett et al., 2009; Carrilho et al., 2007b; Hebling et al., 2005; Ricci et al., 2010). For self-etch adhesives, CHX was incorporated to obtain therapeutic primers (De Munck et al., 2009; Zhou et al., 2010) and prevent the degradation of HL. However, CHX is water soluble and electrostatically binds to demineralized dentin matrix. When incorporated into adhesive, CHX may diffuse out of the dentin collagen matrix via a competitive desorption mechanism in the presence of other cations, leading to a decrease in its long-term anti-MMP effectiveness (Tezvergil-Mutluay et al., 2011a). With the loss of CHX, the protective effect on the bonded interface was reduced after 9 months and severe degradation was detected in HL at 18 months (Sadek et al., 2010a). Therefore, improved approaches are needed for long-term protection of the dentin–resin bonded interface.

Another nonspecific MMP inhibitor, GM 6001 (galardin), is often used as a reference inhibitor in generic MMP assay kits, which has a collagenlike backbone that binds to the MMP active site and a hydroxamate structure that chelates the MMP catalytic domain zinc (Auge et al., 2003). It has been used as an experimental primer to prevent degradation of the HL (Breschi et al., 2010). Polyvinylphosphonic acid (Tezvergil-Mutluay et al., 2010), benzalkonium chloride (Tezvergil-Mutluay et al., 2011b), and proanthocyanidin (PAC) (Epasinghe et al., 2013) were also shown to possess anti-MMP activities.

Other studies showed that QAMs, including MDPB, were effective in inhibiting both soluble recombinant MMPs and matrix-bound dentin MMPs (Tezvergil-Mutluay et al., 2011a). Novel antibacterial monomer DMADDM and DMAE-CB have also been proved to be MMP-inhibitive (Li et al., 2015; Liu et al., 2013). MMPs contain at least a prodomain and a catalytic domain (Visse and Nagase, 2003). The protease domain has one catalytic zinc, one structural zinc, and three calcium ions. The catalytic zinc coordinates with three histidines. One of the three histidine molecules is adjacent to a glutamic acid residue that contains a negative charge (Tezvergil-Mutluay et al., 2011a). The cationic QAM may alter the configuration of the catalytic site of MMPs via electrostatically binding to the negative charges of glutamic acid residue. This QAM–MMP complex would make MMPs unable to hydrolyze the specific peptide bond of collagen (Tezvergil-Mutluay et al., 2011a). Contrary to the unstable anti-MMP effect of CHX-containing adhesive system, QAMs can be copolymerized and immobilized in HL, which can potentially provide durable MMP inhibition and would be beneficial to the durability of dentin bonding. Therefore, a polymerizable anti-MMP monomer may be an ideal candidate for bioactive resin-based material to yield a durable dentin–resin bonded interface.

6.4.3.2 Protein cross-linker agents

The intermolecular cross-linking of collagen is the basis for the stability, tensile strength, and viscoelasticity of the collagen fibrils. The slope of the elastic stress–strain curve for collagen fibers increases with increased degree of cross-linking (Silver et al., 2001). The biodegradability and thermal stability of dentin is also controlled by the amount and type of collagen cross-linking. Increasing the degree of cross-linking of collagen in dentin may improve the mechanical properties of the HL and the resistance against proteolytic degradation, thereby enhancing the dentin–resin bonding durability. Some researchers argued that since dentin collagen was already highly cross-linked, it was doubtful if the increase in resin–dentin bond longevity could be explained by the augmentation in cross-linking density alone (Liu et al., 2011c). Current literature suggests that the enhancement of bonding durability might be due to the silencing of exogenous collagenase, such as MMPs and cysteine cathepsins (Busenlehner and Armstrong, 2005). Covalent cross-links produced with external cross-linkers could inactivate dentin proteases. The reasons would be the reduction of the molecular mobility or conformational changes in the three-dimensional structure of the enzyme (Busenlehner and Armstrong, 2005). By silencing exogenous collagenase, protein cross-linker agents could protect the collagen matrix and thus stabilize the dentin–resin bonding interface.

Glutaraldehyde (GA) is a kind of widely known cross-linker, which is a dialdehyde with high affinity for the free primary amine groups of amino acids (Cheung et al., 1985). GA could reduce the rate of collagen degradation (Cheung et al., 1990; Han et al., 2003) and improve dentin collagen properties (Scheffel et al., 2014). However, the high cytotoxicity limits its clinical applicability. Carbodiimide hydrochloride (EDC) is less toxic than GA (Huang et al., 1990; Petite et al., 1995) and can cross-link the peptides without introducing additional linkage groups. EDC can cross-link both helical and especially telopeptide domains in collagen. Moreover, it may be able to cross-link collagenase to inactivate the active sites of dentin proteases by reducing the molecular mobility, or by changing the negatively charged ionized carboxyl groups into positively charged amides (Tjaderhane et al., 2013). In addition, a study applied 0.1% of riboflavin (nontoxic collagen cross-linking) with ultraviolet-A light irradiation to resin bonding and showed significantly improved durability of the resin–dentin bond (Chiang et al., 2013).

Natural cross-linkers, such as PAC, genipin (GNP) and epigallocatechin gallate (EGCG), have received great attention in the 2000s for their potential use in dentistry. Two of their most attractive characteristics are their very low toxicity when compared with synthetic agents (Han et al., 2003) and their renewable/sustainable resources. PAC, a grape seed polyphenol, is well known as a natural collagen cross-linker, which can enhance the mechanical stability of collagen matrix and resist caries progression (Bedran-Russo et al., 2007, 2011; Castellan et al., 2010; Han et al., 2003; Walter et al., 2008). GNP is a hydrolytic product of geniposide, which is found in the fruit of *Gardenia jasminoides* Ellis and has been reported as an excellent natural cross-linker with low toxicity (Bedran-Russo et al., 2007; Sung et al., 1999, 2003; Walter et al., 2008). EGCG, a green tea polyphenol, has been proved to have such an inhibitory effect against MMPs (Demeule et al., 2000; Sartor et al., 2002). These natural cross-linkers have been used to modify dentin bonding systems and have achieved promising results in improving the bonding durability.

6.4.3.3 Biomineralization of nude collagen fibrils

The protease inhibitor could inactivate MMPs and cathepsin to protect the denuded collagen fibers. However, even if there were no enzymatic degradation, the denuded collagen fiber is still the weakest link of the dentin–resin bond. The elastic modulus of denuded collagen is less than 8 MPa (Carrilho et al., 2009). Even with the strengthening effect of the cross-linking agent, its mechanical property is still far less than that of the collagen–resin mixture (3–5 GPa) and mineralized dentin (20 GPa). Under the long-term functions in vivo, the exposed collagen fibers in the bonded interface will be damaged with fatigue stresses, eventually leading to bonding failure (Fung et al., 2009).

Biomimetic remineralization is an approach to solve this problem by attempting to backfill the denuded collagen fibers with liquidlike amorphous calcium phosphate (ACP) nanoprecursor particles that are stabilized by biomimetic analogs of noncollagenous proteins (Kim et al., 2010a; Tay and Pashley, 2008, 2009). The biomimetic remineralization strategy is based on the nonclassical crystallization pathway, which is particle mediated and involves a mesoscopic transformation process (Colfen and Mann, 2003; Kim et al., 2010a). Biomimetic mineralization of type I collagen may be envisaged to proceed in several stages (Colfen, 2010; Niu et al., 2014). (1) The collagen fibril serves as an active template for hierarchical intrafibrillar mineralization. (2) Calcium and phosphate ions in the calcifying medium self-assemble into stable particulate units known as prenucleation clusters. In the presence of a polyanionic analog of matrix proteins such as poly(aspartic acid), these prenucleation clusters further condense into larger particles of fluidic amorphous ACP precursors (in the range of 10–30 nm) that are capable of diffusing into the intrafibrillar compartments of type I collagen. (3) The negatively charged and polyanion-stabilized ACP precursors interact with the positively charged sites along the collagen molecules, inducing solidification and nucleation of the ACP inside collagen. (4) These nucleated amorphous mineral precursor phases further grow and maturate into apatite nanocrystals along the intrafibrillar space of collagen via nonclassical crystallization pathways. (5) Growth of the intrafibrillar apatite results in heavy intrafibrillar mineralization by apatite crystallites, with concomitant extrafibrillar mineralization between adjacent collagen fibrils.

Previous studies showed that biomimetic mineralization of collagen was achieved via a dual biomimetic analog strategy (Dai et al., 2011; Gu et al., 2010, 2011a,b; Kim et al., 2010c; Liu et al., 2011a). Polyacrylic acid or polyaspartic acid was used as an analog for sequestering the calcium ions. These analogs function by acting as surfactants to prevent fluidic ACP nanoparticles from aggregating into larger particles, and to inhibit autotransformation of the ACP nanoparticles into apatite (ie, apatite nucleation inhibitor) prior to their entry into the intrafibrillar water compartments of the collagen fibril (Kim et al., 2010c; Liu et al., 2011a). In addition, a polyphosphate-containing biomimetic analog such as polyvinylphosphonic acid, sodium trimetaphosphate, or sodium ascorbyl phosphate was employed as a templating biomimetic analog of matrix phosphoproteins. These phosphoprotein analogs were allowed to bind to the collagen fibrils prior to immersion of the fibrillar matrices in the poly(anionic) acid–containing mineralization medium (Gu et al., 2010, 2011a,b). Moreover, polyvinylphosphonic acid was shown to possess matrix metalloproteinase–inhibiting properties, which could prevent collagen degradation during the 3- to 4-month period of remineralization (Tezvergil-Mutluay et al., 2010).

Using this biomimetic remineralization strategy, both HLs created by etch-and-rinse adhesives (Mai et al., 2009, 2010; Tay and Pashley, 2009) and moderately aggressive self-etch adhesives (Kim et al., 2010b; Liu et al., 2011b) were remineralized. This bottom-up remineralization strategy does not rely on seed crystallites. This strategy is useful in extending the longevity of the resin–dentin bond (Kim et al., 2010d) via restoring the dynamic mechanical properties of the denuded collagen and fossilizing the collagenase within the HL (Ryou et al., 2011).

For etch-and-rinse adhesives (Fig. 6.8(a)) (Niu et al., 2014), apatite crystallites were detected in both extrafibrillar and intrafibrillar spaces after remineralization, which could also be seen with moderately aggressive (Fig. 6.8(b)) and aggressive self-etching adhesives (Niu et al., 2014). The remineralized regions corresponded well to water-rich, resin-sparse regions of the HLs, whereas regions that were well-infiltrated by adhesive resin monomers did not undergo remineralization. After biomineralization with the aid of dual biomimetic analogs, the denuded collagen fibrils along the surface of the HL could be remineralized in the form of continuous intrafibrillar strands (Fig. 6.8(c)) (Niu et al., 2014). This phenomenon might be due to the ingress of poly(anionic) acid–stabilized ACP nanoprecursors into the loosened microfibrillar gap and the enlarged water compartments along the overlap zones of the collagen molecules. Conversely, collagen fibrils that were remineralized within the middle part of the HL contained discrete intrafibrillar apatite platelets (Fig. 6.8(d)) (Niu et al., 2014).

For self-etch adhesives, remineralization was not usually apparent in mild self-etching versions of these adhesives. Mild self-etch adhesives that contained the functional monomer 10-methacryloxydecyl dihydrogen phosphate (MDP) were capable of nanolayering with hydroxyapatite (Yoshida et al., 2012b; Yoshihara et al., 2011). For other mild self-etch adhesives not containing MDP, or those containing HEMA that inhibited nanolayering of MDP (Yoshida et al., 2012a), remineralization could only be seen in partially demineralized collagen matrices, probably by epitaxial growth via a top-down crystallization approach (Kim et al., 2010a). For moderately aggressive versions of self-etch adhesives, apatite deposition was almost exclusively identified from the completely demineralized part of the HLs (Niu et al., 2014). For the aggressive versions of self-etch adhesives, remineralization had been observed within the surface, middle, or bottom parts of those thick Hls, depending on the status of resin infiltration and the amount of water present within those HLs (Niu et al., 2014).

Although the biomineralization patterns for the nude collagen matrix might vary with different types of adhesive systems, the biomimetic remineralization of resin–dentin bonds had become an acknowledged concept for bonding durability improvement. There have been attempts to try to translate this concept into a clinically applicable technique (Niu et al., 2014). ACP nanoparticle–containing dentin adhesive was tested for biomimetic remineralizing faulty dentin–resin bond (Niu et al., 2014). This method could only remineralize partially demineralized dentin by epitaxial deposition of calcium and phosphate phases over remnant apatite seed crystallites. Moreover, intrafibrillar remineralization of dentin collagen could not be observed with this solid-state ACP nanoparticles–containing adhesive. Recently, a potential delivery strategy has been proposed to produce poly(anionic) acid–stabilized ACP prenucleation clusters and store them as "cargos" in mesoporous silica

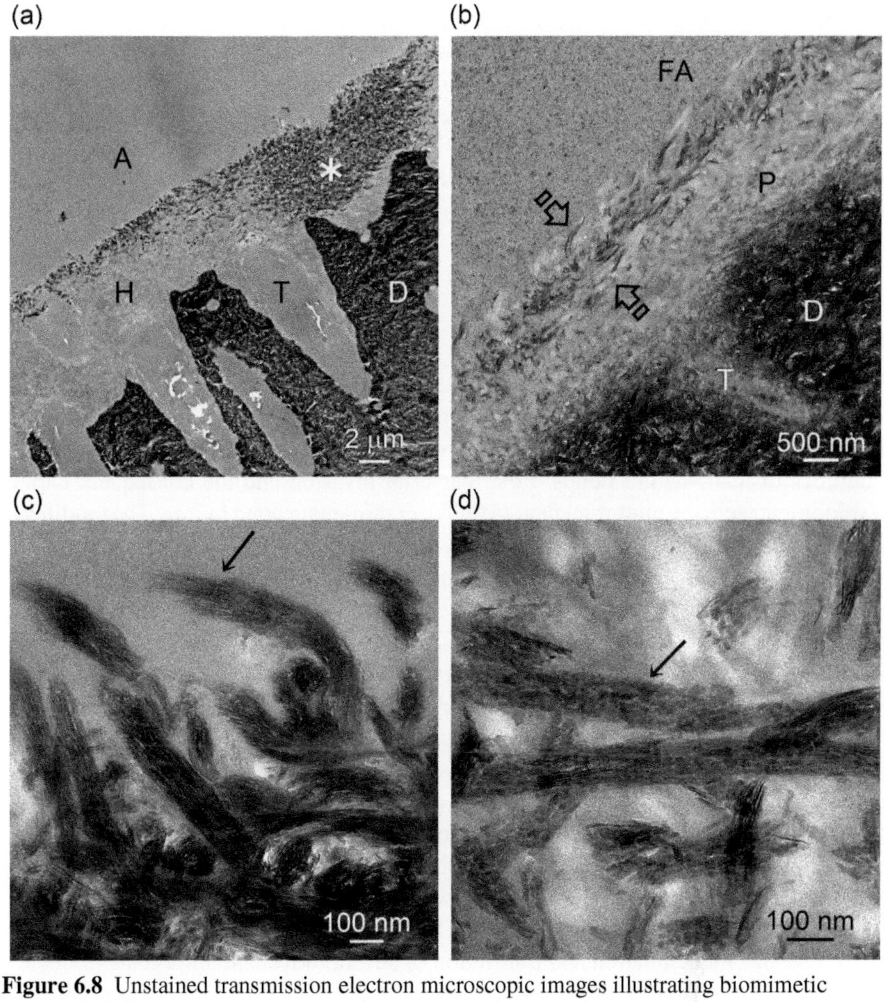

Figure 6.8 Unstained transmission electron microscopic images illustrating biomimetic remineralization of hybrid layers created by (a) an etch-and-rinse adhesive. *A*, adhesive; *H*, apatite-depleted hybrid layer created by phosphoric acid etching for 15 s; *T*, dentinal tubule; *D*, mineralized dentin; *Asterisk*, water-rich part of the hybrid layer remineralized by apatite crystallites. (b) A moderately aggressive self-etch adhesive. *FA*, filled adhesive; *P*, partially demineralized base of the hybrid layer; *T*, dentinal tubule; *D*, mineralized dentin; *between open arrows*, water-rich surface of the hybrid layer remineralized by apatite crystallites. (c) High magnification of the surface of a remineralized hybrid layer showing partially unraveled surface collagen fibrils in which their intrafibrillar compartments were filled with continuous strands of apatite mineral. (d) High-magnification image taken from the middle part of a remineralized hybrid layer showing collagen fibrils that were remineralized with discrete intrafibrillar apatite platelets.
Adapted from Niu LN, Zhang W, Pashley DH, Breschi L, Mao J, Chen JH, et al. Biomimetic remineralization of dentin. Dent Mater 2014;30(1):77–96, with permission.

nanofillers (Niu et al., 2014). These mesoporous silica nanofillers may be incorporated in dentin adhesives as controlled-release devices for the delivery of the ACP prenucleation clusters, or coalesced ACP fluidic polymer-induced liquid-precursor (PILP) phases, into faulty HLs or caries-affected dentin. Another potential strategy is the use of calcium- and phosphate-containing mesoporous bioactive glass nanoparticles to load and deliver biomimetic analogs (Niu et al., 2014). This system could serve as a reservoir for calcium, phosphate and biomimetic analogs to generate prenucleation clusters in situ and therefore facilitate biomimetic remineralization.

6.5 Conclusions

Due to the unique characteristics of dentin, contemporary dentin bonding is not as durable as what has previously been assumed. Three major factors compromised the durability of resin–dentin bonds. First, bacterial invasion and the consequent caries development were the microbial factors for the dentin–resin bond failure. The modification of the HL with antibacterial bonding system, such as QAM-containing adhesives, was extensively studied to deal with the microbiological factor. Second, hydrolysis, inadequate monomer conversion, and incomplete infiltration of the adhesive resin were the material factors for dentin–resin bond failure. Methacrylate side chains were selectively modified to improve the esterase resistance of dentin adhesives. Moreover, water-compatible photoinitiators were developed to promote polymer conversion, and ethanol-wet bonding technique was used to improve resin infiltration. Third, the degradation of the mineral-depleted, resin-sparse, water-rich collagen fibrils along the bonded interface was the biological factor of dentin–resin bond failure. To deal with this problem, three main methods were proposed: the inhibition of endogenous proteases, the biomineralization of denuded collagen fibrils, and the biomodification of collagen. These three factors (microbial, material, and biological) coexist and synergize with each other to be responsible for the degradation of the dentin–resin bond. Therefore, the amalgamation and translation of several novel and important strategies discussed in this chapter is promising to overcome the critical barriers currently facing dentin bonding, and to yield strong dentin–resin bonded interfaces with long-term durability and clinical longevity.

Acknowledgments

We thank Drs. Joseph M. Antonucci, Nancy J. Lin, and Sheng Lin-Gibson of the National Institute of Standards and Technology (NIST) for fruitful discussions. This study was supported by NIH R01DE17974 (HX), National Natural Science Foundation of China 81100772 (FL), National Natural Science Foundation of China 51373198 (LZ), China Scholarship Council (LZ), and a bridge funding and a seed grant from the University of Maryland School of Dentistry (HX).

References

Aida M, Odaki M, Fujita K, Kitagawa T, Teshima I, Suzuki K, et al. Degradation-stage effect of self-etching primer on dentin bond durability. J Dent Res 2009;88(5):443–8.
Auge F, Hornebeck W, Decarme M, Laronze JY. Improved gelatinase a selectivity by novel zinc binding groups containing galardin derivatives. Bioorg Med Chem Lett 2003;13(10):1783–6.
Bedran-Russo AK, Pereira PN, Duarte WR, Drummond JL, Yamauchi M. Application of cross-linkers to dentin collagen enhances the ultimate tensile strength. J Biomed Mater Res B Appl Biomater 2007;80(1):268–72.
Bedran-Russo AK, Castellan CS, Shinohara MS, Hassan L, Antunes A. Characterization of biomodified dentin matrices for potential preventive and reparative therapies. Acta Biomater 2011;7(4):1735–41.
Beyth N, Yudovin-Farber I, Bahir R, Domb AJ, Weiss EI. Antibacterial activity of dental composites containing quaternary ammonium polyethylenimine nanoparticles against *Streptococcus mutans*. Biomaterials 2006;27(21):3995–4002.
Beyth N, Domb AJ, Weiss EI. An in vitro quantitative antibacterial analysis of amalgam and composite resins. J Dent 2007;35(3):201–6.
Boukpessi T, Menashi S, Camoin L, Tencate JM, Goldberg M, Chaussain-Miller C. The effect of stromelysin-1 (MMP-3) on non-collagenous extracellular matrix proteins of demineralized dentin and the adhesive properties of restorative resins. Biomaterials 2008;29(33):4367–73.
Brackett MG, Tay FR, Brackett WW, Dib A, Dipp FA, Mai S, et al. In vivo chlorhexidine stabilization of hybrid layers of an acetone-based dentin adhesive. Oper Dent 2009;34(4):379–83.
Breschi L, Mazzoni A, Ruggeri A, Cadenaro M, Di Lenarda R, De Stefano Dorigo E. Dental adhesion review: aging and stability of the bonded interface. Dent Mater 2008;24(1):90–101.
Breschi L, Martin P, Mazzoni A, Nato F, Carrilho M, Tjaderhane L, et al. Use of a specific MMP-inhibitor (galardin) for preservation of hybrid layer. Dent Mater 2010;26(6):571–8.
Buffet-Bataillon S, Tattevin P, Bonnaure-Mallet M, Jolivet-Gougeon A. Emergence of resistance to antibacterial agents: the role of quaternary ammonium compounds–a critical review. Int J Antimicrob Agents 2012;39(5):381–9.
Busenlehner LS, Armstrong RN. Insights into enzyme structure and dynamics elucidated by amide H/D exchange mass spectrometry. Arch Biochem Biophys 2005;433(1):34–46.
Cadenaro M, Breschi L, Rueggeberg FA, Agee K, Di Lenarda R, Carrilho M, et al. Effect of adhesive hydrophilicity and curing time on the permeability of resins bonded to water vs. ethanol-saturated acid-etched dentin. Dent Mater 2009;25(1):39–47.
Carrilho MR, Carvalho RM, de Goes MF, di Hipolito V, Geraldeli S, Tay FR, et al. Chlorhexidine preserves dentin bond in vitro. J Dent Res 2007a;86(1):90–4.
Carrilho MR, Geraldeli S, Tay F, de Goes MF, Carvalho RM, Tjaderhane L, et al. In vivo preservation of the hybrid layer by chlorhexidine. J Dent Res 2007b;86(6):529–33.
Carrilho MR, Tay FR, Donnelly AM, Agee KA, Tjaderhane L, Mazzoni A, et al. Host-derived loss of dentin matrix stiffness associated with solubilization of collagen. J Biomed Mater Res B Appl Biomater 2009;90(1):373–80.
Carvalho RM, Manso AP, Geraldeli S, Tay FR, Pashley DH. Durability of bonds and clinical success of adhesive restorations. Dent Mater 2012;28(1):72–86.
Castellan CS, Pereira PN, Grande RH, Bedran-Russo AK. Mechanical characterization of proanthocyanidin-dentin matrix interaction. Dent Mater 2010;26(10):968–73.
Chaussain-Miller C, Fioretti F, Goldberg M, Menashi S. The role of matrix metalloproteinases (MMPs) in human caries. J Dent Res 2006;85(1):22–32.

Cheng L, Weir MD, Xu HH, Antonucci JM, Lin NJ, Lin-Gibson S, et al. Effect of amorphous calcium phosphate and silver nanocomposites on dental plaque microcosm biofilms. J Biomed Mater Res B Appl Biomater 2012a;100(5):1378–86.

Cheng L, Zhang K, Melo MA, Weir MD, Zhou X, Xu HH. Anti-biofilm dentin primer with quaternary ammonium and silver nanoparticles. J Dent Res 2012b;91(6):598–604.

Cheng L, Weir MD, Zhang K, Arola DD, Zhou X, Xu HH. Dental primer and adhesive containing a new antibacterial quaternary ammonium monomer dimethylaminododecyl methacrylate. J Dent 2013a;41(4):345–55.

Cheng L, Zhang K, Weir MD, Liu H, Zhou X, Xu HH. Effects of antibacterial primers with quaternary ammonium and nano-silver on *Streptococcus mutans* impregnated in human dentin blocks. Dent Mater 2013b;29(4):462–72.

Cheng YJ, Zeiger DN, Howarter JA, Zhang X, Lin NJ, Antonucci JM, et al. In situ formation of silver nanoparticles in photocrosslinking polymers. J Biomed Mater Res B Appl Biomater 2011;97(1):124–31.

Cheung DT, Perelman N, Ko EC, Nimni ME. Mechanism of crosslinking of proteins by glutaraldehyde III. Reaction with collagen in tissues. Connect Tissue Res 1985;13(2):109–15.

Cheung DT, Tong D, Perelman N, Ertl D, Nimni ME. Mechanism of crosslinking of proteins by glutaraldehyde. IV: in vitro and in vivo stability of a crosslinked collagen matrix. Connect Tissue Res 1990;25(1):27–34.

Chiang YS, Chen YL, Chuang SF, Wu CM, Wei PJ, Han CF, et al. Riboflavin-ultraviolet-A-induced collagen cross-linking treatments in improving dentin bonding. Dent Mater 2013;29(6):682–92.

Colfen H, Mann S. Higher-order organization by mesoscale self-assembly and transformation of hybrid nanostructures. Angew Chem Int Ed Engl 2003;42(21):2350–65.

Colfen H. Biomineralization: a crystal-clear view. Nat Mater 2010;9(12):960–1.

Cox SW, Eley BM, Kiili M, Asikainen A, Tervahartiala T, Sorsa T. Collagen degradation by interleukin-1beta-stimulated gingival fibroblasts is accompanied by release and activation of multiple matrix metalloproteinases and cysteine proteinases. Oral Dis 2006;12(1):34–40.

Dai L, Qi YP, Niu LN, Liu Y, Pucci CR, Looney SW, et al. Inorganic-organic nanocomposite assembly using collagen as template and sodium tripolyphosphate as a biomimetic analog of matrix phosphoprotein. Cryst Growth Des 2011;11(8):3504–11.

Dammaschke T. Rat molar teeth as a study model for direct pulp capping research in dentistry. Lab Anim 2010;44(1):1–6.

De Munck J, Van Landuyt K, Peumans M, Poitevin A, Lambrechts P, Braem M, et al. A critical review of the durability of adhesion to tooth tissue: methods and results. J Dent Res 2005;84(2):118–32.

De Munck J, Van den Steen PE, Mine A, Van Landuyt KL, Poitevin A, Opdenakker G, et al. Inhibition of enzymatic degradation of adhesive-dentin interfaces. J Dent Res 2009;88(12):1101–6.

Delaviz Y, Finer Y, Santerre JP. Biodegradation of resin composites and adhesives by oral bacteria and saliva: a rationale for new material designs that consider the clinical environment and treatment challenges. Dent Mater 2014;30(1):16–32.

Demeule M, Brossard M, Page M, Gingras D, Beliveau R. Matrix metalloproteinase inhibition by green tea catechins. Biochim Biophys Acta 2000;1478(1):51–60.

Dickens SH, Flaim GM, Takagi S. Mechanical properties and biochemical activity of remineralizing resin-based Ca-PO_4 cements. Dent Mater 2003;19(6):558–66.

Ebi N, Imazato S, Noiri Y, Ebisu S. Inhibitory effects of resin composite containing bactericide-immobilized filler on plaque accumulation. Dent Mater 2001;17(6):485–91.

Eick JD. Smear layer–materials surface. Proc Finn Dent Soc 1992;88(Suppl. 1):225–42.

Eliades G, Watts DC, Eliades T. Dental hard tissues and bonding: interfacial phenomena and related properties. Heidelberg: Springer; 2005.

Epasinghe DJ, Yiu CK, Burrow MF, Hiraishi N, Tay FR. The inhibitory effect of proanthocyanidin on soluble and collagen-bound proteases. J Dent 2013;41(9):832–9.

Feng QL, Wu J, Chen GQ, Cui FZ, Kim TN, Kim JO. A mechanistic study of the antibacterial effect of silver ions on *Escherichia coli* and *Staphylococcus aureus*. J Biomed Mater Res 2000;52(4):662–8.

Ferracane JL, Hilton TJ, Sakaguchi RL. Introduction to and outcomes of the conference on adhesion in dentistry. Dent Mater 2010;26(2):105–7.

Ferracane JL. Resin composite–state of the art. Dent Mater 2011;27(1):29–38.

Fruits TJ, Knapp JA, Khajotia SS. Microleakage in the proximal walls of direct and indirect posterior resin slot restorations. Oper Dent 2006;31(6):719–27.

Fung DT, Wang VM, Laudier DM, Shine JH, Basta-Pljakic J, Jepsen KJ, et al. Subrupture tendon fatigue damage. J Orthop Res 2009;27(2):264–73.

Gendron R, Grenier D, Sorsa T, Mayrand D. Inhibition of the activities of matrix metalloproteinases 2, 8, and 9 by chlorhexidine. Clin Diagn Lab Immunol 1999;6(3):437–9.

Gu LS, Kim J, Kim YK, Liu Y, Dickens SH, Pashley DH, et al. A chemical phosphorylation-inspired design for Type I collagen biomimetic remineralization. Dent Mater 2010;26(11):1077–89.

Gu LS, Kim YK, Liu Y, Ryou H, Wimmer CE, Dai L, et al. Biomimetic analogs for collagen biomineralization. J Dent Res 2011a;90(1):82–7.

Gu LS, Kim YK, Liu Y, Takahashi K, Arun S, Wimmer CE, et al. Immobilization of a phosphonated analog of matrix phosphoproteins within cross-linked collagen as a templating mechanism for biomimetic mineralization. Acta Biomater 2011b;7(1):268–77.

Guo X, Wang Y, Spencer P, Ye Q, Yao X. Effects of water content and initiator composition on photopolymerization of a model BisGMA/HEMA resin. Dent Mater 2008;24(6):824–31.

Guo X, Peng Z, Spencer P, Wang Y. Effect of initiator on photopolymerization of acidic, aqueous dental model adhesives. J Biomed Mater Res A 2009;90(4):1120–7.

Gupta A, Matsui K, Lo JF, Silver S. Molecular basis for resistance to silver cations in *Salmonella*. Nat Med 1999;5(2):183–8.

Han B, Jaurequi J, Tang BW, Nimni ME. Proanthocyanidin: a natural crosslinking reagent for stabilizing collagen matrices. J Biomed Mater Res A 2003;65(1):118–24.

Hebling J, Pashley DH, Tjaderhane L, Tay FR. Chlorhexidine arrests subclinical degradation of dentin hybrid layers in vivo. J Dent Res 2005;84(8):741–6.

Hosaka K, Nishitani Y, Tagami J, Yoshiyama M, Brackett WW, Agee KA, et al. Durability of resin-dentin bonds to water- vs. ethanol-saturated dentin. J Dent Res 2009;88(2):146–51.

Huang L, Xiao YH, Xing XD, Li F, Ma S, Qi LL, et al. Antibacterial activity and cytotoxicity of two novel cross-linking antibacterial monomers on oral pathogens. Arch Oral Biol 2011;56(4):367–73.

Huang L, Sun X, Xiao YH, Dong Y, Tong ZC, Xing XD, et al. Antibacterial effect of a resin incorporating a novel polymerizable quaternary ammonium salt MAE-DB against *Streptococcus mutans*. J Biomed Mater Res B Appl Biomater 2012;100(5):1353–8.

Huang YP, Kimura M, Tawada K. Covalent crosslinking of myosin subfragment-1 and heavy meromyosin to actin at various molar ratios: different correlations between ATPase activity and crosslinking extent. J Muscle Res Cell Motil 1990;11(4):313–22.

Imazato S, Torii M, Tsuchitani Y, McCabe JF, Russell RR. Incorporation of bacterial inhibitor into resin composite. J Dent Res 1994;73(8):1437–43.

Imazato S, Kinomoto Y, Tarumi H, Torii M, Russell RR, McCabe JF. Incorporation of antibacterial monomer MDPB into dentin primer. J Dent Res 1997;76(3):768–72.

Imazato S, Ehara A, Torii M, Ebisu S. Antibacterial activity of dentine primer containing MDPB after curing. J Dent 1998a;26(3):267–71.

Imazato S, Imai T, Russell RR, Torii M, Ebisu S. Antibacterial activity of cured dental resin incorporating the antibacterial monomer MDPB and an adhesion-promoting monomer. J Biomed Mater Res 1998b;39(4):511–5.

Imazato S, Ebi N, Tarumi H, Russell RR, Kaneko T, Ebisu S. Bactericidal activity and cytotoxicity of antibacterial monomer MDPB. Biomaterials 1999;20(9):899–903.

Imazato S, Tarumi H, Ebi N, Ebisu S. Cytotoxic effects of composite restorations employing self-etching primers or experimental antibacterial primers. J Dent 2000;28(1):61–7.

Imazato S, Torii Y, Takatsuka T, Inoue K, Ebi N, Ebisu S. Bactericidal effect of dentin primer containing antibacterial monomer methacryloyloxydodecylpyridinium bromide (MDPB) against bacteria in human carious dentin. J Oral Rehabil 2001;28(4):314–9.

Imazato S, Walls AW, Kuramoto A, Ebisu S. Penetration of an antibacterial dentine-bonding system into demineralized human root dentine in vitro. Eur J Oral Sci 2002;110(2):168–74.

Imazato S. Antibacterial properties of resin composites and dentin bonding systems. Dent Mater 2003;19(6):449–57.

Imazato S, Ebi N, Takahashi Y, Kaneko T, Ebisu S, Russell RR. Antibacterial activity of bactericide-immobilized filler for resin-based restoratives. Biomaterials 2003a;24(20):3605–9.

Imazato S, Kinomoto Y, Tarumi H, Ebisu S, Tay FR. Antibacterial activity and bonding characteristics of an adhesive resin containing antibacterial monomer MDPB. Dent Mater 2003b;19(4):313–9.

Imazato S, Kaneko T, Takahashi Y, Noiri Y, Ebisu S. In vivo antibacterial effects of dentin primer incorporating MDPB. Oper Dent 2004;29(4):369–75.

Imazato S, Kuramoto A, Takahashi Y, Ebisu S, Peters MC. In vitro antibacterial effects of the dentin primer of Clearfil Protect Bond. Dent Mater 2006;22(6):527–32.

Imazato S, Tay FR, Kaneshiro AV, Takahashi Y, Ebisu S. An in vivo evaluation of bonding ability of comprehensive antibacterial adhesive system incorporating MDPB. Dent Mater 2007;23(2):170–6.

Imazato S, Ma S, Chen JH, Xu HH. Therapeutic polymers for dental adhesives: loading resins with bio-active components. Dent Mater 2014;30(1):97–104.

Inoue S, Vargas MA, Abe Y, Yoshida Y, Lambrechts P, Vanherle G, et al. Microtensile bond strength of eleven contemporary adhesives to dentin. J Adhes Dent 2001;3(3):237–45.

Ishiguro K, Yamashita K, Nakagaki H, Iwata K, Hayakawa T. Identification of tissue inhibitor of metalloproteinases-1 (TIMP-1) in human teeth and its distribution in cementum and dentine. Arch Oral Biol 1994;39(4):345–9.

Kanca 3rd J. Improving bond strength through acid etching of dentin and bonding to wet dentin surfaces. J Am Dent Assoc 1992;123(9):35–43.

Katoh Y, Suzuki M, Kato C, Shinkai K, Ogawa M, Yamauchi J. Observation of calcium phosphate powder mixed with an adhesive monomer experimentally developed for direct pulp capping and as a bonding agent. Dent Mater J 2010;29(1):15–24.

Kim J, Arola DD, Gu L, Kim YK, Mai S, Liu Y, et al. Functional biomimetic analogs help remineralize apatite-depleted demineralized resin-infiltrated dentin via a bottom-up approach. Acta Biomater 2010a;6(7):2740–50.

Kim J, Vaughn RM, Gu L, Rockman RA, Arola DD, Schafer TE, et al. Imperfect hybrid layers created by an aggressive one-step self-etch adhesive in primary dentin are amendable to biomimetic remineralization in vitro. J Biomed Mater Res A 2010b;93(4):1225–34.

Kim YK, Gu LS, Bryan TE, Kim JR, Chen L, Liu Y, et al. Mineralisation of reconstituted collagen using polyvinylphosphonic acid/polyacrylic acid templating matrix protein analogues in the presence of calcium, phosphate and hydroxyl ions. Biomaterials 2010c;31(25):6618–27.

Kim YK, Mai S, Mazzoni A, Liu Y, Tezvergil-Mutluay A, Takahashi K, et al. Biomimetic remineralization as a progressive dehydration mechanism of collagen matrices–implications in the aging of resin-dentin bonds. Acta Biomater 2010d;6(9):3729–39.

Kong H, Jang J. Antibacterial properties of novel poly(methyl methacrylate) nanofiber containing silver nanoparticles. Langmuir 2008;24(5):2051–6.

Langhorst SE, O'Donnell JN, Skrtic D. In vitro remineralization of enamel by polymeric amorphous calcium phosphate composite: quantitative microradiographic study. Dent Mater 2009;25(7):884–91.

Lehmann N, Debret R, Romeas A, Magloire H, Degrange M, Bleicher F, et al. Self-etching increases matrix metalloproteinase expression in the dentin-pulp complex. J Dent Res 2009;88(1):77–82.

Lendenmann U, Grogan J, Oppenheim FG. Saliva and dental pellicle–a review. Adv Dent Res 2000;14:22–8.

Li F, Chai ZG, Sun MN, Wang F, Ma S, Zhang L, et al. Anti-biofilm effect of dental adhesive with cationic monomer. J Dent Res 2009a;88(4):372–6.

Li F, Chen J, Chai Z, Zhang L, Xiao Y, Fang M, et al. Effects of a dental adhesive incorporating antibacterial monomer on the growth, adherence and membrane integrity of *Streptococcus mutans*. J Dent 2009b;37(4):289–96.

Li F, Weir MD, Chen J, Xu HH. Comparison of quaternary ammonium-containing with nano-silver-containing adhesive in antibacterial properties and cytotoxicity. Dent Mater 2013a;29(4):450–61.

Li F, Weir MD, Fouad AF, Xu HH. Time-kill behaviour against eight bacterial species and cytotoxicity of antibacterial monomers. J Dent 2013b;41(10):881–91.

Li F, Weir MD, Xu HH. Effects of quaternary ammonium chain length on antibacterial bonding agents. J Dent Res 2013c;92(10):932–8.

Li F, Wang P, Weir MD, Fouad AF, Xu HH. Evaluation of antibacterial and remineralizing nanocomposite and adhesive in rat tooth cavity model. Acta Biomater 2014a;10(6):2804–13.

Li F, Weir MD, Chen J, Xu HH. Effect of charge density of bonding agent containing a new quaternary ammonium methacrylate on antibacterial and bonding properties. Dent Mater 2014b;30(4):433–41.

Li F, Weir MD, Fouad AF, Xu HH. Effect of salivary pellicle on antibacterial activity of novel antibacterial dental adhesives using a dental plaque microcosm biofilm model. Dent Mater 2014c;30(2):182–91.

Li F, Majd H, Weir MD, Arola DD, Xu HH. Inhibition of matrix metalloproteinase activity in human dentin via novel antibacterial monomer. Dent Mater 2015;31(3):284–92.

Liu N, Li F, Chen YJ, Zhang L, Lu S, Kang JJ, et al. The inhibitory effect of a polymerisable cationic monomer on functional matrix metalloproteinases. J Dent 2013;41(11):1101–8.

Liu Y, Li N, Qi YP, Dai L, Bryan TE, Mao J, et al. Intrafibrillar collagen mineralization produced by biomimetic hierarchical nanoapatite assembly. Adv Mater 2011a;23(8):975–80.

Liu Y, Mai S, Li N, Yiu CK, Mao J, Pashley DH, et al. Differences between top-down and bottom-up approaches in mineralizing thick, partially demineralized collagen scaffolds. Acta Biomater 2011b;7(4):1742–51.

Liu Y, Tjaderhane L, Breschi L, Mazzoni A, Li N, Mao J, et al. Limitations in bonding to dentin and experimental strategies to prevent bond degradation. J Dent Res 2011c;90(8):953–68.

Mai S, Kim YK, Toledano M, Breschi L, Ling JQ, Pashley DH, et al. Phosphoric acid esters cannot replace polyvinylphosphonic acid as phosphoprotein analogs in biomimetic remineralization of resin-bonded dentin. Dent Mater 2009;25(10):1230–9.

Mai S, Kim YK, Kim J, Yiu CK, Ling J, Pashley DH, et al. In vitro remineralization of severely compromised bonded dentin. J Dent Res 2010;89(4):405–10.

Manuja N, Nagpal R, Pandit IK. Dental adhesion: mechanism, techniques and durability. J Clin Pediatr Dent 2012;36(3):223–34.

Mazzoni A, Pashley DH, Nishitani Y, Breschi L, Mannello F, Tjaderhane L, et al. Reactivation of inactivated endogenous proteolytic activities in phosphoric acid-etched dentine by etch-and-rinse adhesives. Biomaterials 2006;27(25):4470–6.

Mazzoni A, Mannello F, Tay FR, Tonti GA, Papa S, Mazzotti G, et al. Zymographic analysis and characterization of MMP-2 and -9 forms in human sound dentin. J Dent Res 2007;86(5):436–40.

Mazzoni A, Scaffa P, Carrilho M, Tjaderhane L, Di Lenarda R, Polimeni A, et al. Effects of etch-and-rinse and self-etch adhesives on dentin MMP-2 and MMP-9. J Dent Res 2013;92(1):82–6.

Mazzoni A, Tjaderhane L, Checchi V, Di Lenarda R, Salo T, Tay FR, et al. Role of dentin MMPs in caries progression and bond stability. J Dent Res 2015;94(2):241–51.

McCabe JF, Walls AWG, editors. Applied dental materials. Oxford: Blackwell Publishing; 2008.

Melo MA, Cheng L, Weir MD, Hsia RC, Rodrigues LK, Xu HH. Novel dental adhesive containing antibacterial agents and calcium phosphate nanoparticles. J Biomed Mater Res B Appl Biomater 2013a;101(4):620–9.

Melo MA, Cheng L, Zhang K, Weir MD, Rodrigues LK, Xu HH. Novel dental adhesives containing nanoparticles of silver and amorphous calcium phosphate. Dent Mater 2013b;29(2):199–210.

Mjor IA, Toffenetti F. Secondary caries: a literature review with case reports. Quintessence Int 2000;31(3):165–79.

Moore WE, Moore LV. The bacteria of periodontal diseases. Periodontol 2000 1994;5:66–77.

Morones JR, Elechiguerra JL, Camacho A, Holt K, Kouri JB, Ramirez JT, et al. The bactericidal effect of silver nanoparticles. Nanotechnology 2005;16(10):2346–53.

Mount GJ, Ngo H. Minimal intervention: advanced lesions. Quintessence Int 2000;31(9):621–9.

Muller R, Eidt A, Hiller KA, Katzur V, Subat M, Schweikl H, et al. Influences of protein films on antibacterial or bacteria-repellent surface coatings in a model system using silicon wafers. Biomaterials 2009;30(28):4921–9.

Nakabayashi N, Pashley DH, editors. Hybridization of dental hard tissues. 1998.

Namba N, Yoshida Y, Nagaoka N, Takashima S, Matsuura-Yoshimoto K, Maeda H, et al. Antibacterial effect of bactericide immobilized in resin matrix. Dent Mater 2009;25(4):424–30.

Nishida M, Imazato S, Takahashi Y, Ebisu S, Ishimoto T, Nakano T, et al. The influence of the antibacterial monomer 12-methacryloyloxydodecylpyridinium bromide on the proliferation, differentiation and mineralization of odontoblast-like cells. Biomaterials 2010;31(7):1518–32.

Nishitani Y, Yoshiyama M, Wadgaonkar B, Breschi L, Mannello F, Mazzoni A, et al. Activation of gelatinolytic/collagenolytic activity in dentin by self-etching adhesives. Eur J Oral Sci 2006;114(2):160–6.

Niu LN, Zhang W, Pashley DH, Breschi L, Mao J, Chen JH, et al. Biomimetic remineralization of dentin. Dent Mater 2014;30(1):77–96.

Oyarzun A, Rathkamp H, Dreyer E. Immunohistochemical and ultrastructural evaluation of the effects of phosphoric acid etching on dentin proteoglycans. Eur J Oral Sci 2000;108(6):546–54.

Pallavicini P, Taglietti A, Dacarro G, Diaz-Fernandez YA, Galli M, Grisoli P, et al. Self-assembled monolayers of silver nanoparticles firmly grafted on glass surfaces: low Ag^+ release for an efficient antibacterial activity. J Colloid Interface Sci 2010;350(1):110–6.

Park JG, Ye Q, Topp EM, Kostoryz EL, Wang Y, Kieweg SL, et al. Preparation and properties of novel dentin adhesives with esterase resistance. J Appl Polym Sci Symp 2008;107(6):3588–97.

Park JG, Ye Q, Topp EM, Spencer P. Enzyme-catalyzed hydrolysis of dentin adhesives containing a new urethane-based trimethacrylate monomer. J Biomed Mater Res B Appl Biomater 2009;91(2):562–71.

Park JG, Ye Q, Topp EM, Misra A, Kieweg SL, Spencer P. Effect of photoinitiator system and water content on dynamic mechanical properties of a light-cured bisGMA/HEMA dental resin. J Biomed Mater Res A 2010;93(4):1245–51.

Parthasarathy R, Misra A, Park J, Ye Q, Spencer P. Diffusion coefficients of water and leachables in methacrylate-based crosslinked polymers using absorption experiments. J Mater Sci Mater Med 2012;23(5):1157–72.

Pashley DH, Tay FR, Yiu C, Hashimoto M, Breschi L, Carvalho RM, et al. Collagen degradation by host-derived enzymes during aging. J Dent Res 2004;83(3):216–21.

Pashley DH, Tay FR, Carvalho RM, Rueggeberg FA, Agee KA, Carrilho M, et al. From dry bonding to water-wet bonding to ethanol-wet bonding. A review of the interactions between dentin matrix and solvated resins using a macromodel of the hybrid layer. Am J Dent 2007;20(1):7–20.

Pashley DH, Tay FR, Breschi L, Tjaderhane L, Carvalho RM, Carrilho M, et al. State of the art etch-and-rinse adhesives. Dent Mater 2011;27(1):1–16.

Paster BJ, Boches SK, Galvin JL, Ericson RE, Lau CN, Levanos VA, et al. Bacterial diversity in human subgingival plaque. J Bacteriol 2001;183(12):3770–83.

Peng JJ, Botelho MG, Matinlinna JP. Silver compounds used in dentistry for caries management: a review. J Dent 2012;40(7).

Perdigao J. Dentin bonding-variables related to the clinical situation and the substrate treatment. Dent Mater 2010;26(2):e24–37.

Pereira PN, Bedran-de-Castro AK, Duarte WR, Yamauchi M. Removal of noncollagenous components affects dentin bonding. J Biomed Mater Res B Appl Biomater 2007;80(1):86–91.

Petite H, Duval JL, Frei V, Abdul-Malak N, Sigot-Luizard MF, Herbage D. Cytocompatibility of calf pericardium treated by glutaraldehyde and by the acyl azide methods in an organotypic culture model. Biomaterials 1995;16(13):1003–8.

Peumans M, Kanumilli P, De Munck J, Van Landuyt K, Lambrechts P, Van Meerbeek B. Clinical effectiveness of contemporary adhesives: a systematic review of current clinical trials. Dent Mater 2005;21(9):864–81.

Rai M, Yadav A, Gade A. Silver nanoparticles as a new generation of antimicrobials. Biotechnol Adv 2009;27(1):76–83.

Ricci HA, Sanabe ME, de Souza Costa CA, Pashley DH, Hebling J. Chlorhexidine increases the longevity of in vivo resin-dentin bonds. Eur J Oral Sci 2010;118(4):411–6.

Ryou H, Niu LN, Dai L, Pucci CR, Arola DD, Pashley DH, et al. Effect of biomimetic remineralization on the dynamic nanomechanical properties of dentin hybrid layers. J Dent Res 2011;90(9):1122–8.

Sadek FT, Pashley DH, Nishitani Y, Carrilho MR, Donnelly A, Ferrari M, et al. Application of hydrophobic resin adhesives to acid-etched dentin with an alternative wet bonding technique. J Biomed Mater Res A 2008;84(1):19–29.

Sadek FT, Braga RR, Muench A, Liu Y, Pashley DH, Tay FR. Ethanol wet-bonding challenges current anti-degradation strategy. J Dent Res 2010a;89(12):1499–504.

Sadek FT, Castellan CS, Braga RR, Mai S, Tjaderhane L, Pashley DH, et al. One-year stability of resin-dentin bonds created with a hydrophobic ethanol-wet bonding technique. Dent Mater 2010b;26(4):380–6.

Sakaguchi RL. Review of the current status and challenges for dental posterior restorative composites: clinical, chemistry, and physical behavior considerations. Summary of discussion from the Portland Composites Symposium (POCOS) June 17–19, 2004, Oregon Health and Science University, Portland, Oregon. Dent Mater 2005;21(1):3–6.

Sartor L, Pezzato E, Dell'Aica I, Caniato R, Biggin S, Garbisa S. Inhibition of matrix-proteases by polyphenols: chemical insights for anti-inflammatory and anti-invasion drug design. Biochem Pharmacol 2002;64(2):229–37.

Sauro S, Watson TF, Mannocci F, Miyake K, Huffman BP, Tay FR, et al. Two-photon laser confocal microscopy of micropermeability of resin-dentin bonds made with water or ethanol wet bonding. J Biomed Mater Res B Appl Biomater 2009;90(1):327–37.

Scheffel DL, Hebling J, Scheffel RH, Agee KA, Cadenaro M, Turco G, et al. Stabilization of dentin matrix after cross-linking treatments, in vitro. Dent Mater 2014;30(2):227–33.

Schmalz G, Ergucu Z, Hiller KA. Effect of dentin on the antibacterial activity of dentin bonding agents. J Endod 2004;30(5):352–8.

Scott JE, Thomlinson AM. The structure of interfibrillar proteoglycan bridges (shape modules') in extracellular matrix of fibrous connective tissues and their stability in various chemical environments. J Anat 1998;192(Pt 3):391–405.

Shahverdi AR, Fakhimi A, Shahverdi HR, Minaian S. Synthesis and effect of silver nanoparticles on the antibacterial activity of different antibiotics against *Staphylococcus aureus* and *Escherichia coli*. Nanomedicine 2007;3(2):168–71.

Shin TP, Yao X, Huenergardt R, Walker MP, Wang Y. Morphological and chemical characterization of bonding hydrophobic adhesive to dentin using ethanol wet bonding technique. Dent Mater 2009;25(8):1050–7.

Shokati B, Tam LE, Santerre JP, Finer Y. Effect of salivary esterase on the integrity and fracture toughness of the dentin-resin interface. J Biomed Mater Res B Appl Biomater 2010;94(1):230–7.

Silver FH, Horvath I, Foran DJ. Viscoelasticity of the vessel wall: the role of collagen and elastic fibers. Crit Rev Biomed Eng 2001;29(3):279–301.

Simoncic B, Tomcis B. Structures of novel antimicrobial agents for textiles - a review. Text Res J 2010;80:1721–37.

Spencer P, Wang Y. Adhesive phase separation at the dentin interface under wet bonding conditions. J Biomed Mater Res 2002;62(3):447–56.

Spencer P, Ye Q, Park J, Topp EM, Misra A, Marangos O, et al. Adhesive/Dentin interface: the weak link in the composite restoration. Ann Biomed Eng 2010;38(6):1989–2003.

Spencer P, Ye Q, Misra A, Goncalves SE, Laurence JS. Proteins, pathogens, and failure at the composite-tooth interface. J Dent Res 2014;93(12):1243–9.

Stangel I, Ellis TH, Sacher E. Adhesion to tooth structure mediated by contemporary bonding systems. Dent Clin North Am 2007;51(3):677–94. vii.

Sulkala M, Wahlgren J, Larmas M, Sorsa T, Teronen O, Salo T, et al. The effects of MMP inhibitors on human salivary MMP activity and caries progression in rats. J Dent Res 2001;80(6):1545–9.

Sulkala M, Tervahartiala T, Sorsa T, Larmas M, Salo T, Tjaderhane L. Matrix metalloproteinase-8 (MMP-8) is the major collagenase in human dentin. Arch Oral Biol 2007;52(2):121–7.

Sung HW, Huang DM, Chang WH, Huang RN, Hsu JC. Evaluation of gelatin hydrogel crosslinked with various crosslinking agents as bioadhesives: in vitro study. J Biomed Mater Res 1999;46(4):520–30.

Sung HW, Chang WH, Ma CY, Lee MH. Crosslinking of biological tissues using genipin and/or carbodiimide. J Biomed Mater Res A 2003;64(3):427–38.

Tay FR, Pashley DH, Kapur RR, Carrilho MR, Hur YB, Garrett LV, et al. Bonding BisGMA to dentin–a proof of concept for hydrophobic dentin bonding. J Dent Res 2007;86(11):1034–9.

Tay FR, Pashley DH. Guided tissue remineralisation of partially demineralised human dentine. Biomaterials 2008;29(8):1127–37.

Tay FR, Pashley DH. Biomimetic remineralization of resin-bonded acid-etched dentin. J Dent Res 2009;88(8):719–24.

Tersariol IL, Geraldeli S, Minciotti CL, Nascimento FD, Paakkonen V, Martins MT, et al. Cysteine cathepsins in human dentin-pulp complex. J Endod 2010;36(3):475–81.
Tezvergil-Mutluay A, Agee KA, Hoshika T, Tay FR, Pashley DH. The inhibitory effect of polyvinylphosphonic acid on functional matrix metalloproteinase activities in human demineralized dentin. Acta Biomater 2010;6(10):4136–42.
Tezvergil-Mutluay A, Agee KA, Uchiyama T, Imazato S, Mutluay MM, Cadenaro M, et al. The inhibitory effects of quaternary ammonium methacrylates on soluble and matrix-bound MMPs. J Dent Res 2011a;90(4):535–40.
Tezvergil-Mutluay A, Mutluay MM, Gu LS, Zhang K, Agee KA, Carvalho RM, et al. The anti-MMP activity of benzalkonium chloride. J Dent 2011b;39(1):57–64.
Tjaderhane L, Larjava H, Sorsa T, Uitto VJ, Larmas M, Salo T. The activation and function of host matrix metalloproteinases in dentin matrix breakdown in caries lesions. J Dent Res 1998;77(8):1622–9.
Tjaderhane L, Nascimento FD, Breschi L, Mazzoni A, Tersariol IL, Geraldeli S, et al. Strategies to prevent hydrolytic degradation of the hybrid layer-a review. Dent Mater 2013;29(10):999–1011.
Van Landuyt KL, Snauwaert J, De Munck J, Peumans M, Yoshida Y, Poitevin A, et al. Systematic review of the chemical composition of contemporary dental adhesives. Biomaterials 2007;28(26):3757–85.
Van Meerbeek B, Peumans M, Poitevin A, Mine A, Van Ende A, Neves A, et al. Relationship between bond-strength tests and clinical outcomes. Dent Mater 2010;26(2):e100–121.
Van Meerbeek B, Yoshihara K, Yoshida Y, Mine A, De Munck J, Van Landuyt KL. State of the art of self-etch adhesives. Dent Mater 2011;27(1):17–28.
van Strijp AJ, Jansen DC, DeGroot J, ten Cate JM, Everts V. Host-derived proteinases and degradation of dentine collagen in situ. Caries Res 2003;37(1):58–65.
Visse R, Nagase H. Matrix metalloproteinases and tissue inhibitors of metalloproteinases: structure, function, and biochemistry. Circ Res 2003;92(8):827–39.
Walter R, Miguez PA, Arnold RR, Pereira PN, Duarte WR, Yamauchi M. Effects of natural cross-linkers on the stability of dentin collagen and the inhibition of root caries in vitro. Caries Res 2008;42(4):263–8.
Weir MD, Chow LC, Xu HH. Remineralization of demineralized enamel via calcium phosphate nanocomposite. J Dent Res 2012;91(10):979–84.
Xu HH, Sun L, Weir MD, Antonucci JM, Takagi S, Chow LC, et al. Nano DCPA-whisker composites with high strength and Ca and PO(4) release. J Dent Res 2006;85(8):722–7.
Xu HH, Weir MD, Sun L, Moreau JL, Takagi S, Chow LC, et al. Strong nanocomposites with Ca, PO(4), and F release for caries inhibition. J Dent Res 2010;89(1):19–28.
Xu HH, Moreau JL, Sun L, Chow LC. Nanocomposite containing amorphous calcium phosphate nanoparticles for caries inhibition. Dent Mater 2011;27(8):762–9.
Ye Q, Park J, Topp E, Spencer P. Effect of photoinitiators on the in vitro performance of a dentin adhesive exposed to simulated oral environment. Dent Mater 2009;25(4):452–8.
Yoshida K, Tanagawa M, Atsuta M. Characterization and inhibitory effect of antibacterial dental resin composites incorporating silver-supported materials. J Biomed Mater Res 1999;47(4):516–22.
Yoshida Y, Yoshihara K, Hayakawa S, Nagaoka N, Okihara T, Matsumoto T, et al. HEMA inhibits interfacial nano-layering of the functional monomer MDP. J Dent Res 2012a;91(11):1060–5.
Yoshida Y, Yoshihara K, Nagaoka N, Hayakawa S, Torii Y, Ogawa T, et al. Self-assembled nano-layering at the adhesive interface. J Dent Res 2012b;91(4):376–81.
Yoshihara K, Yoshida Y, Hayakawa S, Nagaoka N, Irie M, Ogawa T, et al. Nanolayering of phosphoric acid ester monomer on enamel and dentin. Acta Biomater 2011;7(8):3187–95.

Zhang K, Melo MA, Cheng L, Weir MD, Bai Y, Xu HH. Effect of quaternary ammonium and silver nanoparticle-containing adhesives on dentin bond strength and dental plaque microcosm biofilms. Dent Mater 2012;28(8):842–52.

Zhang K, Cheng L, Wu EJ, Weir MD, Bai Y, Xu HH. Effect of water-ageing on dentine bond strength and anti-biofilm activity of bonding agent containing new monomer dimethylaminododecyl methacrylate. J Dent 2013a;41(6):504–13.

Zhang K, Li F, Imazato S, Cheng L, Liu H, Arola DD, et al. Dual antibacterial agents of nano-silver and 12-methacryloyloxydodecylpyridinium bromide in dental adhesive to inhibit caries. J Biomed Mater Res B Appl Biomater 2013b;101(6):929–38.

Zhou J, Tan J, Yang X, Cheng C, Wang X, Chen L. Effect of chlorhexidine application in a self-etching adhesive on the immediate resin-dentin bond strength. J Adhes Dent 2010;12(1):27–31.

Biology of the oral environment and its impact on the stability of dental and craniofacial reconstructions

7

M.H. Tanaka, G.M.G. Lima, C.Y. Koga Ito
Universidade Estadual Paulista (UNESP), São Paulo, Brazil

7.1 Salivary factors

Saliva is a secretion derived from three-paired major salivary glands (parotid, submandibular, and sublingual glands) and numerous minor salivary glands (Fig. 7.1). This secretion, together with the gingival crevicular fluid, constitutes the oral fluid or whole saliva (Edgar, 1992; Sas and Dawes, 1997; Huang, 2004; Huq et al., 2007; Sun et al., 2008; Amado et al., 2013).

Salivary production is higher in major glands than in minor ones; however, the quality and the type of protection differ (Humphrey and Williamson, 2001). Each type of gland secretes a different type of saliva that can be classified as serous, mucous, or mixed (Pfaffe et al., 2011). Parotid glands produce mainly serous secretions and are located in the subcutaneous tissues in front of the ear and behind the ramus of the mandible. The sublingual glands produce mixed serous and mucous secretions and are situated in the floor of the mouth beneath the sublingual folds of mucous membrane. The submandibular glands produce mixed serous and mucous secretions and are located beneath the lower jaws. The minor glands produce mainly mucous secretions, and they are found throughout the oral cavity (Humphrey and Williamson, 2001; Pfaffe et al., 2011; Schulz et al., 2013).

Despite the diversity of the fluid source, salivary composition also varies in stimulated or nonstimulated (basal flow) samples (Kalk et al., 2002). The contribution of the different salivary glands during basal flow can be described as follows: 20% from parotid, 65% from submandibular, 7–8% from sublingual, and less than 10% from numerous minor glands (Dawes, 2008; Saleh et al., 2015). Stimulated samples are drastically different: parotid contributes more than 50% of the total salivary secretion; submandibular, 35%; sublingual, 7–8%; and the minor glands, 7–8% (Edgar, 1990; Dodds et al., 2005; Dawes, 2008).

The basal salivary flow rate averages 0.3–0.4 mL/min in the oral cavity, but the range is broad (Dawes, 2004, 2008). The salivary flow rate can be modified by systemic diseases, degree of hydration, body position, exposure to light, masticatory stimulus, circadian rhythms, gland size, radiation treatment for head and neck cancer, and drug use (Dawes, 2004, 2008; Dodds et al., 2005). Clock genes are

Material-Tissue Interfacial Phenomena. http://dx.doi.org/10.1016/B978-0-08-100330-5.00007-8

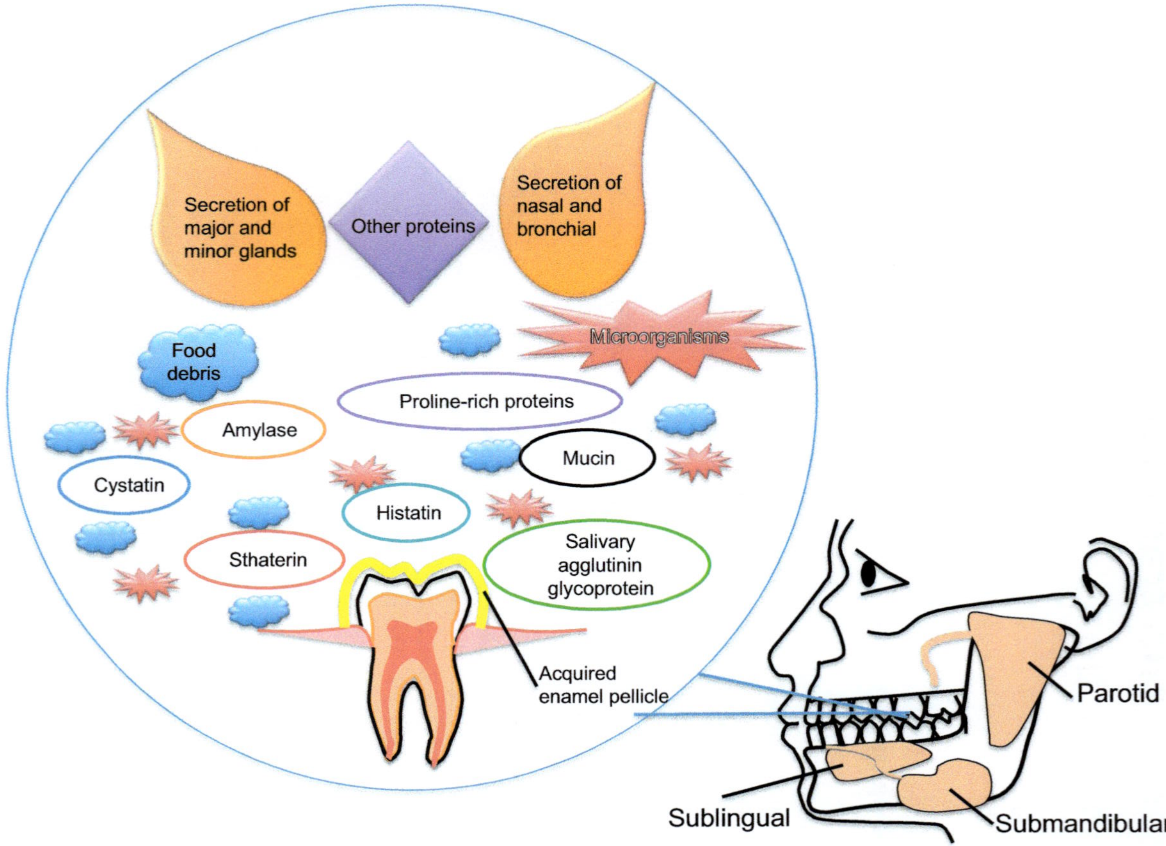

Figure 7.1 The components of whole saliva and the location of major salivary glands. Saliva is composed of secretions of major and minor salivary glands, a mixture of bronchial and nasal secretions, gingival crevicular fluid, as well as products from microorganisms, blood, cells, and food debris. The salivary proteins form the acquired enamel pellicle that is precursor of dental biofilm formation.

expressed in salivary glands, and they are in turn regulated by genes at specific daily times (Zheng et al., 2012). Clock genes are defined by a set of criteria that include circadian rhythm to regulate the type, amount, and content of saliva (Papagerakis et al., 2014).

Saliva is composed of water, a variety of electrolytes (such as sodium, potassium, calcium, magnesium, chloride, and phosphate), proteins, peptides, and other substances (Humphrey and Williamson, 2001; Chiappin et al., 2007; Navazesh et al., 2008; Amado et al., 2013). In addition, the oral fluid is also a mixture derived from expectorated bronchial and nasal secretions, as well as products from microorganism, blood, cells and food debris (Kaufman and Lamster, 2002; Huq et al., 2007). Salivary composition varies according to many factors including age, medications, circadian rhythm, flow rate, buffering capacity, and pH (Humphrey and Williamson, 2001; Zheng et al., 2012). Salivary composition can be modified by disease, such as Sjögren syndrome (Zhang et al., 2013; Delaleu et al., 2015), oral and head/neck cancers (Sivadasan et al., 2015), and systemic diseases including infections by HIV (Pfaffe et al., 2011) and hepatitis C virus (Al Kawas et al., 2012), type 2 diabetes (Desai and Mathews, 2014), insulin resistance (Desai and Mathews, 2014), cystic fibrosis (Livnat et al., 2010; Goncalves et al., 2013; Nie et al., 2015), and ectodermal dysplasia (Nordgarden et al., 2003; Lexner et al., 2007).

The functions of saliva are vital for the sustenance of healthy oral tissues and teeth, and it is necessary for talking, tasting perception, swallowing, oral digestion, lubrication, and microbial growth inhibition. Besides other functions, it also participates in dental and mucosal surface protection, due to the antimicrobial properties of saliva and its function in clearance (Tenovuo, 1998; Huq et al., 2007; Schulz et al., 2013). Salivary buffering system is the mechanism that maintains the pH in the oral cavity near neutral, protecting the teeth against attack from acids produced by microbial biofilms (Humphrey and Williamson, 2001; Moritsuka et al., 2006). The buffering capacity of saliva allows dental enamel remineralization, thus maintaining tooth integrity by inhibiting caries initiation and progression (Humphrey and Williamson, 2001; Moritsuka et al., 2006). Additionally, bicarbonate, phosphate, urea, amphoteric proteins, and enzymes are important for buffering capacity (Humphrey and Williamson, 2001). Also, the salivary clearance helps to maintain the resting pH around 6.0–7.0 and contributes to the removal of food, drinks, and food debris (Humphrey and Williamson, 2001; Dawes, 2008; Dawes et al., 2015).

The protection conferred by saliva is related to multiple components such as proline-rich proteins (PRPs), alpha-amylase, albumin, lysozyme, lactoferrin, lactoperoxidase, histatins (a group of proteins with antimicrobial activities), statherin (for calcium homeostasis), mucins (for lubrication), cystatins (cysteine protease inhibitors), secretory IgA (related to local immunity), and carbonic anhydrase (bicarbonate regulation) (Huang, 2004; Vitorino et al., 2004; Oppenheim et al., 2007; Denny et al., 2008; Al Kawas et al., 2012; Amado et al., 2013; Gibbins et al., 2015).

Most of these proteins have been investigated; however, comprehensive analyses and identification of the other salivary proteins are still necessary to fully understand the oral pathophysiology. This knowledge may also allow the future use of salivary proteins and peptides as biomarkers.

7.2 Overview of salivary proteins

Differences related to synthesis, secretion, and function are observed among the salivary proteins produced by each gland (Carpenter, 2013). For better understanding the salivary proteins, it is important to recognize the structural features of the major salivary protein families, such as amylases, histatins, PRPs, statherin, mucins, and cystatins (Oppenheim et al., 2007; Denny et al., 2008) (Fig. 7.1 and Table 7.1).

Alpha-amylase (α1,4-glucan 4-glucanohydrolase) is the most abundant protein. It is mainly synthesized by the parotid, and it is involved in the initial food digestion. Once a swallowed food bolus is impregnated with acidic gastric, the amylase is inactivated (Oppenheim et al., 2007; Carpenter, 2013; Dawes et al., 2015). This enzyme can cleave starch into maltose, maltotriose, and maltotetrose and provide an abundant source of carbohydrate for oral bacterial nutrition. It may benefit several oral streptococcal species that selectively bind to human salivary amylase (Nikitkova et al., 2013; Dawes et al., 2015; Sabharwal et al., 2015). However, alpha-amylase exhibits inhibitory activity against *Porphyromonas gingivalis* (Ochiai et al., 2014).

Histatins are a group salivary proteins that have the lowest molecular weight and are secreted by major and minor salivary glands (Oppenheim et al., 2007; Siqueira et al., 2008; Vukosavljevic et al., 2014). The most abundant proteins in glandular secretions are histatins 1, 3 and 5 that correspond to 80% of the total. (Oppenheim et al., 2007). Histatins are considered relevant to the innate oral host defense system and show inhibitory activity against *Candida albicans* (Vukosavljevic et al., 2012; Puri and Edgerton, 2014; Puri et al., 2015). Also, histatins can reduce *Streptococcus mutans* adhesion to hydroxyapatite's (HA) surface (Shimotoyodome et al., 2006). Moreover, these proteins have strong molecular adhesive forces to HA, resulting in high affinity

Table 7.1 Major salivary proteins families, main sources, and function

Protein	Main source	Function
α-Amylase	Parotid gland	Involved in the initial food digestion
Histatins	Major and minor salivary glands	Innate oral host defense system and involved in the development of the AEP
PRPs	Parotid saliva	Act as lubricant and are able to bind to bacteria, fungi, and viruses
Statherins	Major and minor salivary glands	Inhibit calcium phosphate precipitation and can inhibit the growth of anaerobic bacteria
Cystatins	Submandibular and sublingual glands than parotid	Regulation of salivary calcium and antimicrobial activity
Mucins	Major glands (except, parotid gland)	Lubricant and antifungal and bactericidal activities
SAG	All salivary glands	Clearance of the microorganisms and inhibit the attachment to AEP

to dental enamel. Histatins, PRPs, and staterin are the main proteins involved in the development of the acquired enamel pellicle (AEP) (Siqueira et al., 2012; Vukosavljevic et al., 2014).

PRPs form a major fraction of salivary proteins, and many of these proteins contain high levels of proline (35–40%). Almost 70% of the total protein comes from parotid saliva (Huq et al., 2007; Oppenheim et al., 2007; Buzalaf et al., 2012; Fabian et al., 2015). PRPs are classified as acidic with calcium hydroxide–binding properties in AEP. They act as a thin protein layer on dental surface and can also bind to bacteria. Basic PRPs are also present in the AEP and show binding interactions with fungi and viruses. Also, basic glycosylated PRPs act as lubricants and are able to bind to bacteria and viruses (Tenovuo, 2002; Huq et al., 2007; Vitorino et al., 2008; Fabian et al., 2015).

Statherins are very similar to histatins due to the low molecular weight. Statherin is also secreted by the major and minor salivary glands (Oppenheim et al., 2007; Xiao et al., 2015). This small salivary protein is rich in tyrosine and proline and contains phosphoserine residues at positions 2 and 3 (Xiao et al., 2015). Levels of statherin in whole saliva are considerably low due to proteolytic degradation and strong affinity to dental surfaces (Oppenheim et al., 2007; Dawes et al., 2015; Xiao et al., 2015). However, statherin is the most effective salivary protein to inhibit calcium phosphate precipitation, and it can also inhibit the growth of anaerobic bacteria. At the same time, it notably contributes to the maintenance of intact tooth enamel (Oppenheim et al., 2007; Gorr, 2009; Buzalaf et al., 2012; Dawes et al., 2015; Xiao et al., 2015).

Cystatins are low-molecular-weight salivary proteins that are constituted by four main families associated with the inhibition of cysteine peptidases (CPs), such as cathepsins (Oppenheim et al., 2007; de Sousa-Pereira et al., 2014). The main cystatins secreted by salivary glands include cystatins S, SA, SN, C, and D. They are secreted more abundantly by the submandibular and sublingual glands than by the parotid glands (Oppenheim et al., 2007; de Sousa-Pereira et al., 2014; Fabian et al., 2015). S-type cystatins inhibit CP. These proteins (such as cystatin-SN and cystatin-S) play a role in the regulation of salivary calcium. They are also present in the AEP, which suggests participation in the maintenance and integrity of the tooth surfaces (Vitorino et al., 2008; de Sousa-Pereira et al., 2014). Additionally, cystatin-SN and cystatin-S can also bind to bacteria, specifically to bacterial lipopolysaccharides (Choi et al., 2011). Besides the inhibition of CPs, other activities have also been detected, such as antimicrobial activity (de Sousa-Pereira et al., 2014).

Mucins are high-molecular-weight glycoproteins, which are synthesized by major glands (except, parotid gland), and various minor salivary glands (eg, located in palatal, buccal, and labial mucosa) (Oppenheim et al., 2007; Kejriwal et al., 2014; Dawes et al., 2015). Two main glycoproteins are identified as MUC5B and MUC7, which are part of AEP and create a thin layer attached to the oral mucosa (Siqueira et al., 2007; Gibbins et al., 2014; Dawes et al., 2015). MUC5B is more effective as a lubricant than MUC7 (Dijkema et al., 2012), whereas MUC7 promotes the binding and clearance of microorganisms, exhibiting antifungal and bactericidal activities (Situ et al., 2003; Wei et al., 2006; Gorr, 2009; Kejriwal et al., 2014).

Another interesting salivary protein is salivary agglutinin glycoprotein (SAG), which has a dual function. They promote clearance of the microorganisms and inhibit the attachment to AEP (Gorr, 2009; Bikker et al., 2013; Spencer et al., 2014; Dawes et al., 2015). This high-molecular-weight glycoprotein is a member of scavenger receptor cysteine-rich superfamily and it is secreted by salivary and lacrimal glands (Gorr, 2009; Leito et al., 2011; Bikker et al., 2013).

7.3 Biofilms

Bacteria usually tend to attach to surfaces to form colonies, and approximately 99% of bacteria live as surface-attached cells. The adhesion process depends on surface characteristics, such as hydrophobicity and coating with adsorbed polymers. The first step of adhesion is the reversible adherence of a planktonic cell to a surface, followed by an irreversible phase mediated by exopolysaccharides. Next, adhered cells start to multiply to form microcolonies immersed in a hydrated matrix of self-produced extracellular polymeric substance, proteins, cell rests, DNA, RNA, and newly adhered cells. This matrix protects the biofilm and allows cell-to-cell and cell-to surface interactions (Costerton et al., 1987; Mancl et al., 2013). However, bacterial cell-surface properties and physiologic adjustment to the local surface is yet to be elucidated (Song et al., 2015). Interestingly, microbial phenotypic behavior may vary during the different phases of biofilm formation (Hall-Stoodley and Stoodley, 2002).

Some variables deeply affect the formation of a sessile biofilm. Microbial aspects such as motility, contributing to surface dispersal of the attached cells, cell binary division, recruitment of cells from the bulk fluid, and physicochemical conditions of the environment are among the most relevant factors (Hall-Stoodley and Stoodley, 2002). Recent evidence showed that cell aggregation can be the precursor behavior to biofilm formation (Alexandre, 2015). Motile cells constantly join and leave the aggregates interacting in a cell-to-cell manner to form new aggregates. This process is a result of chemotaxis signaling in a transient behavior in which the cells are not permanently adhered (Alexandre, 2015).

The microbial permanent attachment is mostly due to microbial metabolism and environmental changes that lead to cell surface interaction and biofilm formation. The interaction between microorganisms and extracellular environment, represented by extracellular polysaccharide (EPS) and surface adhesins, directly trigger the permanent attachment of cells (Alexandre, 2015).

Biofilm formation is a microbial survival strategy that provides equilibrium and stability to heterogenic communities to form clusters, mature, and disseminate in a dynamic environment (Hall-Stoodley and Stoodley, 2005). To date, it is known that the biofilm formation is a dynamic process involving microbial reversible cell attachment, cell aggregation, growth of the cells into a sessile biofilm colony, and then, detachment of matrix-enclosed aggregates, which contributes to biological dispersal and biofilm renovation (Hall-Stoodley and Stoodley, 2002; Emerenini et al., 2015).

Usually, pathogens in a biofilm are more prone to cause disease than planktonic cells. The heterogeneity of the microbial communities, cell density, and the ability to allow more efficient cell dissemination are important factors. Also, the differential expression of virulence-related genes in biofilms should be considered (Hall-Stoodley and Stoodley, 2005). Biofilm favors microbial antibiotic resistance mainly due to the presence of extracellular matrix and increase of microbial genetic competence (Fux et al., 2005). It is estimated that bacteria in biofilms are 100–1000 times more tolerant to antimicrobials than the corresponding planktonic cells (Olsen, 2015).

Surface properties, such as charge, roughness, energy, stiffness, and topography, show high influence on biofilm formation (Song et al., 2015). Considering that the bacterial cell is commonly negatively charged, positive surfaces can favor biofilm formation. Although nonviable cells can form a barrier that reduces charges, bacteria show the ability to resist surface changes and can break through this factor (Song et al., 2015). Although superhydrophobic, superhydrophilic, and nanometerscale roughness seem to reduce bacterial adhesion, other factors such as the AEP may help bacteria to overcome these factors and succeed in biofilm formation (Song et al., 2015).

The success of the biofilm formation is not only confined to metabolic consortia with compound exchange between species. Biofilm also provides mechanisms for intraspecies cooperation that are necessary for their survival. Bacteria can communicate regulating the gene expression of the whole population in a process called quorum sensing (QS). This process is responsible for not only modulating different activities on the bacterial community itself (such as metabolite production, motility, biofilm maturation, and virulence) but also between these communities and the environment. These complementary processes contribute to the environmental adaptation of the biofilm (Joint et al., 2007).

QS depends on the microbial density. When there is an increment in cell density, an increase in the concentration of chemical signaling molecules, called autoinducers (AIs) is observed. As the levels of these molecules reach a threshold, gene expression alteration is activated, which synchronizes collective behavior (Joint et al., 2007; Hall-Stoodley and Stoodley, 2009; Emerenini et al., 2015). QS leads to a stronger biofilm inducing continuous dispersal that balances the growth of the biofilm. It also provides a potential mechanism for the biofilm to regulate dispersal depending on its size to ensure the maintenance of the integrity (Emerenini et al., 2015). Moreover, evidence is emerging that QS may provide means for bacteria to directly interact with eukaryotes (Nobbs and Jenkinson, 2015). *N*-acyl-L-homoserine lactones (AHLs) are an important class of freely diffusible AIs produced exclusively by gram-negative bacteria (Karavolos, 2015). AHLs produced by *Pseudomonas aeruginosa* are able to inhibit *C. albicans* filamentation (Hogan et al., 2004). Previous studies have also shown that bacteria express adrenergic receptor. There is evidence that adrenergic hormones can characterize a cross-talk between host and bacteria. Pathogen exposure to adrenaline alerts the bacterial defenses against oxidative stress, whereas the same stimulus can act to support host defenses by reducing bacterial antimicrobial peptide resistance (Karavolos, 2015) (Fig. 7.2).

7.4 Oral biofilm

Oral biofilm can be regarded as a transition of bacteria from the planktonic microbiome to the adhering microbiome on oral hard and soft surfaces, mediated by ligand–receptor interactions and nonspecific Lifshitz-van der Waals, acid–base, and electrostatic forces (Wessel et al., 2014).

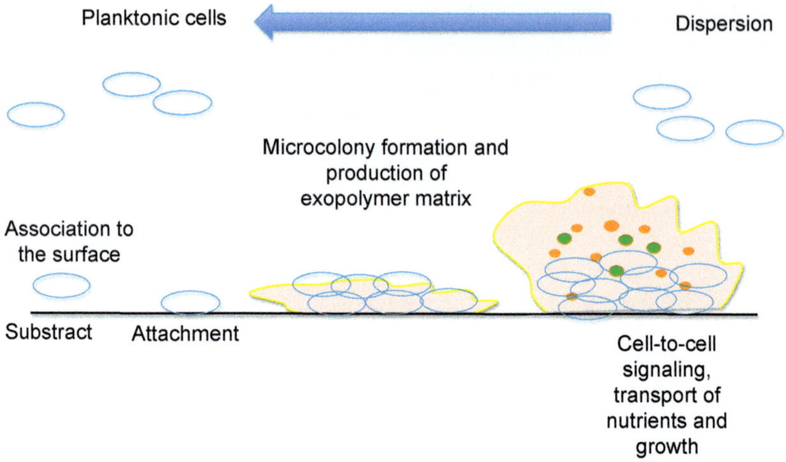

Figure 7.2 Steps of biofilm formation. In the first step, planktonic cells associate with a surface in a reversible stage. Thereafter, microbial cells attach to the surface in a stable stage. Cell division starts, and a microcolony is formed. At this stage, microbial cells start to be involved by exopolymer matrix. The biofilm gets into a maturation process, and cell-to-cell signaling (quorum sensing) starts. Nutrients and signaling molecules are transported inside the biofilm through the water channels. Maturation of biofilm is achieved, and new cells are continuously formed. The efficient cell-to-cell signaling and the protection offered by the matrix bring important ecological advantages to biofilm microbial community. Dispersion occurs by detachment of new cells from the biofilm. Those cells are able to colonize other surfaces.

In the oral environment, the AEP is formed both on biotic and abiotic oral surfaces. Teeth constitute approximately 20% of the oral surface area and consist of a crown and a root. Enamel is the hard and more mineralized part and involves the dentin which is formed and supported by the dental pulp. Teeth are attached to the bone of the jaw by the periodontium, consisting of the cementum, periodontal ligament, and alveolar bone (Nanci, 2013) (Fig. 7.3).

The AEP is formed by the selective adsorption of proteins, peptides, and other molecules, which are present in the oral fluid, onto the enamel surface (Lendenmann et al., 2000). It represents a source of receptors for primary colonizers, such as oral streptococci. The initial colonizers can attach to the oral surfaces mainly via adhesion receptor and charge interactions. Subsequently, late colonizers arrive and a multispecies biofilm is formed (Mancl et al., 2013; Wang et al., 2014; Song et al., 2015). Differences in the composition of planktonic and adhering oral microbiome on oral hard surfaces are related to the forces by which different bacterial species adhere to the tooth surface, ie, saliva-coated enamel (Wessel et al., 2014).

Biofilms are three-dimensional structures of several microbial species embedded in an exopolysaccharide matrix. In the oral cavity, biofilm formation starts with the AEP, formed by salivary components including glucosyltransferase (Gtfs) and fructosyltransferase, the primary sources of extracellular polysaccharide; salivary proteins, such as glycoprotein 340 (gp340); and bacterial components, which are the basis for the biofilm formation (Bowen and Koo, 2011; Krzysciak et al., 2014; Spencer et al., 2014).

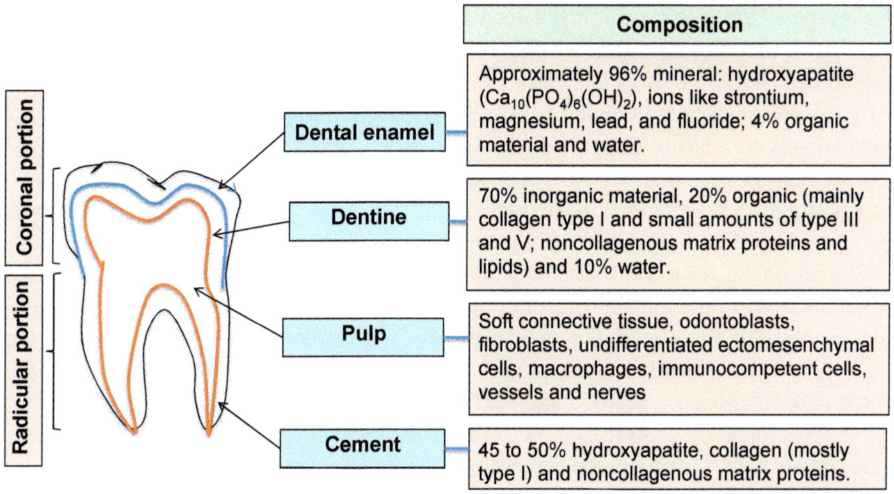

Figure 7.3 Dental structure and composition. The tooth is formed by mineralized tissues (dental enamel, dentine and cement) and pulp.
Based on Nanci A. Ten cate's oral histology: development, structure and function. 8th ed. 2013.

The main components of the biofilm formed on the dental surface include glucan (10–20% of dry weight), fructan (1–2% of dry weight), and proteins (40% dry matter) (Krzysciak et al., 2014). The structure of polysaccharide matrix influences the physical and biochemical properties of biofilm affecting microorganism-related factors, as well as the transport of substances through the biofilm and Gtfs (Krzysciak et al., 2014; Bowen and Koo, 2011).

Gtfs is adsorbed to saliva-coated HA. They facilitate the formation of glucan from sucrose and provide bacterial adhesion to tooth enamel (Bowen and Koo, 2011). *Streptococcus sanguinis*, *S. mutans*, *Streptococcus sobrinus*, *Actinomyces* spp., *Streptococcus salivarius*, and *Lactobacillus* spp. are the main Gtfs producers (Bowen and Koo, 2011). The effect of material properties on pellicle formation and the underlying mechanisms are not well understood (Song et al., 2015).

The oral biofilm formation is a multistep process where interactions between agglutinins of saliva and microorganisms cause the aggregation of early colonizers with *Actinomyces* spp., *Streptococcus* spp., *Lactobacillus* spp., and *Candida* spp. (Krzysciak et al., 2014). Within the first 24 h after dental cleaning, streptococci and Gram-positive pleomorphic rods colonize the oral surfaces. *Streptococcus sanguinis* corresponds to 6–18% of the early colonizers; *Streptococcus mitis* and *Streptococcus oralis* varied between 24% and 42% and 1% and 27%, respectively (Wang et al., 2014). Some species such as *S. mutans* and *Lactobacillus* sp., were only found in the adhering microbiome on oral hard surfaces (Wessel et al., 2014).

More than 350 genomes have been fully sequenced, and the abundant groups found in biofilm include: *Streptococcus*, *Actinomyces*, *Granulicatella*, *Gemella*, *Rothia*, *Neisseria*, *Haemophilus*, *Lautropia*, *Prevotella*, *Angustibacter*, *Kineococcus*, *Neisseria*, *Kingella*, *Alysiella*, *Paenibacillus*, *Veillonella*, *Capnocytophaga*, and *Fusobacterium*.

However, no clear association between bacterial composition and biofilm development stage was detected (Benítez-Páez et al., 2014; Nobbs and Jenkinson, 2015).

The oral microbiome is different among individuals, and it is specific in different sites and materials (Wessel et al., 2014). Metatranscriptomic and pyrosequencing analyses comparing individual profiles before and after a carbohydrate-rich meal showed that for each sample there was no specific pattern of biofilm composition. The results suggest that changes in the biofilm, after a meal, depend on the original host microbial population (Benítez-Páez et al., 2014).

Studies on the genetic expression in oral biofilm formation from 6 to 48 h showed that genes involved in the metabolism of carbohydrates, energy, amino acids, cofactor/vitamins, and xenobiotic degradation were expressed to a greater extent in early biofilms. On the contrary, in late biofilms, the expression of ABC transporters, cell motility genes associated with chemotaxis (K02676 and K02390), and genes involved in repair and homologous recombination was predominant (Benítez-Páez et al., 2014). Also, in late biofilms, genes involved in controlling the expression of proteins along the full oral biofilm process (*mnmC, yfiC, cmoA, tadA, queE, trmK, and dusC*), as well as genes involved in competition between bacterial species (*comFC, comFA, comGB, comGC, and comGA*) and in QS response, and DNA uptake were also up-regulated (Benítez-Páez et al., 2014).

In the biofilm, cell–cell, intraspecies, interspecies, and microbial–host interactions are intricately involved in shaping the oral microbiome. Cell–cell interactions between biofilm colonizers seem to be a start to coaggregation (Nobbs and Jenkinson, 2015). The literature shows examples of those interactions resulting in mixed biofilm formation. *Fusobacterium nucleatum* expresses at least one adhesin that recognizes streptococci, and a galactose-specific lectin that interacts with *P. gingivalis* (Nobbs and Jenkinson, 2015). Yet, proteomics and quantitative PCR studies showed that expression of *GapC* in *S. oralis* was increased after its interaction with *P. gingivalis*, which is likely related to mixed biofilm formation (Maeda et al., 2015). Additionally, *C. albicans* hyphal morphotype and presence of commensal *S. oralis* strongly affect the architecture and virulence characteristics of mucosal fungal biofilms (Bertolini et al., 2015).

Small-molecule signals produced by oral microorganisms and detected by human cells, or vice versa, have been shown to interfere in QS and to mediate a range of microbe–microbe and microbe–host interactions. These interactions are imperative to biofilm and disease development. For instance, farnesol, produced by *C. albicans*, inhibits fungal filamentation and at the same time upregulates host epithelial TLR2 increasing the production of interleukin-6 and defensins (Nobbs and Jenkinson, 2015).

7.5 Biofilm–bacteria interaction

7.5.1 *Influence on the stability of dental and craniofacial reconstructions*

Interactions between microbial biofilms and oral milieu have essential influence on the stability of dental and craniofacial reconstructions. Owing to the different structural features of each reconstruction, as well as their anatomic location, specific microbiome is involved in each case. The microbiome in each biomaterial depends on several factors including surface roughness, energy, and chemical composition (Oilo and Bakken, 2015).

Secondary caries is cited as one of the major reasons for failure of posterior resin composite restorations (Ástvaldsdóttir et al., 2015). Amalgam restorations are also susceptible to secondary caries (Rasinez Alcaraz et al., 2014). The occurrence of secondary caries is directly influenced by the individual caries risk (Demarco et al., 2012). In this context, the oral microbiota influencing the stability of dental restorations is mainly composed by species involved in caries pathogenesis.

The knowledge on caries pathogenesis had great advances in the past years, and identifying precisely the involved species is not an easy task. In fact, these reports point to a polymicrobial and tissue-dependent disease that does not have a unique etiology (Simón-Soro et al., 2015). These results will have a major impact on planning preventive protocols.

The microbial ecology on the surface of primary lesions differs from that on lesions next to composite restorations. These findings suggest that the secondary caries next to composite may differ from the primary caries process. Higher proportion of combined mutans streptococci and lactobacilli was more frequently observed in restored dental tissue. An association between lesion depth and lactobacilli was also found (Thomas et al., 2008).

Three hypotheses were related to the etiopathogeny of dental caries throughout history: specific plaque hypothesis, nonspecific plaque hypothesis, and ecological plaque hypothesis (Marsh, 1994). More recently, the role of microbial species in the caries process has been described by the so-called extended caries ecological hypothesis (Tahakashi and Nyvad, 2011). In the first stage of the process, the sound enamel surface is colonized by non-mutans streptococci and *Actinomyces*. As acidification is rare, the mineral balance in the enamel is in dynamic stability stage. Under the presence of fermentable carbohydrates, acidogenicity and acidurance of the nonmutans streptococci are favored. The low-pH environment will lead to an imbalance in the demineralization/mineralization process of dental enamel, leading to initiation of dental caries. This second phase is called the acidogenic stage. In the last stage, acidogenic and aciduric bacteria is the most frequently found, eg, mutans streptococci, lactobacilli, *Actinomyces*, *Bifidobacteria*, and aciduric non-mutans streptococci (Takahashi and Nyvad, 2011) (Fig. 7.4).

Recent DNA- and RNA-based studies pointed to a consortia formed by multiple microorganisms acting synergistically in caries initiation and progress (Simón-Soro and Mira, 2015). Microbiota isolated from caries lesions includes several species that are able to proliferate in cariogenic environment, such as lactobacilii, *Actinomyces gerencseriae, S. mutans*, *S. sobrinus*, yeasts, and *Bifidobacteria* (Mantzourani et al., 2009; Peterson et al., 2011).

Despite great advances in the study of caries pathogeny, there is much that is unknown. For example, there is very limited understanding of the metabolic capabilities of most species found in the oral microbial community (Peterson et al., 2011).

For decades, *S. mutans* has been considered the main causative agent of caries. The extended caries ecological hypothesis associated with data generated by genomics/proteomic studies has generated questions regarding the role of *S. mutans* in caries

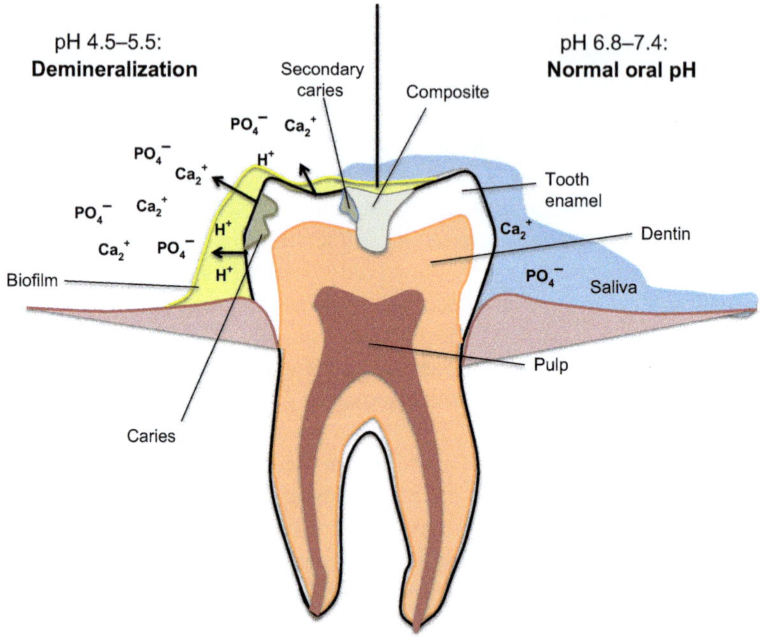

Figure 7.4 Dynamics of demineralization and remineralization in dental enamel and secondary caries formation. At normal oral pH (6.8–7.4), represented at the right side of the figure, the concentrations of Ca^{2+} and $PO_4^{\ -}$ of the dental enamel are in equilibrium with saliva. Demineralization of dental enamel does not occur in this condition. When biofilm is formed, the microorganisms start to produce acid as a result of carbohydrate metabolism. Oral milieu starts to become acidic, and when critical pH is reached (pH 5.5), dental enamel looses Ca^{2+} and $PO_4^{\ -}$ (demineralization process). The maintenance of this condition leads to initial caries formation. Lesions in dental enamel are classified as primary, whereas those formed in the tooth-composite interface are called secondary caries. The evolution of caries results in progressive dental tissue loss affecting the mineralized portions (enamel, dentine) and can reach the pulpar region.

pathogenesis. A cross-sectional study, using sequencing analyses, indicated that 10% of patients with rampant caries in permanent teeth had no detectable levels of *S. mutans* (Aas et al., 2008). Another study reported that streptococci accounted for 40% of the total active community in caries lesions; however, *S. mutans* represented a very low proportion (0.02–0.73%) of the total bacterial community (Simón-Soro et al., 2014). Interestingly, the proportion of *S. mutans* varies considerably depending on the type of lesion. A metatranscriptomic study revealed that *S. mutans* accounted for 0.02% of active microbiota in hidden dentin cavities, and this value was 0.48% and 0.73% in open dentin cavities and enamel lesions, respectively (Simón-Soro et al., 2014).

Studies suggest that the participation of *S. mutans* in caries pathogenesis is not hegemonic; however, undoubtedly, this species shows important cariogenic features. For example, *S. mutans* has the ability to adhere to dental enamel and to metabolize dietary producing acids (Banas, 2004). Other essential features include the ability to survive in an acidic environment and to interact specifically with other microorganisms colonizing the oral ecosystem (Krzsciak et al., 2014). Also, the ability of *S. mutans* to form biofilms has to be highlighted. Previous studies reported that *S. mutans* isolates showed greater ability to form biofilm when compared with other streptococci found in the oral cavity (Tamura et al., 2009). Biofilms are constituted by microbial-derived extracellular matrix, and *S. mutans* has the ability to produce important extracellular polymeric substances. The extracellular polysaccharides (EPS)-rich matrix provides mechanical stability and contributes to the development of acidic environments (Klein et al., 2015). Gtfs produced by *S. mutans* influence the development of virulence of dental biofilm, providing sites for microbial colonization and an insoluble matrix (Bowen and Koo, 2011). Cariogenicity features of *S. mutans* are highly influenced by competence stimulating peptide-mediated QS system (Senadheera and Cvitkovitch, 2008).

Streptococcus sobrinus has also been implicated in caries pathogenesis, in particular when caries development appears to be independent of *S. mutans* (Peterson et al., 2011). However, frequently, this species has been found together with *S. mutans* in more severe caries (Lindquist and Emilson, 2004). *Streptococcus sobrinus* is able to grow and sustain acidogenic and aciduric activity at low pH, and interestingly, the mechanisms of acid tolerance are different from those observed in *S. mutans* (Nascimento et al., 2004). The ability to penetrate dental enamel has been recently reported (Kneist et al., 2015).

Lactobacilli have been correlated to the progression of dental caries, and levels of these microorganisms are widely used as caries risk predictor. They produce high concentrations of acid from carbohydrates and show exceptional acid tolerance (Klinke et al., 2009; Jalasvuori et al., 2012). *Lactobacillus fermentum, Lactobacillus rhamnosus*, and *Lactobacillus crispatus* are the main species found in low-pH areas of caries lesions (Kianoush et al., 2014).

Bifidobacteria have been cited as a potential cariogenic species in the latest polymicrobial etiology scenario. *Bifidobacterium dentium*, *Scardovia inopicata*, and *Parascardovia denticolens* were isolated from dentinal and occlusal caries lesions and supragingival biofilm (Hoshino, 1985; Modesto et al., 2006; Mantzourani et al., 2009). Additionally, studies using molecular methodologies reported the isolation of *Bifidobacteria* from carious lesions (Aas et al., 2005; Chhour et al., 2005). Also, molecular studies identified increased levels of *Bifidobacteria* in patients with early childhood caries (Becker et al., 2002). *Bifidobacteria* are able to produce lactic and acetic acids in the molar proportion of 1:2.9 and 1:2, respectively (Crociani et al., 1996). Also, they show acid tolerance levels comparable to *S. mutans* (Nakajo et al., 2010).

Studies have also associated *Candida* species with dental caries. *Candida* oral levels are frequently used as indicators of caries risk evaluation (Raja et al., 2010). These yeasts particularly actively take part in the dentinal caries progress (Szabó et al., 2014). *Candida* spp. are very efficient at producing acid from carbohydrate sources (Parahitiyawa et al., 2006; Thein et al., 2007). Moreover, secreted aspartyl proteinases gene I expression level was higher in early childhood caries samples compared with control (Li et al., 2014). The cariogenic capacity seems to be favored when *C. albicans* appears in combination with *S. mutans*, such as in cases of early childhood caries (Koo and Bowen, 2014; Falsetta et al., 2014).

In summary, considering that current theories sustain the idea of a multispecies involvement on caries etiopathogeny, preventive and therapeutic strategies that focus on specific and isolated species seem to have limited application.

7.6 Biofilm and dental devices

Dental implants have been in the market for more than 40 years. Dental implants are artificial devices that are generally made of titanium and used to replace one or more missing natural teeth (Charalampakis and Belibasakis, 2015). Diverse surface treatments, such as nanometer-sized pores and surface energy–changing processes, have been proposed as a means of mitigating biofilm attachment.

Peri-implantitis is one important factor in the failure of dental implants. The literature shows that the peri-implantitis microbiome is similar to that found on periodontitis where habitat with low oxygen conditions does not favor the growth of aerobic bacteria. *Aggregatibacter actinomycetemcomitans*, *P. gingivalis*, *Prevotella intermedia*, *Tannerella forsythia*, *Treponema denticola*, and *Fusobacterium* spp. can be found. Interestingly, higher counts of *S. aureus* are frequently detected in implants when compared with dental surfaces (Charalampakis and Belibasakis, 2015).

Dentures, palatal orthodontic appliances or palatal obturators create new niches for biofilm formation that can lead to infections and therapeutic failure. These devices are made by resin, and the nature of the material, as well as the surface roughness and surface free energy, can influence the microbial adherence (Koch et al., 2013).

The occurrence of denture-related stomatitis is one of the main reasons for failure among patients with removable prosthetic devices. Denture-related stomatitis is caused by nighttime wearing of dentures, poor hygiene, and biofilm formation. Poor-fitting dentures can also cause additional trauma in the oral mucosa (Gendreau and Loewy, 2011). Microbial flora diverges between healthy patients and those with denture-related stomatitis. Biofilm from palatal tissue and from the corresponding fitting surface of the denture showed the presence of *Streptococcus, Gemella, Selenomonas*, and *Veillonella*, *Proteobacteria* (eg, *Neisseria* spp.), and *Bacteroides* (eg, species of *Prevotella* and *Capnocytophaga*) in healthy denture wearers. *Prevotella* sp. was found only in the stomatitis group, whereas *Veillonella* sp., *Atopobium* sp., and *C. albicans* were found in both groups. *Non-albicans Candida* (*Candida glabrata* and *Candida tropicalis*) could be detected only on the denture stomatitis group (Campos et al., 2008). In the presence of predisposing factors, *C. albicans* can colonize both denture and mucosal surface (Gendreau and Loewy, 2011) and may invade the host's tissue and cause infection.

7.7 Introduction to factors known to impact salivary protein–bacteria interactions with reconstructions

The main factors that can impact interactions between salivary protein and bacteria and reconstructions are related to the features of the material and the integrity of the interface between the biofilm and restoration.

In this context, the interaction of the biofilm with the dental restoration is an important point to be discussed. Both the enamel HA coated by saliva and dentin tubules are able to attract oral colonizers. Ceramic composites allow less biofilm accumulation than natural tooth surface and gold and amalgam restorations (Wang et al., 2014). Biofilms on gold and amalgam are thick and fully covering, but barely viable (Busscher et al., 2010; Wang et al., 2014).

The composition of the material interferes directly in biofilm formation. Titanium and zirconia surfaces of the implants are less prone to bacterial adhesion when compared with dental enamel surfaces. Titanium and zirconia discs showed reduced *P. gingivalis* and *S. mutans* adhesion when compared with bovine enamel discs after 16- and 48-h biofilm contact (Avila et al., 2015). In fact, no *S. mutans* was found on the titanium surfaces when recovered specimens were examined using confocal microscopy (Avila et al., 2015). Yet, *S. mutans*, *Actinomyces viscosus*, and *P. gingivalis* biofilm formation on the surface of tantalum nitride–decorated titanium (Ti) were reduced when compared with pure Ti and titanium nitride coating samples immersed in artificial saliva (Zhang et al., 2015).

Denture surface treatments, modifying the resin or even disinfecting its surface, show good results in reducing biofilm formation. The application of a diamond-like carbon thin film–coated acrylic resin reduced *C. albicans* biofilm formation (Queiroz et al., 2013). Also, surface treatment with atmospheric cold plasma showed promising disinfection power against *C. albicans* (Kostov et al., 2015; Pan et al., 2015).

Resin composites, widely used as restorative material, facilitate microbial aggregation, especially of *S. mutans*. This aggregation may be favored by the surface roughness and chemical properties such as the release of ethylene glycol dimethylacrylate and triethylene glycol dimethacrylate from resins with limited monomer-to-polymer conversion; the release of these components can induce *Streptococcus* and *Lactobacillus* species aggregation (Wang et al., 2014; Spencer et al., 2014).

As resin composites are too viscous to bond directly to the tooth, a low-viscosity adhesive must be used to bond composite to the tooth. However, if this step is not adequately done, gaps between the tooth and the composite can be penetrated by oral fluids, bacterial enzymes, and bacteria (Spencer et al., 2014). In fact, the interface between restoration and dental surface is considered the site most vulnerable to the occurrence of secondary caries (Donmez et al., 2005).

Bis-GMA–containing (Bisphenol A glycidylmethacrylate-containing) resin composites and adhesives may undergo biodegradation by esterases from the saliva, contributing to the development of recurrent caries (Kermanshahi et al., 2010). Model esterases, such as cholesterol esterase-like and pseudocholinesterase hydrolase activities, have been widely used to show the degradation of resin components (Jaffer et al., 2002; Delaviz et al., 2014). Esterase is an enzymatic hydrolase that has different sources, such as salivary glands, inflammatory responses, and microorganisms (Delaviz et al., 2014). Saliva can infiltrate the defects produced by degradation and bring microorganisms into the margins between tooth and restoration. Two processes can occur at this point: (1) oral microorganisms are able to demineralize the dental surface at these margins and (2) matrix metalloproteinases may promote the degradation of the exposed collagen at the dentin adhesive interface (Delaviz et al., 2014). *Streptococcus mutans* has a higher affinity for resin composites when compared with enamel, metal, and ceramics (Delaviz et al., 2014).

In the presence of resin composite, protein gp340 binds to *S. mutans* surface protein and supports its attachment to the HA surface (Spencer et al., 2014). This SAG is encoded by *DMBT1* gene, and one of the main protein produced is gp340 (Madsen et al., 2010; Leito et al., 2011; Bikker et al., 2013). Furthermore, this glycoprotein shows a wide binding variety, for instance, inducing the aggregation with Gram-negative (such as *Escherichia coli* and *Helicobacter pylori*) and Gram-positive species (such as *S. mutans* and *Streptococcus gordonii*). It can also bind to influenza virus and HIV (Gorr, 2009; Madsen et al., 2010; Bikker et al., 2013; Spencer et al., 2014).

7.8 Summary

In conclusion, to achieve better stability of dental and craniofacial reconstructions, all the factors that compose the complex oral environment should be considered. The factors discussed in this chapter, such as salivary factors, microbial biofilms, and factors related to reconstructions compose a unique and interdependent dynamic and complex system. Novel technologies should be developed and applied to overcome the challenges imposed by this system.

References

Aas JA, Paster BJ, Stokes LN, Olsen I, Dewhirst FE. Defining the normal bacterial flora of the oral cavity. J Clin Microbiol 2005;43(11):5721–32.

Aas JA, Griffen AL, Dardis SR, Lee AM, Olsen I, Dewhirst FE, et al. Bacteria of dental caries in primary and permanent teeth in children and young adults. J Clin Microbiol April 2008;46(4):1407–17.

Al Kawas S, Rahim ZH, Ferguson DB. Potential uses of human salivary protein and peptide analysis in the diagnosis of disease. Arch Oral Biol 2012;57:1–9.

Alexandre G. Minireview: chemotaxis control of transient cell aggregation. J Bacteriol 2015 Oct;197(20):3230–7.

Amado FM, Ferreira RP, Vitorino R. One decade of salivary proteomics: current approaches and outstanding challenges. Clin Biochem 2013;46:506–17.

Ástvaldsdóttir Á, Dagerhamn J, Van Dijken JW, Naimi-Akbar A, Sandborgh-Englund G, Tranæus S, et al. Longevity of posterior resin composite restorations in adults - a systematic review. J Dent August 2015;43(8):934–54.

Avila É, Molon RS, Lima B, Lux R, Shi W, Junior MJ, et al. The impact of physical chemical characteristics of implant abutment surfaces on bacteria adhesion. J Oral Implantol 2015;42(2).

Banas JA. Virulence properties of *Streptococcus mutans*. Front Biosci May 2004;1(9):1267–77.

Becker MR, Paster BJ, Leys EJ, Moeschberger ML, Kenyon SG, Galvin JL, et al. Molecular analysis of bacterial species associated with childhood caries. J Clin Microbiol 2002;40(3):1001–9.

Benítez-Páez A, Belda-Ferre P, Simón-Soro A, Mira A. Microbiota diversity and gene expression dynamics in human oral biofilms. BMC Genomics 2014;15:311.

Bertolini MM, Xu H, Sobue T, Nobile CJ, Del Bel Cury AA, Dongari-Bagtzoglou A. *Candida*-streptococcal mucosal biofilms display distinct structural and virulence characteristics depending on growth conditions and hyphal morphotypes. Mol Oral Microbiol 2015;30:307–22.

Bikker FJ, Cukkemane N, Nazmi K, Veerman EC. Identification of the hydroxyapatite-binding domain of salivary agglutinin. Eur J Oral Sci 2013;121:7–12.

Bowen WH, Koo H. Biology of *Streptococcus mutans*-derived glucosyltransferases: role in extracellular matrix formation of cariogenic biofilms. Caries Res 2011;45(1):69–86.

Busscher HJ, Rinastiti M, Siswomihardjo W, Van Der Mei HC. Biofilm formation on dental restorative and implant materials. J Dent Res 2010;89:657–65.

Buzalaf MA, Hannas AR, Kato MT. Saliva and dental erosion. J Appl Oral Sci 2012;20:493–502.

Campos MS, Marchini L, Bernardes LA, Paulino LC, Nobrega FG. Biofilm microbial communities of denture stomatitis. Oral Microbiol Immunol 2008;23:419–24.

Carpenter GH. The secretion, components, and properties of saliva. Annu Rev Food Sci Technol 2013;4:267–76.

Charalampakis G, Belibasakis GN. Microbiome of peri-implant infections: lessons from conventional, molecular and metagenomic analyses. Virulence 2015;6:183–7.

Chhour KL, Nadkarni MA, Byun R, Martin FE, Jacques NA, Hunter N. Molecular analysis of microbial diversity in advanced caries. J Clin Microbiol 2005;43(2):843–9.

Chiappin S, Antonelli G, Gatti R, De Palo EF. Saliva specimen: a new laboratory tool for diagnostic and basic investigation. Clin Chim Acta 2007;383:30–40.

Choi S, Baik JE, Jeon JH, Cho K, Seo DG, Kum KY, et al. Identification of *Porphyromonas gingivalis* lipopolysaccharide-binding proteins in human saliva. Mol Immunol 2011;48:2207–13.

Costerton JW, Cheng KJ, Geesey GG, Ladd TI, Nickel JC, Dasgupta M, et al. Bacterial biofilms in nature and disease. Annu Rev Microbiol 1987;41:435–64.

Crociani F, Biavati B, Alessandrini A, Chiarini C, Scardovi V. *Bifidobacterium inopinatum* sp. nov. and *denticolens* sp. nov., two new species human dental caries. Int J Syst Bacteriol 1996;46(2):564–71.

Dawes C, Pedersen AM, Villa A, Ekstrom J, Proctor GB, Vissink A, et al. The functions of human saliva: a review sponsored by the World Workshop on Oral Medicine VI. Arch Oral Biol 2015;60:863–74.

Dawes C. How much saliva is enough for avoidance of xerostomia? Caries Res 2004;38:236–40.

Dawes C. Salivary flow patterns and the health of hard and soft oral tissues. J Am Dent Assoc 2008;139(Suppl.):18S–24S.

de Sousa-Pereira P, Abrantes J, Pinheiro A, Colaco B, Vitorino R, Esteves PJ. Evolution of C, D and S-type cystatins in mammals: an extensive gene duplication in primates. PLoS One 2014;9:e109050.

Delaleu N, Mydel P, Kwee I, Brun JG, Jonsson MV, Jonsson R. High fidelity between saliva proteomics and the biologic state of salivary glands defines biomarker signatures for primary Sjogren's syndrome. Arthritis Rheumatol 2015;67:1084–95.

Delaviz Y, Finer Y, Santerre JP. Biodegradation of resin composites and adhesives by oral bacteria and saliva: a rationale for new material designs that consider the clinical environment and treatment challenges. Dent Mater January 2014;30(1):16–32.

Demarco FF, Corrêa MB, Cenci MS, Moraes RR, Opdam NJ. Longevity of posterior composite restorations: not only a matter of materials. Dent Mater January 2012;28(1):87–101.

Denny P, Hagen FK, Hardt M, Liao L, Yan W, Arellanno M, et al. The proteomes of human parotid and submandibular/sublingual gland salivas collected as the ductal secretions. J Proteome Res 2008;7:1994–2006.

Desai GS, Mathews ST. Saliva as a non-invasive diagnostic tool for inflammation and insulin-resistance. World J Diabetes 2014;5:730–8.

Dijkema T, Terhaard CH, Roesink JM, Raaijmakers CP, Van Den Keijbus PA, Brand HS, et al. MUC5B levels in submandibular gland saliva of patients treated with radiotherapy for head-and-neck cancer: a pilot study. Radiat Oncol 2012;7:91.

Dodds MW, Johnson DA, Yeh CK. Health benefits of saliva: a review. J Dent 2005;33:223–33.

Donmez N, Belli S, Pashley DH, Tay FR. Ultrastructural correlates of in vivo/in vitro bond degradation in self-etch adhesives. J Dent Res April 2005;84(4):355–9.

Edgar WM. Saliva and dental health. Clinical implications of saliva: report of a consensus meeting. Br Dent J 1990;169:96–8.

Edgar WM. Saliva: its secretion, composition and functions. Br Dent J 1992;172:305–12.

Emerenini BO, Hense BA, Kuttler C, Eberl HJ. A mathematical model of quorum sensing induced biofilm detachment. PLoS One 2015;10:e0132385.

Fabian TK, Beck A, Fejerdy P, Hermann P, Fabian G. Molecular mechanisms of taste recognition: considerations about the role of saliva. Int J Mol Sci 2015;16:5945–74.

Falsetta ML, Klein MI, Colonne PM, Scott-Anne K, Gregoire S, Pai CH, et al. Symbiotic relationship between *Streptococcus mutans* and *Candida* albicans synergizes virulence of plaque biofilms in vivo. Infect Immun May 2014;82(5):1968–81.

Fux CA, Costerton JW, Stewart PS, Stoodley P. Survival strategies of infectious biofilms. Trends Microbiol 2005;13:34–40.

Gendreau L, Loewy ZG. Epidemiology and etiology of denture stomatitis. J Prosthodont 2011;20:251–60.

Gibbins HL, Proctor GB, Yakubov GE, Wilson S, Carpenter GH. Concentration of salivary protective proteins within the bound oral mucosal pellicle. Oral Dis 2014;20:707–13.

Gibbins HL, Proctor GB, Yakubov GE, Wilson S, Carpenter GH. SIgA binding to mucosal surfaces is mediated by mucin-mucin interactions. PLoS One 2015;10:e0119677.

Goncalves AC, Marson FA, Mendonca RM, Ribeiro JD, Ribeiro AF, Paschoal IA, et al. Saliva as a potential tool for cystic fibrosis diagnosis. Diagn Pathol 2013;8:46.

Gorr SU. Antimicrobial peptides of the oral cavity. Periodontology 2000 2009;51:152–80.

Hall-Stoodley L, Stoodley P. Developmental regulation of microbial biofilms. Curr Opin Biotechnol 2002;13:228–33.

Hall-Stoodley L, Stoodley P. Biofilm formation and dispersal and the transmission of human pathogens. Trends Microbiol 2005;13:7–10.

Hall-Stoodley L, Stoodley P. Evolving concepts in biofilm infections. Cell Microbiol 2009;11:1034–43.

Hogan DA, Vik A, Kolter R. A *Pseudomonas aeruginosa* quorum-sensing molecule influences *Candida albicans* morphology. Mol Microbiol 2004;54:1212–23.

Hoshino E. Predominant obligate anaerobes in human carious dentin. J Dent Res 1985;64(10):1195–8.

Huang CM. Comparative proteomic analysis of human whole saliva. Arch Oral Biol 2004;49:951–62.

Humphrey SP, Williamson RT. A review of saliva: normal composition, flow, and function. J Prosthet Dent 2001;85:162–9.

Huq NL, Cross KJ, Ung M, Myroforidis M, Veith PD, Chen D, et al. A review of the salivary proteome and peptidome and saliva-derived peptide therapeutics. Int J Peptide Res Ther 2007;13:547–64.

Jaffer F, Finer Y, Santerre JP. Interactions between resin monomers and commercial composite resins with human saliva derived esterases. Biomaterials 2002;23:1707–19.

Jalasvuori H, Haukioja A, Tenovuo J. Probiotic *Lactobacillus reuteri* strains ATCC PTA 5289 and ATCC 55730 differ in their cariogenic properties in vitro. Arch Oral Biol December 2012;57(12):1633–8.

Joint I, Allan Downie J, Williams P. Bacterial conversations: talking, listening and eavesdropping. An introduction. Philos Trans R Soc Lond B Biol Sci 2007;362:1115–7.

Kalk WW, Vissink A, Stegenga B, Bootsma H, Nieuw Amerongen AV, Kallenberg CG. Sialometry and sialochemistry: a non-invasive approach for diagnosing Sjogren's syndrome. Ann Rheum Dis 2002;61:137–44.

Karavolos MH. Host microbe interactions: a licence to interfere? Curr Pharm Biotechnol 2015;16:87–93.

Kaufman E, Lamster IB. The diagnostic applications of saliva–a review. Crit Rev Oral Biol Med 2002;13:197–212.

Kejriwal S, Bhandary R, Thomas B, Kumari S. Estimation of levels of salivary mucin, amylase and total protein in gingivitis and chronic periodontitis patients. J Clin Diagn Res 2014;8:ZC56–60.

Kermanshahi S, Santerre JP, Cvitkovitch DG, Finer Y. Biodegradation of resin-dentin interfaces increases bacterial microleakage. J Dent Res September 2010;89(9):996–1001.

Kianoush N, Adler CJ, Nguyen KA, Browne GV, Simonian M, Hunter N. Bacterial profile of dentine caries and the impact of pH on bacterial population diversity. PLoS One March 27, 2014;9(3):e92940.

Klein MI, Hwang G, Santos PH, Campanella OH, Koo H. *Streptococcus mutans*-derived extracellular matrix in cariogenic oral biofilms. Front Cell Infect Microbiol February 13, 2015;5:10.

Klinke T, Kneist S, de Soet JJ, Kuhlisch E, Mauersberger S, Forster A, Klimm W. Acid production by oral strains of Candida albicans and lactobacilli. Caries Res. 2009;43(2):83–91.

Kneist S, Nietzsche S, Küpper H, Raser G, Willershausen B, Callaway A. Penetration of *Streptococcus sobrinus* and *Streptococcus sanguinis* into dental enamel. Anaerobe March 21, 2015. http://dx.doi.org/10.1016/j.anaerobe.2015.01.013. pii:S1075–9964(15)00033-5; [Epub ahead of print].

Koch C, Burgers R, Hahnel S. *Candida albicans* adherence and proliferation on the surface of denture base materials. Gerodontology 2013;30:309–13.

Koo H, Bowen WH. *Candida albicans* and *Streptococcus mutans*: a potential synergistic alliance to cause virulent tooth decay in children. Future Microbiol 2014;9(12):1295–7.

Kostov KG, Borges AC, Koga-Ito CY, Nishime TMC, Prysiazhnyi V, Honda RY. Inactivation of *Candida albicans* by cold atmospheric pressure plasma jet. IEEE Trans Plasma Sci 2015;43(3). http://dx.doi.org/10.1109/TPS.2014.2360645.

Krzysciak W, Jurczak A, Koscielniak D, Bystrowska B, Skalniak A. The virulence of *Streptococcus mutans* and the ability to form biofilms. Eur J Clin Microbiol Infect Dis 2014;33:499–515.

Leito JT, Ligtenberg AJ, Van Houdt M, Van Den Berg TK, Wouters D. The bacteria binding glycoprotein salivary agglutinin (SAG/gp340) activates complement via the lectin pathway. Mol Immunol 2011;49:185–90.

Lendenmann U, Grogan J, Oppenheim FG. Saliva and dental pellicle–a review. Adv Dent Res 2000;14:22–8.

Lexner MO, Bardow A, Hertz JM, Almer L, Nauntofte B, Kreiborg S. Whole saliva in X-linked hypohidrotic ectodermal dysplasia. Int J Paediatr Dent 2007;17:155–62.

Li W, Yu D, Gao S, Lin J, Chen Z, Zhao W. Role of *Candida albicans*-secreted aspartyl proteinases (Saps) in severe early childhood caries. Int J Mol Sci June 13, 2014;15(6): 10766–10779.

Lindquist B, Emilson CG. Colonization of *Streptococcus mutans* and *Streptococcus sobrinus* genotypes and caries development in children to mothers harboring both species. Caries Res 2004;38:95–103.

Livnat G, Bentur L, Kuzmisnsky E, Nagler RM. Salivary profile and oxidative stress in children and adolescents with cystic fibrosis. J Oral Pathol Med 2010;39:16–21.

Madsen J, Mollenhauer J, Holmskov U. Review: gp-340/DMBT1 in mucosal innate immunity. Innate Immun 2010;16:160–7.

Maeda K, Nagata H, Ojima M, Amano A. Proteomic and transcriptional analysis of interaction between oral microbiota *Porphyromonas gingivalis* and *Streptococcus oralis*. J Proteome Res 2015;14:82–94.

Mancl KA, Kirsner RS, Ajdic D. Wound biofilms: lessons learned from oral biofilms. Wound Repair Regen 2013;21:352–62.

Mantzourani M, Gilbert SC, Sulong HNH, Sheehy EC, Tank S, Fenlon M, et al. The isolation of *Bifidobacteria* from occlusal carious lesions in children and adults. Caries Res 2009;43(4):308–13.

Marsh PD. Microbial ecology of dental plaque and its significance in health and disease. Adv Dent Res July 1994;8(2):263–71.

Modesto M, Biavati B, Mattarelli P. Occurrence of the family Bifidobacteriaceae in human dental caries and plaque. Caries Res 2006;40(3):271–6.

Moritsuka M, Kitasako Y, Burrow MF, Ikeda M, Tagami J. The pH change after HCl titration into resting and stimulated saliva for a buffering capacity test. Aust Dent J 2006;51:170–4.

Nakajo K, Takahashi N, Beighton D. Resistance to acidic environments of caries-associated bacteria: *Bifidobacterium dentium* and *Bifidobacterium longum*. Caries Res 2010;44(5):431–7.

Nanci A. Ten cate's oral histology: development, structure and function. 2013.

Nascimento MM, Lemos JA, Abranches J, Gonçalves RB, Burne RA. Adaptive acid tolerance response of *Streptococcus sobrinus*. J Bacteriol October 2004;186(19):6383–90.

Navazesh M, Kumar SK, University of Southern California School of Dentistry. Measuring salivary flow: challenges and opportunities. J Am Dent Assoc 2008;139(Suppl.):35S–40S.

Nie S, Zhang H, Mayer KM, Oppenheim FG, Little FF, Greenberg J, et al. Correlations of salivary biomarkers with clinical assessments in patients with cystic fibrosis. PLoS One 2015;10:e0135237.

Nikitkova AE, Haase EM, Scannapieco FA. Taking the starch out of oral biofilm formation: molecular basis and functional significance of salivary alpha-amylase binding to oral streptococci. Appl Environ Microbiol 2013;79:416–23.

Nobbs AH, Jenkinson HF. Interkingdom networking within the oral microbiome. Microbes Infect 2015;17:484–92.

Nordgarden H, Storhaug K, Lyngstadaas SP, Jensen JL. Salivary gland function in persons with ectodermal dysplasias. Eur J Oral Sci 2003;111:371–6.

Ochiai A, Harada K, Hashimoto K, Shibata K, Ishiyama Y, Mitsui T, et al. α-Amylase is a potential growth inhibitor of *Porphyromonas gingivalis*, a periodontal pathogenic bacterium. J Periodontal Res 2014;49:62–8.

Oilo M, Bakken V. Biofilm and dental biomaterials. Materials 2015;8(6):2887–900.

Olsen I. Biofilm-specific antibiotic tolerance and resistance. Eur J Clin Microbiol Infect Dis 2015;34:877–86.

Oppenheim FG, Salih E, Siqueira WL, Zhang W, Helmerhorst EJ. Salivary proteome and its genetic polymorphisms. Ann NY Acad Sci 2007;1098:22–50.

Pan H, Wang G, Pan J, Ye G, Sun K, Zhang J, et al. Cold plasma-induced surface modification of heat-polymerized acrylic resin and prevention of early adherence of *Candida albicans*. Dent Mater J 2015;34:529–36.

Papagerakis S, Zheng L, Schnell S, Sartor MA, Somers E, Marder W, et al. The circadian clock in oral health and diseases. J Dent Res 2014;93:27–35.

Parahitiyawa NB, Samaranayake YH, Samaranayake LP, Ye J, Tsang PW, Cheung BP, Yau JY, Yeung SK. Interspecies variation in *Candida* biofilm formation studied using the Calgary biofilm device. APMIS 2006 Apr;114(4):298–306.

Peterson SN, Snesrud E, Schork NJ, Bretz WA. Dental caries pathogenicity: a genomic and metagenomic perspective. Int Dent J August 2011;61(Suppl. 1):11–22.
Pfaffe T, Cooper-White J, Beyerlein P, Kostner K, Punyadeera C. Diagnostic potential of saliva: current state and future applications. Clin Chem 2011;57:675–87.
Puri S, Edgerton M. How does it kill?: understanding the candidacidal mechanism of salivary histatin 5. Eukaryot Cell 2014;13:958–64.
Puri S, Li R, Ruszaj D, Tati S, Edgerton M. Iron binding modulates candidacidal properties of salivary histatin 5. J Dent Res 2015;94:201–8.
Queiroz JR, Fissmer SF, Koga-Ito CY, Salvia AC, Massi M, Sobrinho AS, et al. Effect of diamond-like carbon thin film coated acrylic resin on *Candida albicans* biofilm formation. J Prosthodont 2013;22:451–5.
Raja M, Hannan A, Ali K. Association of oral candidal carriage with dental caries in children. Caries Res 2010;44(3):272–6.
Rasines Alcaraz MG, Veitz-Keenan A, Sahrmann P, Schmidlin PR, Davis D, Iheozor-Ejiofor Z. Direct composite resin fillings versus amalgam fillings for permanent or adult posterior teeth. Cochrane Database Syst Rev March 31, 2014;3:CD005620.
Sabharwal A, Liao YC, Lin HH, Haase EM, Scannapieco FA. Draft genome sequences of 18 oral streptococcus strains that encode amylase-binding proteins. Genome Announc 2015;3.
Saleh J, Figueiredo MA, Cherubini K, Salum FG. Salivary hypofunction: an update on aetiology, diagnosis and therapeutics. Arch Oral Biol 2015;60:242–55.
Sas R, Dawes C. The intra-oral distribution of unstimulated and chewing-gum-stimulated parotid saliva. Arch Oral Biol 1997;42:469–74.
Schulz BL, Cooper-White J, Punyadeera CK. Saliva proteome research: current status and future outlook. Crit Rev Biotechnol 2013;33:246–59.
Senadheera D, Cvitkovitch DG. Quorum sensing and biofilm formation by *Streptococcus mutans*. Adv Exp Med Biol 2008;631:178–88.
Shimotoyodome A, Kobayashi H, Tokimitsu I, Matsukubo T, Takaesu Y. Statherin and histatin 1 reduce parotid saliva-promoted *Streptococcus mutans* strain MT8148 adhesion to hydroxyapatite surfaces. Caries Res 2006;40:403–11.
Simón-Soro A, Mira A. Solving the etiology of dental caries. Trends Microbiol February 2015;23(2):76–82.
Simón-Soro A, Guillen-Navarro M, Mira A. Metatranscriptomics reveals overall active bacterial composition in caries lesions. J Oral Microbiol October 24, 2014;6:25443.
Siqueira WL, Zhang W, Helmerhorst EJ, Gygi SP, Oppenheim FG. Identification of protein components in in vivo human acquired enamel pellicle using LC-ESI-MS/MS. J Proteome Res 2007;6:2152–60.
Siqueira WL, Salih E, Wan DL, Helmerhorst EJ, Oppenheim FG. Proteome of human minor salivary gland secretion. J Dent Res 2008;87:445–50.
Siqueira WL, Lee YH, Xiao Y, Held K, Wong W. Identification and characterization of histatin 1 salivary complexes by using mass spectrometry. Proteomics 2012;12:3426–35.
Situ H, Wei G, Smith CJ, Mashhoon S, Bobek LA. Human salivary MUC7 mucin peptides: effect of size, charge and cysteine residues on antifungal activity. Biochem J 2003;375:175–82.
Sivadasan P, Gupta MK, Sathe GJ, Balakrishnan L, Palit P, Gowda H, et al. Human salivary proteome - a resource of potential biomarkers for oral cancer. J Proteomics 2015;127.
Song F, Koo H, Ren D. Effects of material properties on bacterial adhesion and biofilm formation. J Dent Res 2015;94:1027–34.
Spencer P, Ye Q, Misra A, Goncalves SE, Laurence JS. Proteins, pathogens, and failure at the composite-tooth interface. J Dent Res 2014;93:1243–9.

Sun QF, Sun QH, Du J, Wang S. Differential gene expression profiles of normal human parotid and submandibular glands. Oral Dis 2008;14:500–9.

Szabó B, Majoros L, Papp-Falusi E, Szabó Z, Szabó J, Márton I, et al. Studies on the possible aetiological role of different *Candida* species in pathogenesis of dentine caries by monitoring the calcium release from tooth particles. Acta Microbiol Immunol Hung March 2014;61(1):11–7.

Takahashi N, Nyvad B. The role of bacteria in the caries process: ecological perspectives. J Dent Res March 2011;90(3):294–303.

Tamura S, Yonezawa H, Motegi M, Nakao R, Yoneda S, Watanabe H, et al. Inhibiting effects of *Streptococcus salivarius* on competence-stimulating peptide-dependent biofilm formation by *Streptococcus mutans*. Oral Microbiol Immunol April 2009;24(2):152–61.

Tenovuo J. Antimicrobial function of human saliva–how important is it for oral health? Acta Odontol Scand 1998;56:250–6.

Tenovuo J. Antimicrobial agents in saliva–protection for the whole body. J Dent Res 2002;81:807–9.

Thein ZM, Samaranayake YH, Samaranayake LP. Dietary sugars, serum and the biocide chlorhexidine digluconate modify the population and structural dynamics of mixed *Candida albicans* and *Escherichia coli* biofilms. APMIS 2007 Nov;115(11):1241–51.

Thomas RZ, van der Mei HC, van der Veen MH, de Soet JJ, Huysmans MC. Bacterial composition and red fluorescence of plaque in relation to primary and secondary caries next to composite: an in situ study. Oral Microbiol Immunol 2008 Feb;23(1):7–13.

Vitorino R, Lobo MJ, Ferrer-Correira AJ, Dubin JR, Tomer KB, Domingues PM, et al. Identification of human whole saliva protein components using proteomics. Proteomics 2004;4:1109–15.

Vitorino R, Calheiros-Lobo MJ, Duarte JA, Domingues PM, Amado FM. Peptide profile of human acquired enamel pellicle using MALDI tandem MS. J Sep Sci 2008;31:523–37.

Vukosavljevic D, Custodio W, Del Bel Cury AA, Siqueira WL. The effect of histatin 5, adsorbed on PMMA and hydroxyapatite, on *Candida albicans* colonization. Yeast 2012;29:459–66.

Vukosavljevic D, Hutter JL, Helmerhorst EJ, Xiao Y, Custodio W, Zaidan FC, et al. Nanoscale adhesion forces between enamel pellicle proteins and hydroxyapatite. J Dent Res 2014;93:514–9.

Wang Z, Shen Y, Haapasalo M. Dental materials with antibiofilm properties. Dent Mater 2014;30:e1–16.

Wei GX, Campagna AN, Bobek LA. Effect of MUC7 peptides on the growth of bacteria and on *Streptococcus mutans* biofilm. J Antimicrob Chemother 2006;57:1100–9.

Wessel SW, Chen Y, Maitra A, Van Den Heuvel ER, Slomp AM, Busscher HJ, et al. Adhesion forces and composition of planktonic and adhering oral microbiomes. J Dent Res 2014;93:84–8.

Xiao Y, Karttunen M, Jalkanen J, Mussi MC, Liao Y, Grohe B, et al. Hydroxyapatite growth inhibition effect of pellicle statherin peptides. J Dent Res 2015;94:1106–12.

Zhang A, Sun H, Wang P, Wang X. Salivary proteomics in biomedical research. Clin Chim Acta 2013;415:261–5.

Zhang Y, Zheng Y, Li Y, Wang L, Bai Y, Zhao Q, et al. Tantalum nitride-decorated titanium with enhanced resistance to microbiologically induced corrosion and mechanical property for dental application. PLoS One 2015;10:e0130774.

Zheng L, Seon YJ, Mchugh J, Papagerakis S, Papagerakis P. Clock genes show circadian rhythms in salivary glands. J Dent Res 2012;91:783–8.

Part Three

Characterization of material-tissue interfaces in dental and craniofacial reconstructions

Morphologic and structural analysis of material-tissue interfaces relevant to dental reconstruction

8

J.H. Purk
University of Missouri-Kansas City, Kansas City, MO, United States

8.1 Introduction

Resin-based composite is rapidly becoming the most popular material for direct restorative dentistry. The reconstruction of teeth using resin-based composite offers considerable promise in terms of esthetics and conservation of tooth structure. Unfortunately, its durability does not match that of dental amalgam. The overall clinical lifetime of amalgam (11 years) usually exceeds that of resin-based composite (5–6 years) [1], and currently, dental amalgam remains the most low-cost, forgiving, and durable posterior restorative material. As an example, in children aged 6–10 years, up to seven times more repairs were required for composite restorations when compared with amalgam restorations [2]. There was a 3.5 times greater risk for recurrent caries for composite as opposed to amalgam restorations in children aged 8–12 years [3].

Patients often request for tooth-colored composite as opposed to the less-esthetic amalgam; however, depending on a myriad of factors the tooth-colored composite restoration may not be the best treatment option. Factors that impact the clinical lifetime of the composite restoration include patient's caries index, extent of the caries, location of the tooth, the available materials, management of the patient, and moisture control as well as the skill of the dentist [4]. There are also multiple challenges with bonding the composite resin to tooth structure. Even the gold standard of "bonding to enamel" in posterior teeth has not been entirely successful. Variability in the morphology and structure of enamel at different locations within the tooth preparation is one factor limiting routine success with enamel bonding. Developing a durable bond to dentin is even more challenging.

Much of what we know about bonding to tooth structure comes from laboratory studies. For example, in vitro static dentin bond strength testing is a routine screening method for comparing between commercial products. There is, however, considerable disparity between the bond strength values reported for the same product tested in different laboratories. There are also distinct differences between in vitro and in vivo performance [5,6]. When materials were placed in a manner similar to clinical in vivo placement, they behaved totally different from materials placed in the laboratory [6–8].

Samples in the laboratory can be manipulated in ways that are impossible to duplicate in the patient's mouth, eg, the use of sanding machines instead of burs to prepare the tooth [9]. Temperature and humidity in the laboratory also have an effect and

Material-Tissue Interfacial Phenomena. http://dx.doi.org/10.1016/B978-0-08-100330-5.00008-X

may explain why some materials behave differently in the mouth compared to the laboratory [10–12].

Simulating in vivo bonding to dentin can be difficult for a variety of reasons including pulpal pressure, which can force dentinal fluid onto the bonding surface [5]. Removing the smear layer increased the rate of fluid flow of axial walls as much as 2.4 times over that of occlusal walls under in vitro conditions [13]. When the permeability of dentin in young teeth (aged 19 or younger) was measured, the cervical third was 3.6 times more permeable than the occlusal third. Scanning electron microscopic (SEM) images showed the dentinal tubular openings to be greater in number and smaller in diameter in the cervical third when compared with tubules in the occlusal and middle thirds [14]. Many clinical problems associated with dentin hypersensitivity, microleakage, and recurrent caries have been related to dentin permeability. Greater fluid flow may occur from the pulp, and this pulpal fluid, upon reaching the cut surface of the dentin, could compromise the adaptability of the restorative material. This could be especially detrimental in deeper preparations in which the tubular diameter is much greater [14] or where cavity preparation surfaces approach the pulp chamber [15]. The success of the tooth—adhesive interface, which has been reported under in vitro conditions, has not been replicated when the same interfacial structure is tested under in vivo conditions [6].

There are many factors affecting the clinical success of the posterior resin composite. This chapter will focus on one key parameter, ie, morphologic and structural features of the resin adhesive–tooth interface.

8.2 Structure of enamel and effect on adhesive bonding

Bonding restorative materials to enamel, dentin, or both is a major goal of restorative dentistry. The most common means of bonding adhesive to tooth is through micromechanical bonding, which involves the interlocking of an adhesive to irregularities in the tooth. In the case of dentin and enamel bonding, the restorative resin adhesive either interlocks with the collagen in the dentin or the acid-etched enamel rods [16–19].

Chemically, enamel is a highly mineralized crystalline structure containing 95–98% inorganic matter by weight. Hydroxyapatite, in the form of a crystalline lattice, is the largest mineral constituent and is present at concentrations of 90–92% by volume. The remaining constituents of tooth enamel include an organic phase, which accounts for about 1–2%, and water, which is about 4% by weight.

Enamel rods are densely packed and intertwined in a wavy course, and extend from the dentinoenamel junction (DEJ) to the external surface of the tooth. In general, enamel rods are aligned perpendicular to both the DEJ and tooth surface. The "ends of the enamel rods" are exposed for adhesive bonding after the enamel is treated with an acid conditioner [20]. However, the rods can also be aligned in a parallel arrangement on the internal surface of a tooth preparation where the "sides of the enamel rods" are exposed after acid conditioning.

Adhesive bonding to the ends of enamel rods (Fig. 8.1) is in the range of 20–25 MPa [21–23] and is considered to be the "gold standard" for adhesive bonding to the tooth.

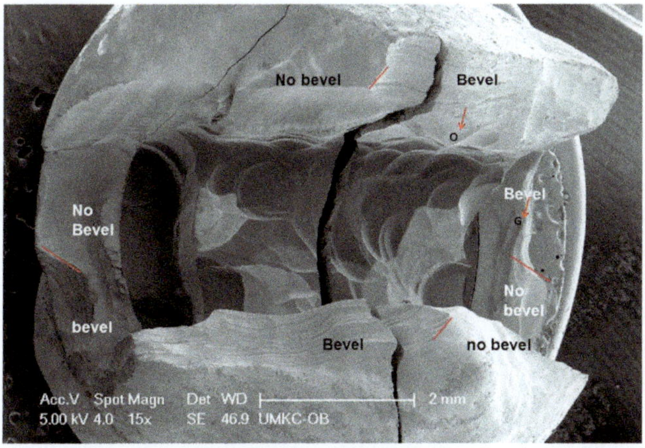

Total etch – 37% phosphoric acid John Purk, DDS, PhD-Vladimir Dusevich PhD

Figure 8.1 Class II preparation with red lines separating beveled and nonbeveled enamel at the occlusal surface and the gingival wall of the preparation.

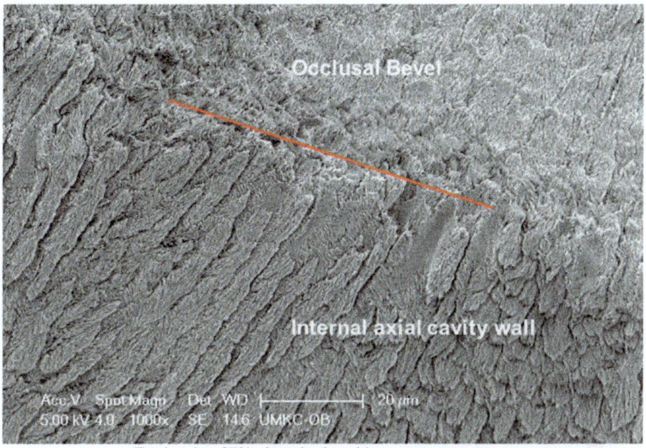

Total etch – 37% phosphoric acid John Purk, DDS, PhD-Vladimir Dusevich PhD

Figure 8.2 Area of Fig. 8.1 labeled O where the occlusal surface above the red line is the enamel cavosurface that has been beveled exposing the ends of the enamel rods (perpendicular-oriented enamel) and the area below the red line is the axial wall of the preparation where the sides of the enamel rods (parallel-oriented enamel) are exposed after etching with 37% phosphoric acid for 30 s.

Adhesive bonding to the sides of the enamel rods (Fig. 8.2) is in the range of 11 MPa [24]. It is no longer sufficient for an operator to just "bond to enamel" and assume that a "gold standard" bond will be obtained. The operator should consider the type of enamel and the direction of the enamel rods in order to obtain the best adhesive bond.

In 1955, Buonocore reported that treatment with 85% phosphoric acid could increase adhesion to the enamel [25]. This acid-etching technique enhanced the retention of class II and V restorations and pit and fissure sealants [26]. Based on recent laboratory investigations, lower concentrations of phosphoric acid, ie, between 30 and 40%, are more effective than higher concentrations; the lower concentrations provide enamel surfaces that have the most retentive appearance [27].

Clinically, cavity preparations leave enamel prisms in various angulations prior to bonding [28]. Most in vitro adhesive studies evaluate bond strengths to the cut ends of the enamel rods, perpendicular to the plane of the crystal. There is, however, a large difference between bonding to the ends of the enamel rods (perpendicular-oriented rods) and bonding to the sides of the enamel rods (parallel-oriented rods). For example, Prime and Bond NT and Herculite XRV yielded microtensile bond strengths to perpendicular and parallel enamel rods of 24.2±9.5 and 7.2±5.5 MPa, respectively. Failure was primarily interfacial for the perpendicular group, whereas debonding occurred in the boundary between enamel prisms for the parallel group [28].

Parallel-oriented enamel is found on the internal walls of occlusal preparations [29] and on the gingival floor of class II preparations [24] (Fig. 8.1). Perpendicular-oriented enamel is found on the occlusal surface of beveled enamel and on the beveled gingival margin of class II preparations (Figs. 8.2 and 8.3). If the bond to the parallel enamel is less than the polymerization shrinkage stress of the resin composite, a gap (Fig. 8.4) can be formed at the gingival margin, even though the adhesive is applied to the enamel.

Perpendicular-oriented enamel can be found on the cavosurface margins of class I preparations [29] and at the bevel of class II preparations [24]. Enamel is a homogeneous material, and enamel bond strengths are very predictable. The bond to enamel remains the best that can be clinically achieved [30]. Preserving adjacent enamel remains one of the most important guidelines when preparing cavities for adhesive restorations [30].

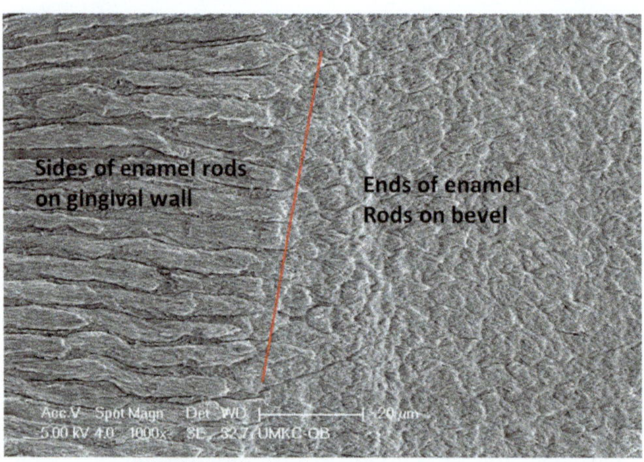

Total etch – 37% phosphoric acid John Purk, DDS, PhD-Vladimir Dusevich PhD

Figure 8.3 Area of Fig. 8.1 labeled G where the gingival floor on the left side of the red line meets the interface of the gingival bevel on the right side of the red line. Notice that the gingival floor on the left side of the enamel rods (parallel-oriented enamel) is exposed and that on the right side of the red line when the gingival floor is beveled, the ends of the enamel rods (perpendicular-oriented enamel) are exposed after etching with 37% phosphoric acid for 30 s.

When self-etch and total-etch adhesives were bonded to beveled and perpendicular (ends of) enamel at the gingival margin of class II resin composite preparations, the adhesive bond strength was ~25.9 MPa with two debonds during specimen preparation. On the contrary, at the nonbeveled location and parallel (sides of) enamel rods, the adhesive bond strength was ~16.0 MPa with 20 debonds during specimen preparation [31]. Clearly, the enamel margin at the gingival floor of the class II preparation is dramatically different if the enamel is not beveled exposing the ends of the enamel rods.

Distinct morphologic differences have also been noted for beveled and nonbeveled cavosurface margins. These distinct differences are highlighted in the following study. A premolar was prepared to receive an MOD (mesial occlusal distal) preparation ~2.0 mm wide from the mesial to distal surface through the center of the tooth. Approximately, half of the cavosurface margins were beveled with a diamond instrument and the other half of the cavosurface margins were left intact and not beveled. (Fig. 8.1). The teeth were observed under environmental (SEM). The ends of the enamel rods were exposed at all the beveled cavosurface margins, whereas the sides of the enamel rods were exposed at all the nonbeveled cavosurface margins (Figs. 8.2 and 8.3). In addition, the proximal walls of the preparation when beveled at the cavosurface exposes the ends of the enamel rods (Figs. 8.5–8.7).

Acid etching removes about 10 μm of the enamel surface and creates a porous layer ranging from 5 to 50 μm in depth [32]. When a low-viscosity resin is applied, it flows into the microporosities of this layer and polymerizes to form a micromechanical bond with the enamel. Etching increases the wettability and surface area of the enamel substrate [33]. Acid etching raises the surface free energy of the enamel [30] to exceed the surface tension of the bonding material, producing spaces (etching patterns) into which the resin may penetrate to form taglike extensions and interlock mechanically when polymerized [34].

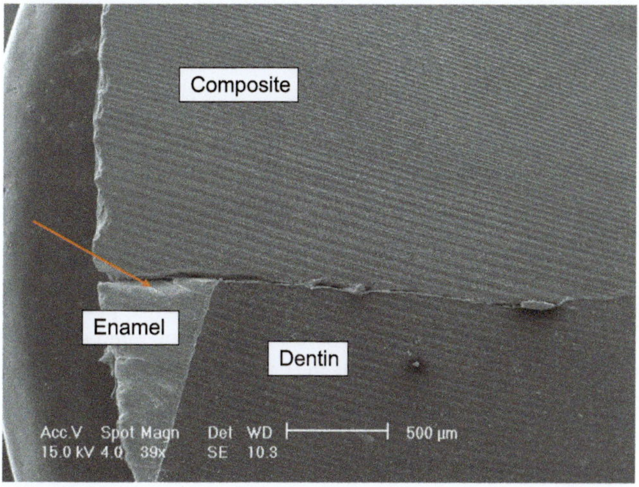

Figure 8.4 Potential gap (*red arrow*) formed at the gingival wall of a class II composite restoration when composite resin is bonded to the sides of the enamel rods. This gap was caused by drying technique in sample preparation when under vacuum environmental scanning electron microscopy preparation.

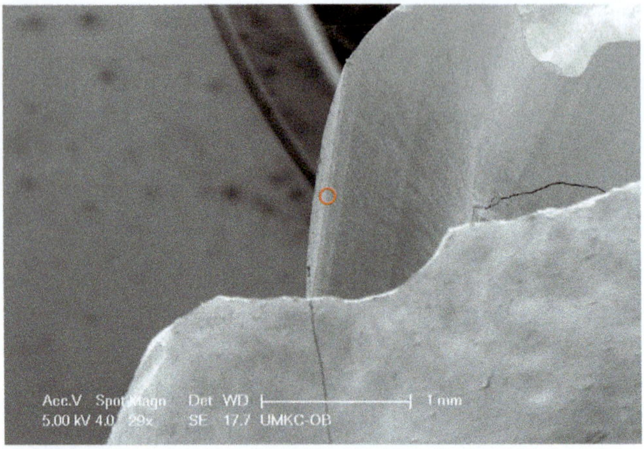

Figure 8.5 Proximal wall of class II preparation exposing proximal enamel that is oriented in a parallel direction to the right of the red circle.

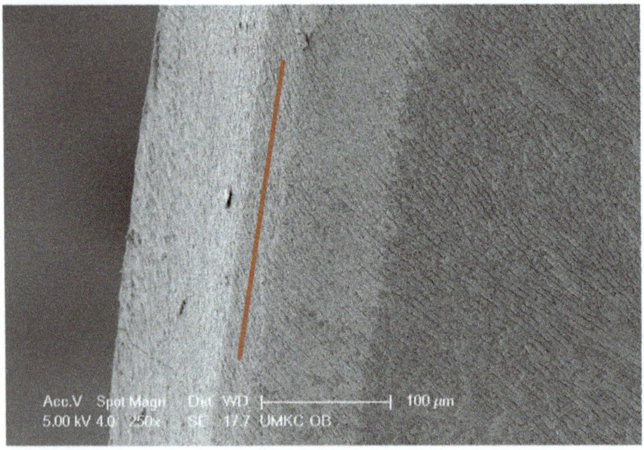

Figure 8.6 The 250 times magnified image of the red circle in Fig. 8.5 showing junction between sides of the enamel rods to the right of the red line and the ends of the enamel rods after the proximal wall has been beveled with a diamond instrument exposing the ends of the enamel rods.

Phosphoric acid applied to enamel creates five different types of microporosities. The most common is type I, which involves removal of enamel prism cores. The prism peripheries remain relatively intact. In type II the peripheries are removed leaving the cores intact. Type III includes areas resembling each of the other patterns as well as regions in which the etching pattern appears unrelated to prism morphology [32,35,36]. Type IV has been characterized as a pitted enamel surface that looks like unfinished puzzles, maps, or networks, and type V looks like a flat smooth surface [37]. The etching patterns on all teeth were similar in occlusal and central parts but differed frequently from cervical areas [37].

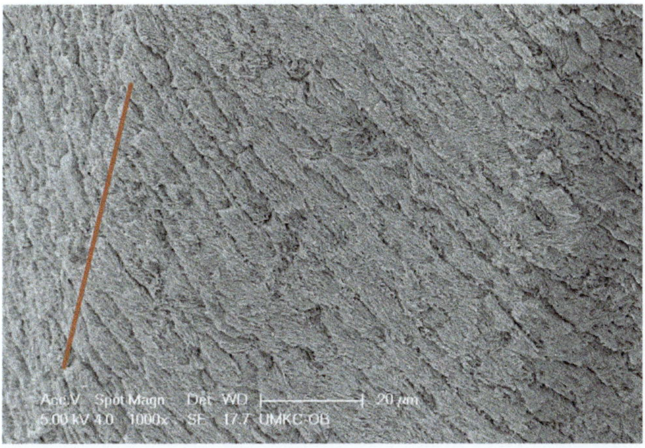

Figure 8.7 The 1000 times magnified image of the red circle in Fig. 8.5 showing junction between sides of the enamel rods to the right of the red line and the ends of the enamel rods after the proximal wall has been beveled with a diamond instrument exposing the ends of the enamel rods.

Cervical areas usually have less prism delineation, primarily due to the presence of prismless enamel [38]. There is more prismless enamel in the gingival third of permanent teeth, and prismless enamel is found in the cervical third of 70% of teeth [39]. The cervical third of a tooth is where the gingival margin of a class II preparation usually ends, if it terminates in enamel. If the dentist removes up to 150 μm of this cervical enamel then the underlying prismatic enamel is exposed which is more amenable to acid etching.

Resin penetration is limited in the cervical regions when compared with the central and occlusal regions. The cervical enamel of acid-etched human premolars have shorter and less numerous adhesive tags than those formed at the central and incisal enamel surface [40]. The highest bond strengths to enamel were obtained on the occlusal third, and the lowest bond strengths were found on the cervical third [41].

Researchers have suggested that bevels in enamel are necessary to reduce microleakage at cervical and ascending walls in class II box-type preparations [42–44]. However, in an in vivo study, there was no difference in failure rate between class II composite preparations with a bevel at the gingival margin and preparations without a gingival bevel. The performance of both groups was found to be equivalent after 5 years of clinical service [27,45]. These results suggest that a bevel does not eliminate the clinical problems associated with bonding at the gingival margin of a composite restoration.

8.3 Structure of dentin and effect on adhesive bonding

Dentin is a biological composite composed of dentin tubules; peritubular dentin, which encircles each tubule; and a collagen matrix of intertubular dentin dispersed between the dentin tubules. In contrast to enamel, the composition of dentin is very heterogeneous. The intertubular collagen matrix is filled with submicrometer- to nanometer-sized, calcium-deficient, carbonate-rich hydroxyapatite crystallites [46–48]. The dentin tubules are parallel micrometer-sized hypermineralized, collagen-poor cylinders lined with inorganic peritubular dentin [47,48]. The peritubular dentin can have a mineral content greater than 90%. In contrast, the intertubular dentin has a mineral content of 70%. Dentin is approximately 55 vol% mineral, 30 vol% organic material (primarily type I collagen), and 15 vol% fluid [46], but dentin composition varies with the age and tooth type. The organic portion of collagen is surrounded by water, and hydrogen bonding exists between the strands of the collagen [48].

Dentin contains continuous tubules that run from the DEJ to the dentin–pulp border. Each tubule is an inverted, elongated cone, with its smallest diameter (c. 0.8 μm) at the DEJ and its largest diameter (c. 3.0 μm) at the pulp. As the tubules converge on the pulp chamber, the surface area of the intertubular dentin decreases and the tubule density increases from about 1.9×10^6 tubules/cm^2 at the DEJ to between 4.5 and 6.5×10^6 tubules/cm^2 at the dentin–pulp border [19].

The surface area occupied by intertubular dentin and dentin tubules varies as a function of the location, ie, close to the pulp or the DEJ. At a location close to the pulp (0.1–0.5 mm from the pulp), the percent of surface area occupied by the intertubular dentin and dentin tubules is about 51% and 12%, respectively. After acid etching, intertubular dentin comprises 70% and the tubules 30%. In comparison, at a location close to the DEJ, the percent of surface area occupied by intertubular dentin and dentin tubules is about 94% and 2%, respectively. After acid etching dentin that is close to the DEJ, 84% of the surface area is intertubular dentin and the tubules make up 16% of the surface area [48,49]. Based on these comparisons, for dentin close to the pulp, intertubular dentin accounts for less surface area, whereas the tubules, which are filled with pulpal fluid, occupy more of the surface area. Close to the pulp and prior to acid etching, dentin tubules account for ~12% of the surface area, whereas after acid etching the tubules account for 30% of the surface area.

The fluid content of the dentin tubules varies by depth, with superficial dentin containing the lowest fluid content and deeper dentin, ie, dentin closest to the pulp, containing more fluid [50]. The amount of collagen in dentin decreases from superficial to deep dentin [51]. Bonding to dentin is variable, depending on the number, density, and size of the tubules. The more the amount of tubules present, the wetter the dentin surface. There is an inverse correlation between the bond strength of the composite resin and that of the superficial and deep dentin, ie, the deeper the dentin, the lower the adhesive bond strength [52–54].

Depending on the location of the cervical wall, the tubule density on the cervical wall of premolars is different from the tubule density on the axial walls. When the cervical tubule density was counted 1.0 mm above the CEJ, there were 149 tubules for every 100 tubules on the axial wall [55]. Incipient to small cavities usually end 1.0–2.0 mm above the CEJ. At these sites, 49% more tubules means that there is less intertubular dentin for bonding on the cervical wall when compared with the axial wall. The increase in tubule density also translates to increased fluid content on the cervical wall. There is an inverse relationship between dentin tubules and intertubular dentin, ie, as the surface area of dentin tubules increases, the surface area of intertubular dentin decreases.

Dentin tubules are filled with pulpal fluid, and after acid etching, more dentinal tubules comprise the total surface area of the dentin. This is true no matter the depth of dentin that is acid etched. The wetter the dentin, the more difficult it is to bond.

Deep dentin with more tubules has a higher fluid content than does superficial dentin, which has less dentin tubules [56]. Pulpal fluid from the dentin tubules may dilute the organic solvents of some bonding agents. Diluting the organic solvent can cause monomers to leave the soluble phase and form resin globules [57].

When a rotating dental bur comes in contact with the tooth surface, it leaves a smear layer over the surface of the dentin [58] and smear plugs over the openings of the dentinal tubules [19]. The composition of the smear layer includes collagen, mineral, and other debris. Based on morphologic studies, it is theorized that acid etching removes the smear layer and smear plugs [19]. There is no chemical evidence to support the theory that acid etchants remove the dentin smear layer [59]. The collagen of the smear layer is not removed by acid etching, and residual mineral is trapped in the denatured, gelatinized collagen. Ultimately, this gelatinous layer could inhibit the formation of an impervious seal at the dentin/adhesive interface; it could act as a weak link in the coupling of adhesive to dentin [59].Acid etching opens the dentinal tubules, increases dentin permeability, and decalcifies the intertubular and peritubular dentin [26]. When dentin is acid etched with phosphoric acid, the apatitic mineral is removed, leaving a collagen fibril network. The collagen is supported by water—the water may either be part of the native structure or be water that has been used to rinse the acid-etched dentin surface [48]. After acid conditioning, the dentin surface is represented as a collagen meshwork 2–4 μm thick [48] that can collapse and shrink due to the loss of support from mineral and/or water [70].When bonded to the cavity surfaces, the polymerizing composite restoration induces the development of stress inside the material, which is transmitted to the tooth structure via bonded interfaces. The magnitude of the polymerization shrinkage stress is influenced by several factors including the volume of material to be polymerized, the filler content and monomer composition, the insertion technique, the flow properties of the composite resin, and the geometry of the cavity [62]. It has been estimated that shear bond strengths of 17–20 MPa are required to resist the contraction forces associated with polymerization shrinkage and to produce gap-free restoration margins [19,63]. If the composite resin cannot bond stronger to the dentin than its polymerization shrinkage stress, then the composite resin can separate from the dentin leaving microgaps [62,64,65]. Leakage of the fluid from the dentin tubules into these microgaps can occur [65,66] (Fig. 8.4). When the patient occludes on the restoration or experiences temperature changes, this fluid movement can cause tooth sensitivity.

8.4 Generations of dentin adhesives

Developing a consistent, reliable, and durable bond to dentin has proven elusive, and bonding to dentin is not as predictable as bonding to enamel is [19,60,61]. The challenges of developing a reliable and durable dentin bond, under in vivo conditions, have prompted a search for better materials. The multiple generations [26,61] of bonding agents are evidence of the research community's ongoing search for materials that can provide a durable dentin bond under clinical conditions.

In the late 1980s, the third generation of bonding resins was introduced, which either modified or removed the smear layer to allow resin penetration in the subjacent dentin [26,67,68]. These three-step total-etch adhesives had hydrophilic low-viscosity resin monomers that were applied as primers after the dentin was etched. The primers wet and infiltrated the dentin smear layer and bonded to the composite resin. The composition of the primers included hydroxyethyl trimellitate anhydride, biphenyl dimethacrylate, and a primer composed of 6% phosphate penta-acrylate, 30% hydroxyethylmethacrylate (HEMA), and 64% ethanol [61].

The fourth generation of bonding agents appeared in the early 1990s [26]. This generation used the total-etch technique, ie, etching enamel and dentin [69] to completely remove the smear layer over the dentin tubules [61]. The bonding mechanism of the fourth-generation adhesive systems is a three-step total-etch process: (1) condition, (2) prime, and (3) bond. After rinsing the acid-etched dentin, the collagen fibril network is primed with a hydrophilic resin monomer, which also contains a solvent, such as water, acetone, or alcohol. This primer aids in displacing water, expanding or reexpanding the collagen network, and thus promoting the infiltration of the monomer into the submicrometer- or nanometer-sized spaces within the collagen fiber network [19]. Primer molecules contain two functional groups—a hydrophilic and a hydrophobic group. The hydrophilic group has an affinity for the dentin surface, and the hydrophobic group has an affinity for the resin. The primer can consist of a hydrophilic monomer such as HEMA. The primer wets and penetrates the demineralized dentin matrix, ie, the collagen network, raising it almost to its original level. The primer also increases the surface energy, and hence the wettability, of the dentin surface. Then a bonding agent consisting of an unfilled resin that consists of a hydrophobic monomer such as bisphenyl-A-glycidyl methacrylate (Bis-GMA), triethyleneglycol dimethacrylate (TEGDMA), and urethane dimethacrylate and hydrophilic monomers such as HEMA is applied [19]. The unfilled resin penetrates into the primed dentin, copolymerizing with the primer to form an intermingled layer of collagen and resin; this collagen–resin structure is commonly called the "hybrid layer" [26]. The formation of the hybrid layer produces increased adhesive bond strengths to dentin [71].

Formation of the hybrid layer was first described by Nakabayashi [48] and is thought to be the primary bonding mechanism of most current adhesives [72]. Many researchers support this hypothesis, ie, that the bond between dentin and the adhesive is due to interdiffusion or micromechanical interlocking/entrapment of the resin within the tissue substrate, yielding a hybrid layer [19,48] of dentin and adhesive resin [19,69]. The mechanical bond of the adhesive to the collagen network and to some extent to the inside of the dentin tubules is what makes it possible for the composite resin to mechanically attach itself to the dentin.

Overetching of the dentin can create problems such as insufficient penetration of the bonding agent, which leaves voids under the hybrid layer. Wet bonding was introduced, which requires a subjective analysis by the clinician; the clinician must determine if the dentin is too wet or too dry. Excessive drying leads to collagen collapse, which will impede penetration of the bonding agent [48].

Using the scanning acoustic microscope, the elastic moduli of dentin was 28 GPa for normal dentin and 13 GPa for demineralized dentin [73]. The demineralized dentinal matrix lacks the stiffness of mineralized dentin [48]. The elastic modulus of wet demineralized dentinal matrix may be about 7 MPa [74], which is more than 1000 times lower than that of mineralized dentin [48]. The clinical implication of this low stiffness is that the collagen fibril network can easily collapse when air-dried and the collapsed collagen may act as a barrier to adhesive infiltration [48].

There are two theories for the major shrinkage of the demineralized dentin matrix when it is air-dried. The passive theory assumes that the collagen network is floating or suspended in water. Each fibril is separated from the other by a water-filled space, which occupies the space previously occupied by apatite crystallites. As the water supporting the collagen network is removed via air-drying, the water that separated the fibrils disappears and the collagen fibrils come closer together in all three dimensions. This results in a passive collapse of the collagen network. The space between the fibrils is lost, and the primer monomer can no longer infiltrate that space [48]. The other theory is as water is evaporated from the collagen network the collagen may shorten slightly and pull down the other collagen with which it is interconnected [75]. Air-drying of demineralized dentin can reduce the volume of dentin by 65%, but it is theorized that the original dimension can be regained after immersion in water [76].

The hybrid layer between adhesive resin and surface demineralized dentin was found to be wider in the area of empty tubules compared with that of the occluded tubules. The hybrid layer was found to be the thinnest at the proximal lateral walls of the cavity where the dentinal tubules run parallel to the cavity surface [77]. Thus the amount of dentin demineralized by acid conditioning as well as the impregnation of resin into the intertubular dentin (forming the hybrid layer) is probably related to the degree of closure and direction of the dentinal tubules [77].

There are differences between a phosphoric acid etching system and a self-etching primer system. A phosphoric acid etching system may open the tubules and allow more dentinal fluid to wet the dentin surface [78]. A self-etching primer system may act on the dentin by modifying the smear layer within the tubules. When the smear layer is modified only partially dissolved smear plugs may remain within the tubules. This lowers the dentin permeability and diminishes the sensitivity to fluid from the pulp chamber [78]. There is more regional variability of adhesive bond strengths to dentin (in vitro) for phosphoric acid systems than for self-etching primer systems [78].

Some collapse of the exposed collagen fibril network due to gentle postconditioning air-drying of the dentin surface, may not have been totally recovered through hybridization by the two step adhesive as opposed to the three-step system. Simplifying the application procedure of adhesives by combining the primer and adhesive resin into a single application step may reduce hybridization effectiveness [79].

Whether self-etching primers etch enamel or phosphoric acid also is debatable. As noted in Fig. 8.8, the depth and definition of the enamel treated with a self-etching HEMA primer (Clear Fil-SE) is much less than that of the tooth treated with a total

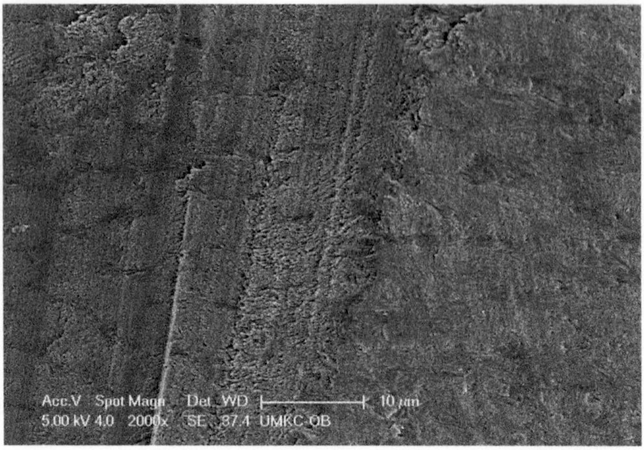

Figure 8.8 Enamel treated with a self-etching primer containing hydroxyethylmethacrylate showing less etching of the enamel with less surface area to form an adhesive–enamel bond.

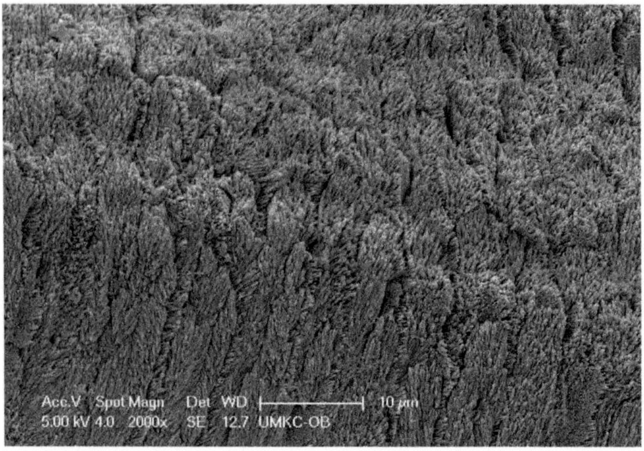

Figure 8.9 Total-etch treatment with 37% phosphoric acid exposing deeper etching of the enamel.

acid-etch technique (Fig. 8.9). Tensile bond strengths of adhesive resins bonded to intact (unground) enamel after etching with self-etching primers were not as high as those of phosphoric acid–etched specimens [80]. However, tensile bond strengths of adhesive resins to ground enamel were similar for self-etching primers and phosphoric acid groups [80]. When using self-etching primers on intact enamel, it may be necessary to double the application time or use multiple layers to achieve sufficient enamel etching [80].

The ideal hybrid layer provides complete resin infiltration within the exposed collagen matrix. Dental bonding systems that have inadequate adhesive penetration can leave exposed collagen at the dentin–adhesive interface [81,82]. The exposed collagen could be degraded by bacterial proteases, compromising the integrity of the dentin–adhesive bond and, ultimately, the restoration [81,83]. The adhesive/dentin interface has been identified as the weak link in most composite restorations [84].

The main factor influencing the pulpal reaction under restorative materials is the presence of bacteria on the cavity walls followed by the remaining dentin thickness [85]. Other factors that can lead to poor outcomes for resin composite in posterior teeth is the ability of the gingival resin increment to be adequately light cured. It was found that a minimum of a 300 mW/cm^2 output was sufficient to cure composite resin 2–3 mm thick when irradiated for 20–30 s [86]. The light should be periodically tested to ensure minimum output light levels [86].

8.5 Bonding to cavity walls

8.5.1 Dentin tubule orientation

The orientation of the dentin tubules to the bonded resin composite can be either perpendicular, parallel, oblique, or mixed [87]. When the shear strength of dentin was determined at different tubule orientations and intratooth locations, there was a difference in shear strength in the central and cusp areas. The shear strength depended on dentin tubule orientation in the central area of the tooth [88]. There is probably a weak dependence on tubule orientation, but the effect is not as dramatic as the microstructural appearance of the dentin might suggest [88].

An in vitro study found that bond strengths after 48 h were not influenced by tubule orientation (parallel or perpendicular) or intratooth (cusp, fissure, cervical root, or midroot) location [89]. Perpendicular- or parallel-oriented dentin tubules had similar bond strengths to resin composite. In comparison, another in vitro study found a difference between regional bond strengths of occlusal (parallel-oriented dental tubules) and gingival dentin (perpendicular-oriented dentin tubules) [90]. Resin bonded to parallel-oriented tubules had higher microtensile bond strengths by ~11–13 MPa than resin bonded to perpendicular-oriented tubules in in-vivo [6] and in-vitro studies [90].

The direction of the dentinal tubules appears to be an important variable determining bond strength to dentin. This may be one of the reasons why the bond strengths of the resin are not uniform inside a cavity [87]. The thickness of the hybrid layer of the parallel group (parallel-oriented tubules) was thicker than that of the perpendicular group. Deeper demineralization of the dentin makes it possible to form a thicker hybrid layer in the parallel than the perpendicular group [87]. In the parallel group, the bonding resin easily penetrates the collagen network of the demineralized dentin as well as the peritubular dentin-free dentinal tubules, which were surrounded by demineralized intertubular dentin [87]. The tubule direction may also determine the intrinsic wetness of the surface [87,91].

8.5.2 Regional bond strength to cavity walls

Tensile bond strength to the gingival wall was significantly lower than that to the occlusal wall in wedge-shaped cavities by more than 11.0 MPa, and this was the same whether single or multiple layers of primer were applied [90]. In a separate study, when resin composite was bonded to occlusal and gingival margins in wedge-shaped in vitro class V preparations, there was no difference in the bond strengths between the regions. Naturally created lesions that had sclerotic dentin had 20–40% lower bond strengths than artificially created wedges [92,93]. The morphology and the effects of acid etching are different on cervical or gingival dentin (oblique, mixed) compared with axial and occlusal dentin (perpendicular), and compared with proximal or lateral wall dentin (parallel) in the class II preparation [93].

It is theorized that a lifting or peeling up of the resin composite that is bonded to the weaker outer 200-μm margin area of the gingival floor, in box preparations below the CEJ, may occur. This lifting could then create a microgap that becomes filled with bacterial sulcular fluid through capillary action. This lifting may produce the same phenomena involved in crack initiation, which permits energy stored in the stressed dentin–resin bond to be dissipated by rapid crack propagation and failure of the substrate [19]. Underfilled or open leaky margins at the cervical region of class II restorations may allow oral fluids, pathogens, and other noxious agents to infiltrate these margins, and this activity could lead to secondary caries [81,94] (Fig. 8.4). The depth of resin penetration at the margins of class II restorations in vital teeth was only a few micrometers [95]. The margins between the tooth and composite are the sites most prone to leakage.

The orientation of dentinal tubules in vitro has a profound effect on the formation of the hybrid layer [96]. In areas with perpendicular tubule orientation, the hybrid layer was $3.2 \pm 0.8\,\mu m$ thick, showing solid 27.2 ± 0.8-μm long resin tags in the dentinal tubules and a network of tiny tags in their side branches [96]. In areas with parallel tubule orientation, the hybrid layer was significantly thinner ($1.3 \pm 0.6\,\mu m$) and resin tags were absent [96]. Yoshiyama has hypothesized that resin engagement of sound dentin to a depth of only one to two collagen fibers may provide retention of the order of 20 MPa; this translates to a thickness of 0.1–0.2 μm [97].

When the cavity margin is below the cementoenamel junction, the presence of a cementum layer of approximately 150–200 μm at the cervical margins of cavities may also pose a serious clinical problem for reliable bonding [98]. It is questionable as to whether cervical margins of class II and class V preparations allow reliable bonding [93]. Cavity floors are primarily composed of perpendicular-oriented dentin and the proximal lateral or axial cavity walls are primarily composed of parallel-oriented dentin [6,93] (Figs. 8.10–8.13).

Clinical researchers have suggested that dentin–adhesive systems should be chosen according to the different types of dentin substrate, such as caries-affected versus unaffected dentin, sclerotic versus nonsclerotic dentin, and young versus old dentin, and the region to be bonded such as close to pulp versus close to the DEJ and cervical versus occlusal walls [78]. Bond strengths can also vary according to the intrinsic wetness of the dentin and what adhesive system is used [78]. Bond strength also varies by the thickness of the increment bonded to dentin, with 1.0-mm increments having higher shear bond strengths than 2.0-mm increments [99]. Bonding to superficial

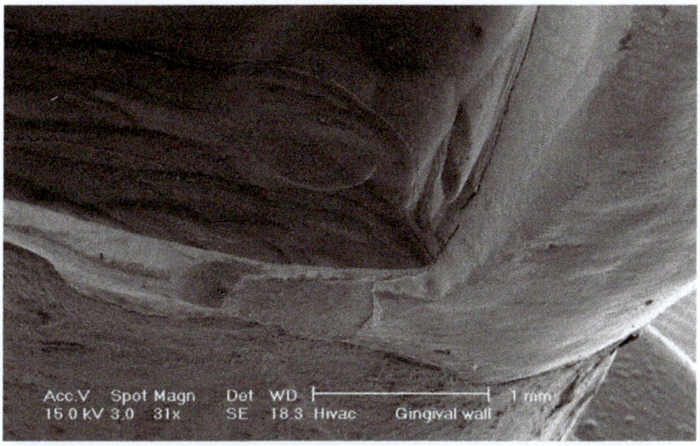

Figure 8.10 Gingival wall of class II resin preparation at proximal box.

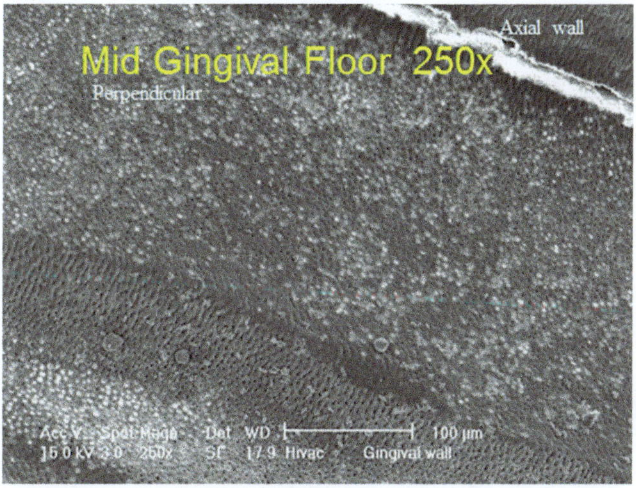

Figure 8.11 Perpendicular-oriented dentin exposing the ends of the dentin tubules at the midgingival floor of class II preparation. Junction of gingival and axial wall of dentin can be seen in the upper right area of picture. Magnification ×250.

dentin, in vitro, also gives higher bond strengths than bonding to deeper dentin which is closer to the pulp [99].

When the microtensile bond strength of dentin–adhesive bonded to flat versus corresponding cavity walls (created with dental burs) from the same teeth were measured, the microtensile bond strength of the adhesive bonded to flat surfaces was significantly higher than that of the adhesive bonded to the corresponding three-dimensional cavity wall. It was concluded that bond strengths on flat dentin surfaces created by 600-grit SiC paper may overestimate the strength that can be achieved under clinically relevant conditions [100].

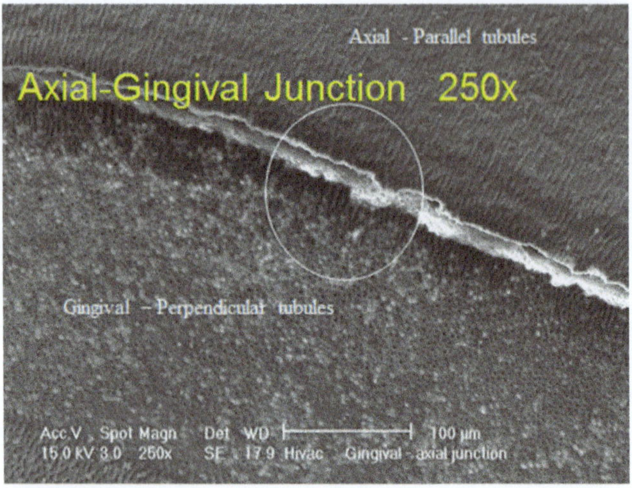

Figure 8.12 Highlighted circle showing junction between the gingival and axial walls. The dentin tubules on the axial wall are in the parallel-oriented direction exposing the sides of the dentin tubules and the tubules at the gingival wall are in the perpendicular-oriented direction exposing the ends of the dentin tubules.

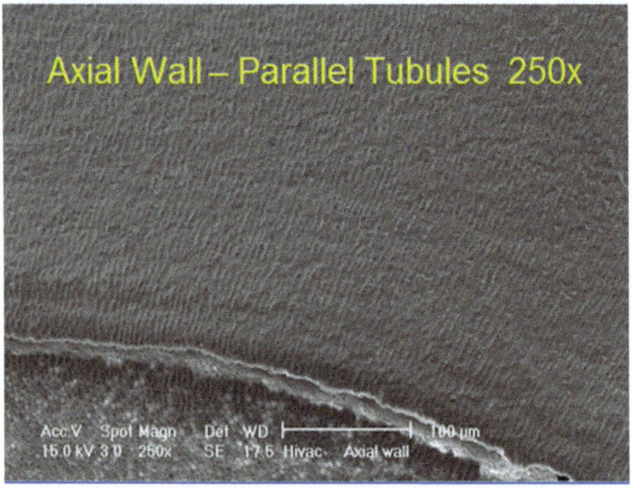

Figure 8.13 Axial wall of preparation showing dentin tubules in a parallel-oriented direction exposing the sides of the dentin tubules.

8.6 Phase separation

The relationship between adhesive thickness and microtensile bond strength may differ as a function of material, eg, Clearfil Liner Bond 2V produced higher bond strengths with an increase in adhesive thickness, whereas Single Bond produced lower values for increased adhesive thickness [101]. It was hypothesized that since

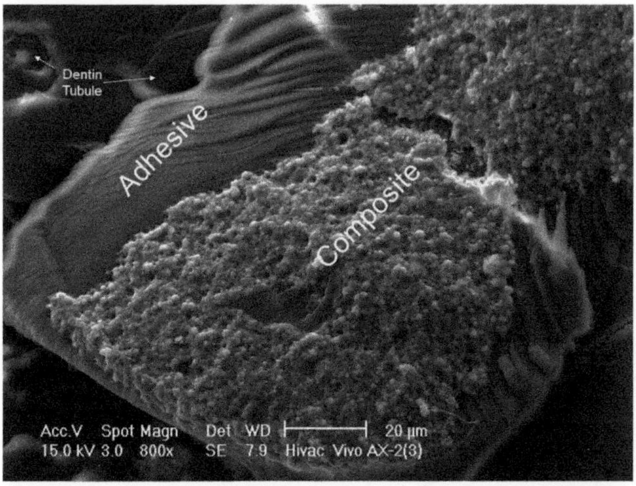

Figure 8.14 Cross-section from the axial wall of a class II resin composite restoration. The tooth was restored under in vivo conditions. The microtensile adhesive bond strength from this sample was 44.1 MPa.

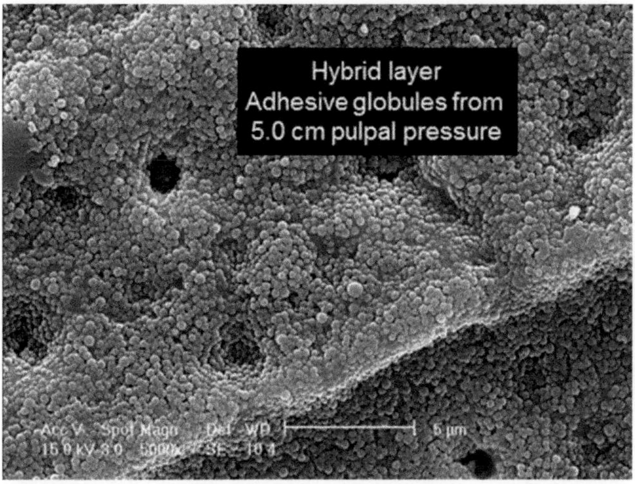

Figure 8.15 Adhesive contaminated with fluid showing phase separation of adhesive. Adhesive was applied on dentin with a pulpal pressure of 5.0 cm water pressure under in vitro conditions.

the Clearfil product did not contain any solvent and Single Bond contained ethanol and water, excess solvents in the bonding agent may have contributed to phase separation between the adhesive and resin composite. Such phase separation could lead to reduced bond strengths as the adhesive layer becomes thicker (Fig. 8.14 no phase separation of adhesive, and Fig. 8.15 showing globules indicating phase separation).

Excess water in the primer or moisture from perpendicular tubules, which have been acid etched, could also contribute to voids at the interface of the dentin and adhesive. These voids could act as stress concentrators—the voids could lead to weak and leaky adhesive bonds (Figs. 8.16–8.19). There were more voids at the gingival margin than at the axial margin for teeth restored under in vivo conditions [91]. It was hypothesized that a major contributor to these voids was excess water at the gingival margin.

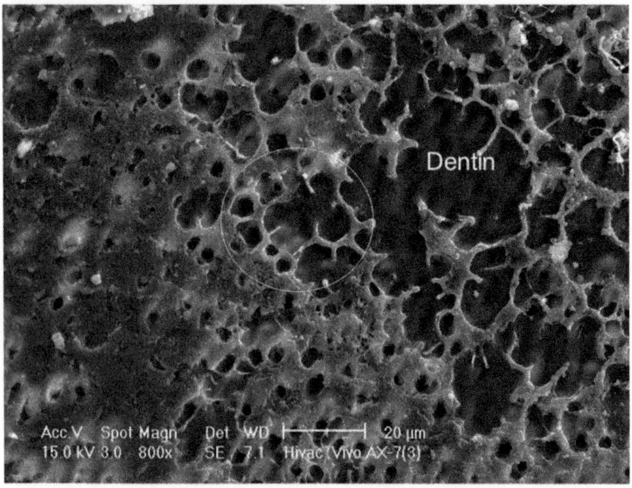

Figure 8.16 Voids through the adhesive junction on dentin from excess water left after washing phosphoric acid or from pulpal fluid from dentin tubules that were opened after acid etching with phosphoric acid. The tooth was prepared under in vivo conditions.

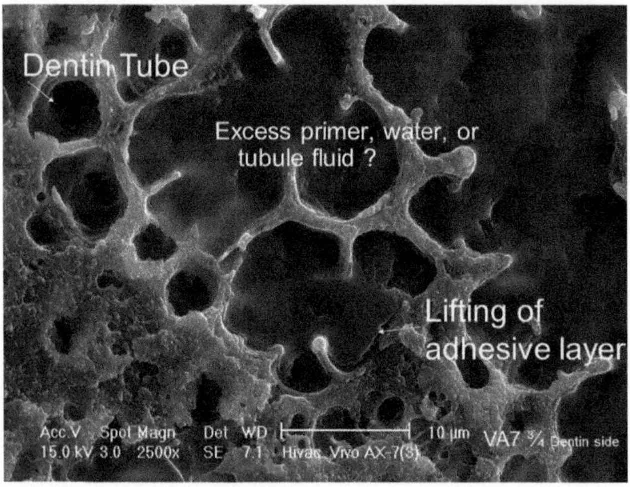

Figure 8.17 Magnified image of the circle in Fig.8 16 showing voids in the adhesive interface on the dentin surface. Voids could be from excess primer, pulpal fluid, or water from the rinsing process during adhesive placement using the total-etch phosphoric acid technique. The microtensile adhesive bond strength of this sample was 10.4 MPa.

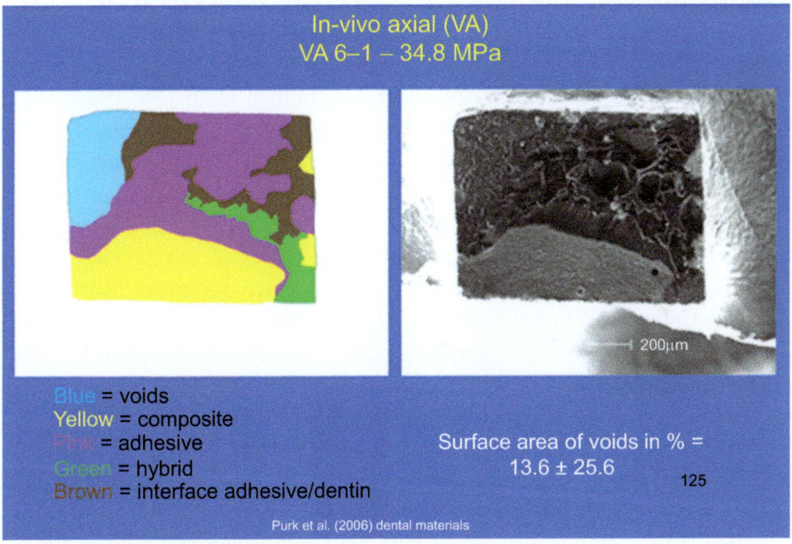

Figure 8.18 Average voids present on dentin axial walls under in vivo conditions. The surface area of voids averaged 13.6 ± 25.6% caused from moisture contamination on dentin axial walls during placement of adhesive in class II resin composite restorations under in vivo conditions. This is a representative sample from this testing group.

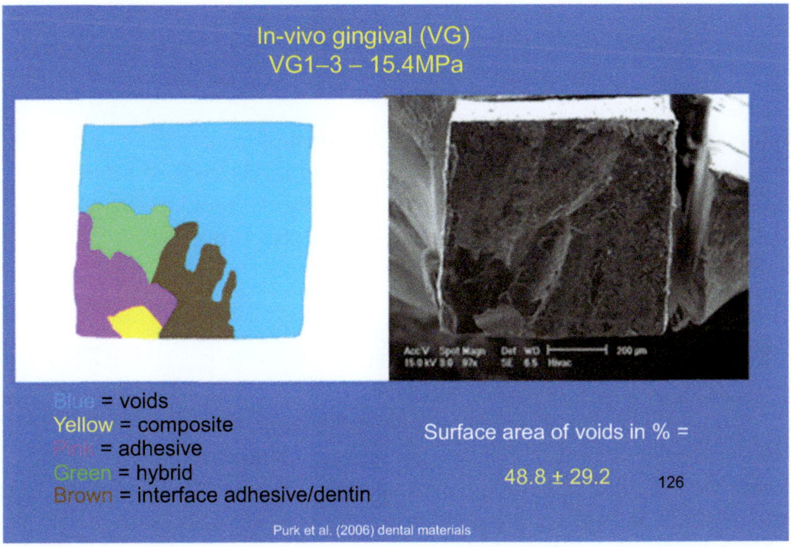

Figure 8.19 Average voids present on dentin gingival walls under in vivo conditions. The surface area of voids averaged 48.8 ± 29.2% caused from moisture contamination on dentin gingival walls during placement of adhesive in class II resin composite restorations under in vivo conditions. This is a representative sample from this testing group.

8.7 Regional bond strength differences in dentin

The location of the dentin can be a factor when performing bond strength studies. Proximal dentin is the most permeable dentin in human teeth [9]. The fluid in the proximal area does not seep from the dentinal tubules until removal of the smear layer with a conditioning agent [9]. Resin composite is also more sensitive to pulpal pressure [52,102]. Bonds made to superficial dentin were greater than those made to deep dentin [103,104]. Some adhesives did not bond well to deep dentin, making them more susceptible to polymerization shrinkage stress, which develops with high C-factors [56]. For bonding systems that purport to remove the smear layer [9,56,105], superficial dentin bonded better than deep dentin. Bond strengths close to the pulp were only 30–40% of the bond strength recorded on superficial dentin [105]. It has been suggested that bonding to deep dentin may require new approaches to blocking the lumina of tubules prior to bonding, or new resin systems that can polymerize well even in high water concentrations may be necessary [19]. For some resin systems, the bond to the deeper dentin was greatly affected by how close one was to the pulp and also by the cavity configuration. Some systems gave reduced bond strengths when they were bonded to more cavity walls compared with just bonding to a flat surface and when bonded to deeper compared with superficial dentin [56].

Bonding to axial wall dentin may be independent of how close it is to the pulp [106,107]. When resin composite was bonded to in vitro occlusal, superficial proximal (the axial wall), middle proximal depth and deep proximal dentin, there was no difference in the bond strengths [107]. When the resin composite was bonded to in vitro occlusal dentin in the outer, middle, and inner areas, there was no difference as well [106]. The tubule orientation at these areas was mixed (perpendicular and parallel) to the resin composite surface, and most of these tests were performed on proximal or axial wall dentin.

In summary, the results of these studies suggest that resin–dentin in vitro bonds are not as homogeneous as enamel bonds that bond to the ends of the enamel rods. Furthermore, resin dentin bonds vary as a function of the adhesive material used [56,108,109], the operator [109], and the cavity wall that is bonded.

8.8 Conclusions

Bonding to the tooth surface in a class II preparation requires the operator to be aware of the myriad of factors that can influence the quality of the bond. These factors include the structure, direction, and morphology of the enamel and dentin. Adhesive bond strength is best when the adhesive is bonded to the ends of the enamel rods (perpendicular-oriented enamel) in the upper two-thirds of the tooth followed by bonding to parallel-oriented dentin, followed by bonding to either the sides of the enamel (parallel-oriented enamel) or perpendicular-oriented dentin.

The site most susceptible to recurrent caries in class II resin composites is the gingival margin. If the gingival margin is close to the cementoenamel junction, the sides of the enamel rods and perpendicular dentin is the type of tooth substrate that is available for bonding. Bonding to gingival dentinal cavity walls is much less predictable and weaker than bonding to axial cavity walls. The strength of the in vivo bond of the resin composite to dentin at the gingival margin may not be sufficient to resist the forces of polymerization shrinkage of the resin composite. In addition, moisture contamination at the gingival margin can inhibit the formation of a durable adhesive bond. Under in vivo conditions, the bond of the resin composite to dentin at the gingival margin is very fragile. Bonding of resin composite to dentin at the gingival wall under in vivo conditions is weaker and more fragile than the previously reported microtensile bond strengths of resin composite bonded to dentin under in vitro conditions.

Studies that combine in vivo application with in vitro testing also confirm a very weak bond at the gingival wall. These studies report a high number of debonds when testing the adhesive strength to the enamel and dentin at this location. It is imperative that researchers report the number of debonds when they perform adhesive bond strength studies. The difficulty of obtaining clinical success with posterior resin composites underscores the importance of recognizing and understanding the numerous factors that can impact the durability of this restoration.

References

[1] Hondrum SO. The longevity of resin-based composite restorations in posterior teeth. [Review, 116 refs] Gen Dent 2000;48(4):398–404.
[2] Soncini JA, et al. The longevity of amalgam versus compomer/composite restorations in posterior primary and permanent teeth: findings from the New England children's amalgam trial. J Am Dent Assoc 2007;138(6):763–72.
[3] Bernardo M, et al. Survival and reasons for failure of amalgam versus composite posterior restorations placed in a randomized clinical trial. J Am Dent Assoc 2007;138(6):775–83.
[4] Liebenberg WH. Assuring restorative integrity in extensive posterior resin composite restorations: pushing the envelope. Quintessence Int 2000;31(3):153–64.
[5] Soderholm KJM. Correlation of in vivo and in vitro performance of adhesive restorative materials: a report of the ASC MD156 task group on test methods for the adhesion of restorative materials. Dent Mater 1991;7:74–83.
[6] Purk J, et al. In-vivo vs. in-vitro microtensile bond strength of axial vs. gingival cavity preparation walls in class II resin-based composite restorations. JADA 2004;135(2):185–93.
[7] Huysmans MC, et al. The influence of simulated clinical handling on the flexural and compressive strength of posterior composite restorative materials. Dent Mater 1996;12(2):116–20.
[8] Hashimoto M, et al. In vivo degradation of resin-dentin bonds in humans over 1 to 3 years. J Dent Res 2000;79(6):1385–91.
[9] Pashley DH. In vitro simulations of in vivo bonding conditions. [Review, 30 refs] Am J Dent 1991;4(5):237–40.
[10] Draughn RA. Effects of temperature on mechanical properties of composite dental restorative materials. J Biomed Mater Res 1981;15(4):489–95.
[11] Burrow MF, et al. Influence of temperature and relative humidity on early bond strengths to dentine. J Dent 1995;23(1):41–5.
[12] Nystrom GP, et al. Temperature and humidity effects on bond strength of a dentinal adhesive. Oper Dent 1998;23(3):454–8.

[13] Pashley D, et al. The effects of acid etching on the in vivo permeability of dentin in the dog. Arch Oral Biol 1983;28:555–9.
[14] Maroli S, Khera SC, Krell KV. Regional variation in permeability of young dentin. Oper Dent 1992;17(3):93–100.
[15] Richardson D, Tao L, Pashley DH. Dentin permeability: effects of crown preparation. Int J Prosthodont 1991;4(3):219–25.
[16] Eliades G, Palaghias G, Vougiouklakis G. Surface reactions of adhesives on dentin. Dent Mater 1990;6(3):208–16.
[17] Spencer P, et al. Chemical characterization of the dentin/adhesive interface by Fourier transform infrared photoacoustic spectroscopy. Dent Mater 1992;8(1):10–5.
[18] Eick JD, et al. Adhesives and nonshrinking dental resins of the future. Quintessence Int 1993;24(9):632–40.
[19] Eick JD, et al. Current concepts on adhesion to dentin. Crit Rev Oral Biol Med 1997;8(3):306–35.
[20] Sturdevant C, et al. The art and science of operative dentistry. 3rd ed. St. Louis, MO: Mosby; 1995. p. 824.
[21] Barkmeier W, Shafer S, Gwinnett A. Effects of 15 vs 60 second enamel acid conditioning on adhesion and morphology. Oper Dent 1986;11:111–6.
[22] Perdigao J, Denehy GE, Swift Jr EJ. Silica contamination of etched dentin and enamel surfaces: a scanning electron microscopic and bond strength study. Quintessence Int 1994;25(5):327–33.
[23] van der Vyver PJ, de Wet FA, Jansen van Rensburg JM. Bonding of composite resin using different enamel etchants. J Dent Assoc S Afr 1997;52(3):169–72.
[24] Carvalho RM, et al. Effects of prism orientation on tensile strength of enamel. J Adhes Dent 2000;2(4):251–7.
[25] Buonocore M. A simple method of increasing the adhesion of acrylic filling materials to enamel surfaces. J Dent Res 1955;34:849–53.
[26] Swift Jr EJ. Bonding systems for restorative materials–a comprehensive review. [Review, 61 refs] Pediatr Dent 1998;20(2):80–4.
[27] Silverstone L. Fissure sealants: laboratory studies. Caries Res 1974;8:2–26.
[28] Vargas M, et al. Microtensile bond strength of composite to different enamel rod angulations. Abstract 1568 J Dent Res January 2001;80(Special Issue):231.
[29] Purk JH, et al. Fracture strength of Class I versus Class II restored premolars tested at the marginal ridge. 2. Cavosurface bonding and cavosurface plus internal enamel bonding. Quintessence Int 1990;21(8):655–62.
[30] Van Meerbeek B, et al. Adhesives and cements to promote preservation dentistry. Oper Dent 2001;(Suppl.):119–44.
[31] Purk J, Thomure J, Dusevich V, Tira D. Beveled vs non-beveled gingival margins in class II composite preparations. J Dent Res April 2011;(Special Issue). p. Abstract # 3186.
[32] Swift Jr EJ, Perdigao J, Heymann HO. Bonding to enamel and dentin: a brief history and state of the art. [Review, 216 refs] Quintessence Int 1995;26(2):95–110.
[33] Retief D. Effect of conditioning the enamel surface with phosphoric acid. J Dent Res 1973;52:333–41.
[34] Retief D. The mechanical bond. Int Dent J 1978;28:18–27.
[35] Silverstone L, et al. Variation in the pattern of acid etching of human dental enamel examined by scanning electron microscopy. Caries Res 1975;9:373–87.
[36] Denys F, Retief D. Variations in enamel etching patterns produced by different concentrations of phosphoric acid. J Dent Assoc S Afr 1982;37:185–9.
[37] Galil K, Wright G. Acid etching patterns on buccal surfaces of permanent teeth. Pediatr Dent 1979;1:230–4.

[38] Gwinnett A. The ultrastructure of the "prismless" enamel of permanent human teeth. Arch Oral Biol 1967;12:381–7.
[39] Ripa LW, Gwinnett AJ, Buonocore MG. The "prismless" outer layer of deciduous and permanent enamel. Arch Oral Biol 1966;11(1):41–8.
[40] Arakawa Y, Takahashi Y, Sebata M. The effect of acid etching on the cervical region of the buccal surface of the human premolar, with special reference to direct bonding techniques. Am J Orthod 1979;76(2):201–8.
[41] Shono Y, et al. Effects of cross-sectional area on resin-enamel tensile bond strength. Dent Mater 1997;13(5):290–6.
[42] Crim G, Shay J. Effect of etchant time on microleakage. J Dent Child 1987;54:339–40.
[43] Shafer S, Barkmeier W, Kelsey W. Effects of reduced acid conditioning time on enamel microleakage. Gen Dent 1987;35:278–80.
[44] Opdam NJ, Roeters JJ, Burgersdijk RC. Microleakage of Class II box-type composite restorations. Am J Dent 1998;11(4):160–4.
[45] Wilson NH, et al. Performance of occlusin in butt-joint and bevel-edged preparations: five-year results. 4. Dent Mater 1991;7(2):92–8.
[46] Marshall G. Dentin: microstructure and characterization. Quintessence Int 1993 ;24:606–17.
[47] Marshall Jr GW, et al. The dentin substrate: structure and properties related to bonding. [Review, 138 refs] J Dent 1997;25(6):441–58.
[48] Nakabayashi N, Pashley DH. Hybridization of dental hard tissues. Tokyo: Quintessence Publishing Co, Ltd; 1998. p. 129.
[49] Gargeroglio R, Brannstrom M. Scanning electron microscopic investigation of human dentinal tubules. Arch Oral Biol 1976;21:355–62.
[50] Pashley DH. Clinical correlations of dentin structure and function. [Review, 51 refs] J Oral Rehabil 1991;66(6):777–81.
[51] Levine RS. The distribution of hydroxyproline in sound human coronal dentine. Arch Oral Biol 1971;16(5):473–8.
[52] Tao L, Pashley D. Dentin perfusion effects on the shear bond strengths of bonding agents to dentin. Dent Mater 1989;5(3):181–4.
[53] Tagami J, Tao L, Pashley DH. Correlation among dentin depth, permeability, and bond strength of adhesive resins. Dent Mater 1990;6(1):45–50.
[54] McGuckin RS, et al. Shear bond strength of Scotchbond in vivo. Dent Mater 1991 ;7(1):50–3.
[55] Garberoglio P. The ratio of the densities of dentinal tubules on the cervical and axial walls in cavities. Quintessence Int 1994;25(1):49–52.
[56] Yoshikawa T, et al. Effects of dentin depth and cavity configuration on bond strength. J Dent Res 1999;78(4):898–905.
[57] Tay FR, Gwinnett JA, Wei SH. Relation between water content in acetone/alcohol-based primer and interfacial ultrastructure. J Dent 1998;26(2):147–56.
[58] Eick JD, et al. Scanning electron microscopy of cut tooth surfaces and identification of debris by use of the electron microprobe. J Dent Res 1970;49(6). Suppl: 1359–1368.
[59] Spencer P, et al. Molecular structure of acid-etched dentin smear layers – in situ study. J Dent Res 2001;80(9):1802–7.
[60] Pashley DH, Carvalho RM. Dentine permeability and dentine adhesion. J Dent 1997;25(5):355–72.
[61] Kugel G, Ferrari M. The science of bonding: from first to sixth generation. [Review, 42 refs] J Am Dent Assoc 2000;131(Suppl.):20S–5S.
[62] Hannig M, Friedrichs C. Comparative in vivo and in vitro investigation of interfacial bond variability. Oper Dent 2001;26(1):3–11.

[63] Davidson CL, de Gee AJ. Relaxation of polymerization contraction stresses by flow in dental composites. J Dent Res 1984;63(2):146–8.
[64] Eick JD, Welch FH. Polymerization shrinkage of posterior composite resins and its possible influence on postoperative sensitivity. Quintessence Int 1986;17(2):103–11.
[65] Barkmeier WW, Cooley RL. Resin adhesive systems: in vitro evaluation of dentin bond strength and marginal microleakage. J Esthet Dent 1989;1(2):67–72.
[66] Pashley DH. Clinical considerations of microleakage. J Endod 1990;16(2):70–7.
[67] Erickson RL. Mechanism and clinical implications of bond formation for two dentin bonding agents. Am J Dent 1989;2(Spec No):117–23.
[68] Prati C, et al. Shear bond strength and SEM evaluation of dentinal bonding systems. Am J Dent 1990;3(6):283–8.
[69] Nakabayashi N, Kojima K, Masuhara E. The promotion of adhesion by the infiltration of monomers into tooth substrates. J Biomed Mater Res 1982;16(3):265–73.
[70] Van Meerbeek B, et al. Morphological aspects of the resin-dentin interdiffusion zone with different dentin adhesive systems. J Dent Res 1992;71(8):1530–40.
[71] Eick JD, et al. The dentinal surface: its influence on dentinal adhesion. Part III Quintessence Int 1993;24(8):571–82.
[72] Gwinnett AJ. Quantitative contribution of resin infiltration/hybridization to dentin bonding. Am J Dent 1993;6(1):7–9.
[73] Katz J, et al. Micromechanics of the dentin/adhesive interface. J Biomed Mater Res Appl Biomater 2001;58:366–71.
[74] Maciel KT, et al. The effects of acetone, ethanol, HEMA, and air on the stiffness of human decalcified dentin matrix. J Dent Res 1996;75(11):1851–8.
[75] Carvalho RM, et al. A review of polymerization contraction: the influence of stress development versus stress relief. Oper Dent 1996;21(1):17–24.
[76] Carvalho RM, et al. In vitro study on the dimensional changes of human dentine after demineralization. Arch Oral Biol 1996;41(4):369–77.
[77] Harnirattisai C, et al. Interfacial morphology of an adhesive composite resin and etched caries-affected dentin. Oper Dent 1992;17(6):222–8.
[78] Pereira PN, et al. Effect of intrinsic wetness and regional difference on dentin bond strength. Dent Mater 1999;15(1):46–53.
[79] Van Meerbeek B, et al. Hybridization effectiveness of a two-step versus a three-step smear layer removing adhesive system examined correlatively by TEM and AFM. J Adhes Dent 1999;1(1):7–23.
[80] Kanemura N, Sano H, Tagami J. Tensile bond strength to and SEM evaluation of ground and intact enamel surfaces. J Dent 1999;27(7):523–30.
[81] Spencer P, Swafford JR. Unprotected protein at the dentin-adhesive interface. Quintessence Int 1999;30(7):501–7.
[82] Spencer P, et al. Interfacial chemistry of the dentin/adhesive bond. J Dent Res 2000;79(7):1458–63.
[83] Hashimoto M, et al. The effect of hybrid layer thickness on bond strength: demineralized dentin zone of the hybrid layer. Dent Mater 2000;16(6):406–11.
[84] Wilson NH. Conference report. Direct adhesive materials: current perceptions and evidence–future solutions. [Review, 49 refs] J Dent 2001;29(5):307–16.
[85] Camps J, et al. Factors influencing pulpal response to cavity restorations. Dent Mater 2000;16(6):432–40.
[86] Barghi N, Berry T, Hatton C. Evaluating intensity output of curing lights in private dental offices. J Am Dent Assoc 1994;125(7):992–6.
[87] Ogata M, et al. Influence of the direction of tubules on bond strength to dentin. Oper Dent 2001;26(1):27–35.

[88] Watanabe LG, Marshall Jr GW, Marshall SJ. Dentin shear strength: effects of tubule orientation and intratooth location. Dent Mater 1996;12(2):109–15.
[89] Phrukkanon S, Burrow MF, Tyas MJ. The effect of dentine location and tubule orientation on the bond strengths between resin and dentine. J Dent 1999;27(4):265–74.
[90] Ogata M, et al. Effect of dentin primer application on regional bond strength to cervical wedge-shaped cavity walls. Oper Dent 1999;24(2):81–8.
[91] Purk JH, et al. Adhesive analysis of voids in class II composite resin restorations at the axial and gingival cavity walls restored under in vivo versus in vitro conditions. Dent Mater 2007;23(7):871–7.
[92] Yoshiyama M, et al. Regional strengths of bonding agents to cervical sclerotic root dentin. J Dent Res 1996;75(6):1404–13.
[93] Cagidiaco MC, et al. Mapping of tubule and intertubule surface areas available for bonding in Class V and Class II preparations. J Dent 1997;25(5):379–89.
[94] Opdam NJ, et al. Necessity of bevels for box only Class II composite restorations. J Prosthet Dent 1998;80(3):274–9.
[95] Ferrari M, Cagidiaco CM, Mason PN. Morphologic aspects of the resin-dentin interdiffusion zone with five different dentin adhesive systems tested in vivo. J Prosthet Dent 1994;71(4):404–8.
[96] Schupbach P, Krejci I, Lutz F. Dentin bonding: effect of tubule orientation on hybrid-layer formation. Eur J Oral Sci 1997;105(4):344–52.
[97] Yoshiyama M, et al. Interfacial morphology and strength of bonds made to superficial versus deep dentin. Am J Dent 1995;8(6):297–302.
[98] Ferrari M, Cagidiaco MC, Davidson CL. Resistance of cementum in Class II and V cavities to penetration by an adhesive system. Dent Mater 1997;13(3):157–62.
[99] Shams SH. The influence of the depth of substrate dentin surface and thickness of the current restorative samples on bond strength. Egypt Dent J 1995;41(4):1513–6.
[100] Bouillaguet S, et al. Bonding characteristics to dentin walls of class II cavities, in vitro. Dent Mater 2001;17(4):316–21.
[101] Zheng L, et al. Relationship between adhesive thickness and microtensile bond strength. Oper Dent 2001;26(1):97–104.
[102] Mitchem JC, Terkla LG, Gronas DG. Bonding of resin dentin adhesives under simulated physiological conditions. Dent Mater 1988;4(6):351–3.
[103] Prati C, Pashley DH. Dentin wetness, permeability and thickness and bond strength of adhesive systems. Am J Dent 1992;5(1):33–8.
[104] Burrow MF, et al. The influence of age and depth of dentin on bonding. Dent Mater 1994;10(4):241–6.
[105] Finger WJ. Dentin bonding agents. Relevance of in vitro investigations. Am J Dent 1988;1(Spec No):184–8.
[106] Chappell R, et al. Pilot Study to determine sample size for micro-tensile testing. J Dent Res 1997:38. Abstract # 193.
[107] Jessop N, Denehy G, Vargas M. Dentin shear strength: effect of depth and location. J Dent Res 1999;78(IADR Abstracts). p. Abstract # 342.
[108] Yoshiyama M, et al. Regional bond strengths of resins to human root dentine. J Dent 1996;24(6):435–42.
[109] Shono Y, et al. Regional measurement of resin-dentin bonding as an array. J Dent Res 1999;78(2):699–705.

Analyses of material-tissue interfaces by Fourier transform infrared, Raman spectroscopy, and chemometrics

9

Q. Ye, P. Spencer
University of Kansas, Lawrence, KS, United States

9.1 Brief introduction to vibrational spectroscopic techniques

Infrared (IR) and Raman spectroscopy are not identical but rather complementary techniques for obtaining information about the structure and properties of molecules from their vibrational transitions. The data from these techniques arise from two different physical effects on the molecule. IR absorption represents a one-photon event, and IR spectra portray vibrational motions that produce a change in the permanent dipole moment of the molecule. In contrast, Raman scattering is a two-photon event, and Raman spectra reflect vibrational motions that cause a change in a source-induced molecular dipole moment. IR spectroscopy is a measurement of a simple absorption process, whereas Raman spectroscopy is the measurement of the reemission of the incident source energy.[1–5] Since IR and Raman spectroscopies were introduced earlier, this chapter will briefly review the fundamental principles. The bulk of the chapter will focus on the application of these techniques for quantitative molecular-level analyses of the adhesive, dentin, and adhesive/dentin (a/d) interface.

9.1.1 *Infrared spectroscopy*

IR spectroscopy is a well-established, well-understood technique. In transmission IR spectroscopy, IR radiation is passed through a sample. Some of the IR radiation is absorbed by the sample and some of it is passed through (transmitted). The resulting spectrum represents the molecular absorption and transmission, creating a molecular fingerprint of the sample. Coupling interferometry, spectral data transformations, and detailed molecular databases, Fourier transform infrared (FTIR) spectroscopy has become ubiquitous within the physical, analytical, and biochemical disciplines. Traditionally, IR spectrometers have been used to analyze solids, liquids, and gases by means of transmission of the IR radiation directly through the sample. Where the sample is in a liquid or solid form the intensity of the spectral features is determined by the thickness of the sample, and typically, this sample thickness cannot be more than a few tens of micrometers. Compared to this, attenuated total reflectance (ATR) FTIR spectrometry is

Material-Tissue Interfacial Phenomena. http://dx.doi.org/10.1016/B978-0-08-100330-5.00009-1

considered a simple, direct, flexible, and sensitive in situ IR technique. ATR technique involves the collection of radiation reflected from the interface between the solution and a prism, in which the evanescent wave penetrated from the prism into the solution is absorbed by substances in the solution. This method may solve many of the problems associated with transmission IR spectroscopy, such as path length and concentration.

9.1.2 Raman spectroscopy

Raman spectroscopy, a complementary vibrational spectroscopic technique for molecular analyses, continues to benefit enormously from advances in laser and array detector developments. A Raman spectrum is a plot of the intensity of Raman scattered radiation as a function of its frequency difference from the incident radiation (usually in units of wavenumbers, cm^{-1}). This difference is called the *Raman shift*. Note that, because it is a difference value, the Raman shift is independent of the frequency of the incident radiation. The energy of a vibrational mode depends on the molecular structure and environment. Atomic mass, bond order, molecular substituents, molecular geometry, and hydrogen bonding all effect the vibrational force constant, which in turn dictates the vibrational energy. Vibrational Raman spectroscopy is not limited to intramolecular vibrations. Crystal lattice vibrations and other motions of extended solids are Raman active. Their spectra are important in such fields as polymers and semiconductors. In the gas phase, rotational structure is resolvable on vibrational transitions. The resulting vibration/rotation spectra are widely used to study combustion and gas-phase reactions generally. Vibrational Raman spectroscopy is an extraordinarily versatile probe into a wide range of phenomena that span diverse disciplines ranging from physical biochemistry to materials science.

Because Raman detects fundamental vibrations, Raman bands have a good signal-to-noise ratio and are nonoverlapping. This allows a Raman spectrum to be used for everything from "fingerprinting" of samples to constructing complex chemical models of reaction processes. The measured intensity of a Raman species is directly proportional to the concentration. This allows a Raman analysis to measure a species concentration from a fraction of 1 to 100% without sample dilution. Traditionally, Raman spectroscopy has had one major disadvantage when studying biological specimens, namely, fluorescence, which leads to a background several orders of magnitude greater than the Raman signal. The advent of near-IR and confocal Raman spectroscopy has made the study of biological specimens more feasible.

Raman scatter is partially polarized, even for molecules in gas or liquid states, where the individual molecules are randomly oriented. The effect is most easily seen with an exciting source that is plane polarized. In isotropic media, polarization arises because the induced electric dipole has components that vary spatially with respect to the coordinates of the molecule. Polarized Raman can be a powerful tool for studying the mechanism of orientation and the final structure of polymeric films and fibers. It is also useful for characterizing single crystals.

The composition of organic materials can be studied using the Raman shifts and relative intensities of all the Raman bands. Changes in individual bands, eg, shifting, narrowing, or varying in intensity, can reveal information about stresses in the sample, variations in crystallinity, and the amount of material. Variations in spectra with position on the sample will reveal changes in the uniformity (homogeneity) of the material. One can analyze at several arbitrary points, or systematically measure an array of points (enabling the production of images of composition, stress, crystallinity, etc.)

Four case studies will be used to illustrate the potential that the developments and advances in vibrational spectroscopy offer to material/tissue interfacial characterization. Examples from our laboratory are used to illustrate both the technique and protocol development.

9.2 Case study 1: in situ monitoring of photopolymerization kinetics using ATR/FTIR spectroscopy

It is challenging for the clinician to determine the appropriate exposure time for different resin chemistries and variable light sources. Investigators frequently use photo–differential scanning calorimetry (DSC) and FTIR spectroscopy to monitor the photocuring processes. DSC is a tool for the analysis of the polymerization behavior of dental resin monomers. The extent and rate of the polymerization of functional vinyl monomers can be analyzed by measuring the caloric value of the exothermal peak, enabling the detection of polymerization behavior by using the DSC method. However, this method is not suitable for the single-solution dental bonding agents that contain acetone and/or ethanol as the hydrophilic carrier; these solvents could easily evaporate during analysis.

ATR technique serves as an important accessory for most current IR spectrometers. This accessory can provide valuable in situ analysis of the chemical structure of complex adhesive solution before, during, and after light curing. Real-time IR including mid-IR or near-IR spectroscopy have been previously used for the characterization of dental resins,[6] which were chosen over DSC for the acrylate polymerization because of the volatility of the sample and the rapid rate of polymerization.[7] Although real-time FTIR-ATR spectroscopy has been used in investigations involving the kinetics of photopolymerization,[8,9] the instrument is more expensive and thus, has not realized widespread application in the study of dental resins.

The preparation of a sample for ATR-FTIR spectroscopy is a crucial step in the process. The sample must be in close contact with the internal reflection element to allow interaction with the evanescent field. In our laboratory, liquid adhesive could be cast on the diamond crystal top plate of the ATR accessory and covered with a mylar film to reduce the potential of oxygen inhibiting the polymerization (Fig. 9.1). The curing light polymerizes the adhesive with the assistance of the mylar film.

The photopolymerization of model adhesives has been monitored in situ using a Perkin–Elmer Spectrum One FT-IR with a resolution of $4\,cm^{-1}$ in the ATR sampling mode. One drop of adhesive solution was placed on the horizontal face of the internal reflectance crystal where total internal reflection occurs. The reflected radiation penetrates the sample to a depth of only a few micrometers. The zinc selenide (ZnSe)

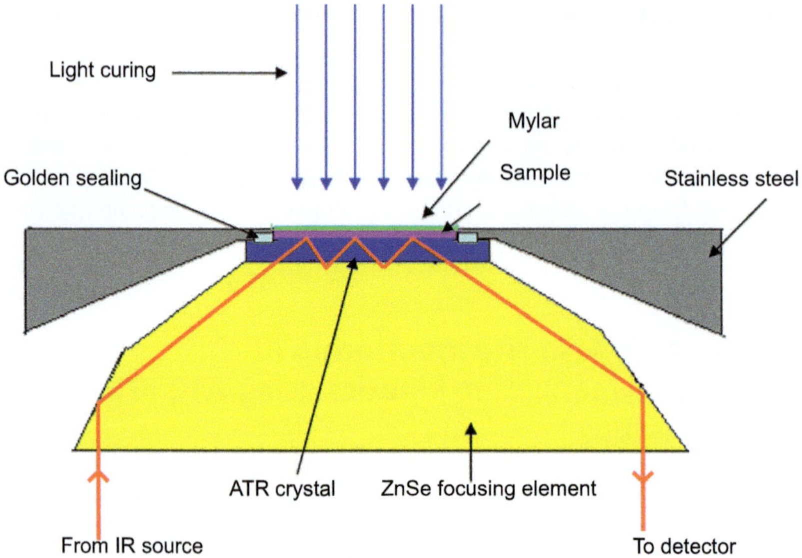

Figure 9.1 Optical layout of attenuated total reflectance sampling accessory and preparation of adhesive sample under a dental curing light.

crystal with a transmission range of 4000–650 cm^{-1} was used in this experiment. The degree of conversion (DC) was calculated based on band ratios of 1637 cm^{-1} (C=C)/1714 cm^{-1}(C=O) or 1608 cm^{-1}(benzyl group) between the polymerized and unpolymerized samples. A novel time-based spectrum collector (PerkinElmerTM Spectrum TimeBase) was also used to provide continuous and automatic collection of the IR spectra of adhesives during photopolymerization. The TimeBase function improves measurement accuracy and offers more spectral data within a designated time. Optimization of the instrument setup enables the collection of 176 spectra in 60 s. This approach enables us to track the photopolymerization reaction in situ. DC was calculated directly from the time-dependent decrease in the absorption intensity band ratios before and after light curing.

An example of Spectrum TimeBase collection of FTIR spectrum of Single Bond adhesive (3M, Dental Products, St. Paul, MN) is shown in Fig. 9.2. Spectrum TimeBase enables one to collect spectra from the sample, either continuously or at regular intervals. A time profile enables one to see how a component of the sample varies as a function of time. For example, if we are monitoring the polymerization reaction where the double bond content is decreasing, it is useful to display a graph of the remaining double bond content against time. The band ratio profile was the time-dependent decrease in the intensity of the ratio of the following spectral features at 1637 cm^{-1} (C=C)/1608 cm^{-1}(benzyl group) (Fig. 9.2):

$$\text{Arb} = \frac{\text{Absorbance}^{\text{sample}}_{1637\ \text{cm}^{-1}} / \text{Absorbance}^{\text{sample}}_{1608\ \text{cm}^{-1}}}{\text{Absorbance}^{\text{monomer}}_{1637\ \text{cm}^{-1}} / \text{Absorbance}^{\text{monomer}}_{1608\ \text{cm}^{-1}}}$$

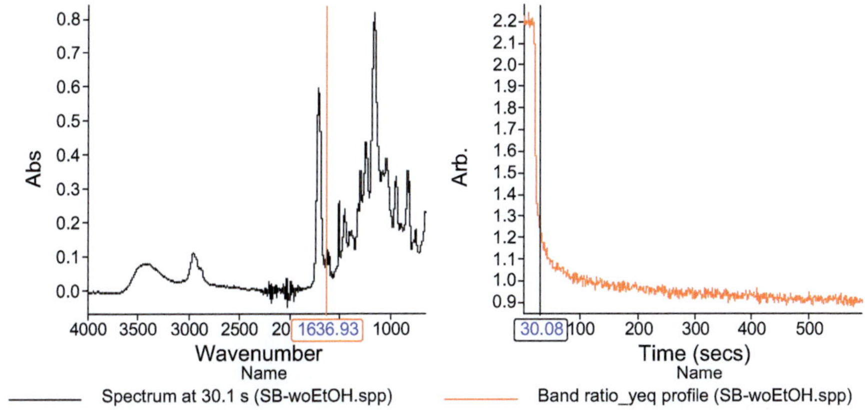

Figure 9.2 Spectrum TimeBase collection of FTIR spectrum of Single Bond adhesive. Band ratio profile showing the time-dependent decrease in the intensity of the ratio of the spectral features at 1637 cm^{-1} (C=C)/1608 cm^{-1} (benzyl group).

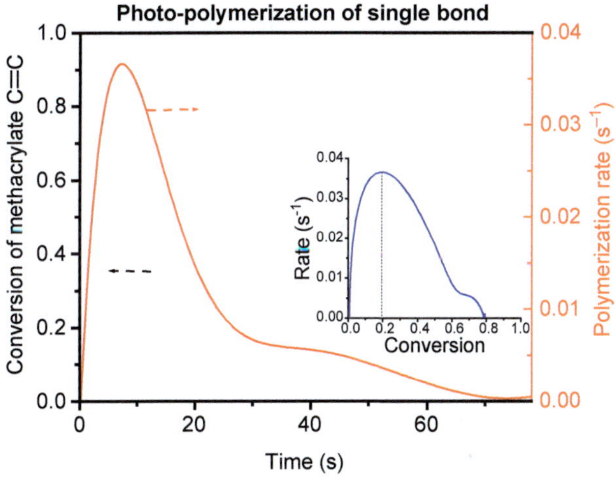

Figure 9.3 The relationship of conversion, curing time, and polymerization rate of Single Bond.

With the help of TimeBase collection, a polymerization conversion versus curing time curve (Fig. 9.3) could be plotted. The kinetic data obtained from this curve were converted to polymerization rate by taking the first derivative of the time versus conversion curve. Conversion was also plotted against the rate of polymerization. The rate of polymerization passes through a maximum at about 20% conversion.

The combination of time-based spectrum collection and ATR sampling method offers an economical means of evaluating new commercial adhesive resin systems. Spectrum TimeBase software also provides the opportunity to batch process spectra, such as ATR correction, baseline correction, and autodifference. As shown in Fig. 9.3, detailed analysis of photopolymerization kinetics can be completed. The rate versus conversion curve displays a bimodal profile, which has been observed by other authors[10] while studying the kinetics of photopolymerization.

9.3 Case study 2: evaluation of the adhesive/dentin interface under aging using Raman microscopy

The hybrid layer (adhesive–collagen composite) has been identified as the weakest link in the bond formed between the adhesive and dentin.[11,12] This characterization is based on laboratory investigations that suggest that the hybrid layer is unstable in aqueous environments.[11,13] It is quite likely that this degradation is related to several factors, including inadequate adhesive infiltration,[14–18] which leads to zones of exposed collagen fibrils within the hybrid layer. The resultant exposed collagen could undergo hydrolytic and enzymatic degradation in the aqueous, oral environment; such degradation would undermine the integrity of the hybrid layer, the adhesive/dentin bond, and ultimately, the composite restoration.

Bond strength measurements and the associated fractographic analyses of specimens stored in aqueous solutions provide evidence of deterioration, but these analyses do not permit direct identification of the degrading components. The loss of bond strength over time could be due to deterioration of the resin or degradation of the collagen that was not fully entrapped by the adhesive resin. Authors of previous publications[19,20] have reported that salivary esterases can degrade methacrylate polymers over time. The purpose of this study was to compare the molecular structure at the adhesive/hybrid layer/dentin interface in class II composite restorations over time in aqueous storage.

The light microscopic image of the a/d interface at the gingival margin of a representative class II composite restoration is shown in Fig. 9.4(b). As noted in this image, the interface is very irregular and gaps are readily identified at the gingival margin. In the photomicrographs of a 5-μm-thick Goldner trichrome–stained section of the a/d interface (Fig. 9.4(c) and (d)), the mineralized dentin is green, whereas the adhesive appears a very pale yellow (Fig. 9.4(d)). An irregular, distinct red region at the gingival margin is visible in Fig. 9.4(d). The red color represents unprotected collagen at the a/d interface; clearly, this exposed collagen was available for reaction with the trichrome stain. Using a 60X water immersion lens, the sample was imaged and Raman spectra were acquired at 1-μm intervals across the composite/adhesive/dentin interface. Representative spectral maps collected from the a/d interface at the gingival margin of specimens stored in aqueous solution for 48 h and 90 days are presented in Figs. 9.5 and 9.6, respectively. All spectra were recorded from 875 to 1785 cm^{-1}, which spans the fingerprint region associated with adhesive, collagen, and mineral. The peaks associated with the adhesive occur at 1720 cm^{-1} (carbonyl), 1609 cm^{-1} (phenyl C=C), and 1113 cm^{-1} (C—O—C), and the major peaks associated with the collagen appear at 1245 cm^{-1} (amide III), 1273 cm^{-1} (amide III), 1453 cm^{-1} (CH_2), and 1667 cm^{-1} (amide I). Additional features associated with the collagen appear at 938 cm^{-1} (backbone) and 921 cm^{-1} (C–C stretch), and the spectral features associated with the mineral occur at 961 cm^{-1} (P–O symmetric stretch) and 1072 cm^{-1} (C–O_3), respectively.

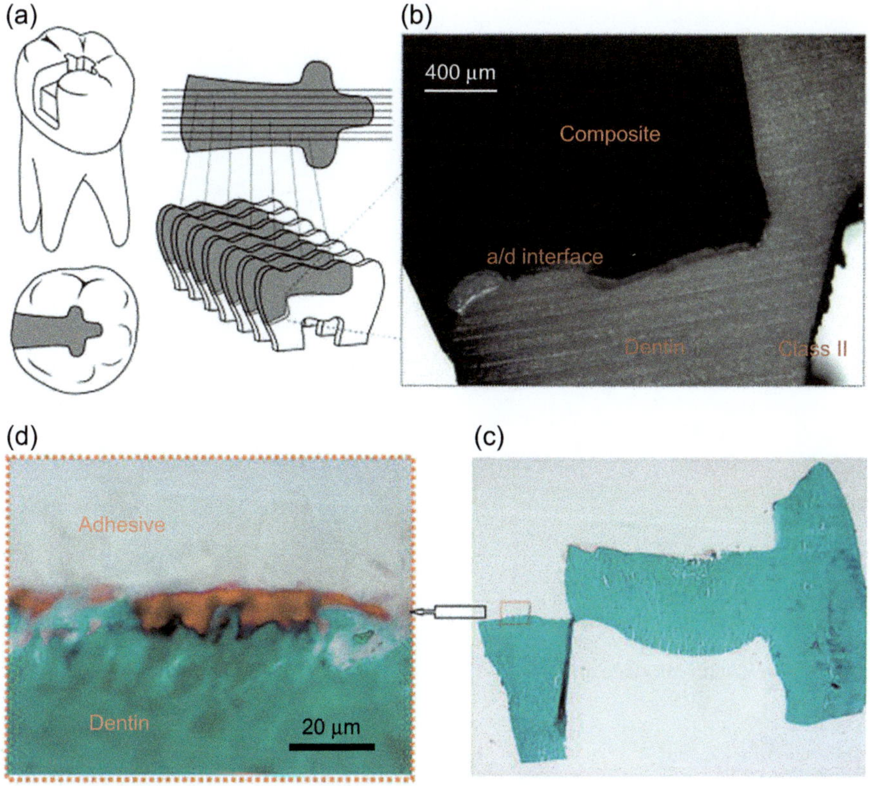

Figure 9.4 Light microscopic picture of the adhesive/dentin interfaces of the proximal and gingival walls of class II composite restorations. (a) the cartoon to show the preparation of the adhesive/dentin interface samples. (b) the light microscopic image of the adhesive/dentin interface at the gingival margin. (c) the photo-micrographs of a 5 micron thick Goldner's trichrome-stained section of the adhesive/dentin interface. (d) the zoomed photo-micrographs from the marked region in (c).

As shown in Figs. 9.5 and 9.6, the first spectrum was acquired from the pure adhesive. Peaks associated with the adhesive and collagen components of dentin were noted in the second spectrum. The Raman peak of the P-O group in the 12th spectrum of the 48-h specimen suggested that this represented the bottom of the demineralized dentin layer. In the 90-day specimens (Fig. 9.6), features associated with demineralized dentin collagen dominate the 2nd through 13th spectra; note the very limited contribution from spectral features associated with the adhesive (1720 and 1609 cm^{-1}) beyond the second micrometer position. The spectra recorded at the second, fourth, and fifth micrometer positions of the interface are presented in detail, and major spectral changes have been marked with arrows (Figs. 9.5 and 9.6). The intensity of the Raman bands associated with the adhesive decreased as a function of depth, indicating the gradual decline of adhesive penetration. At the fifth micrometer position, there is almost no contribution from spectral features associated with the adhesive. After water

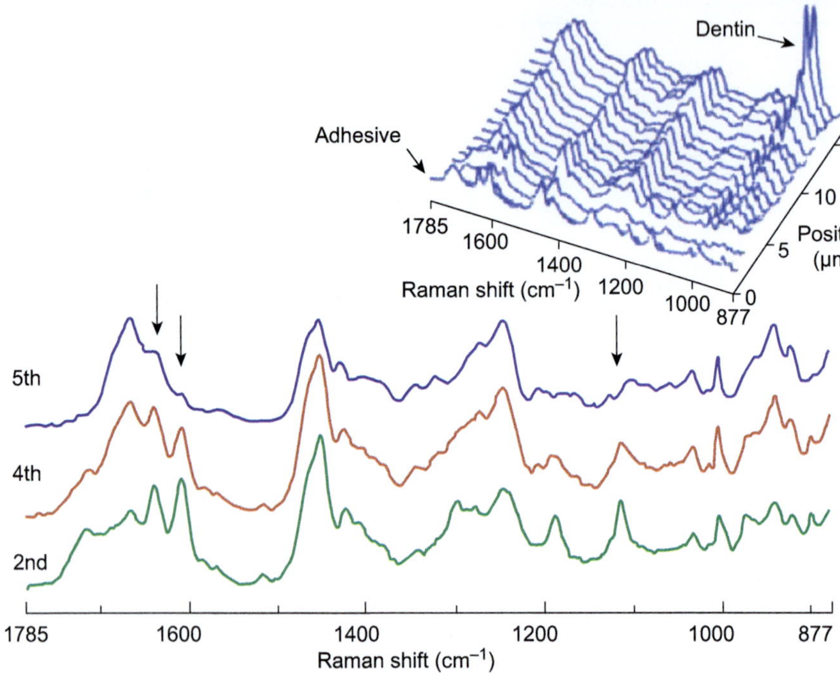

Figure 9.5 Micro-Raman mapping spectra acquired at 1-μm intervals across Single Bond (SB) adhesive/dentin interface at gingival margin (for 48 h of aqueous storage).

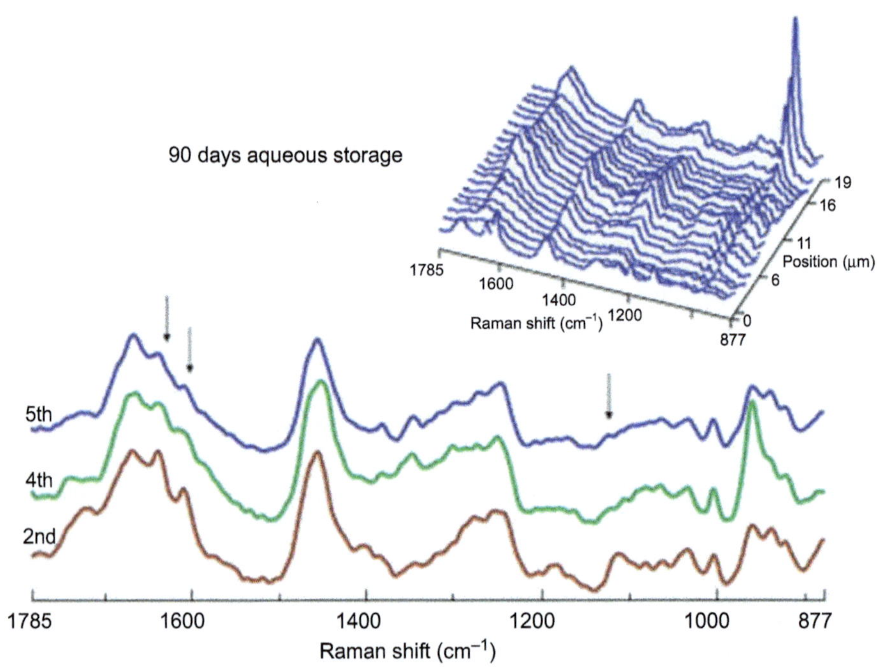

Figure 9.6 Micro-Raman mapping spectra acquired at 1-μm intervals across SB adhesive/dentin interface at gingival margin (for 90 days of aqueous storage).

storage for 90 days, the relative intensity of the adhesive bands is reduced, indicating that there has been leaching of adhesive resin from the interfacial region. It was also noted that the relative intensity of the band at 1640 cm^{-1} in the spectra recorded at the second and fourth micrometer positions was relatively high. This band is associated with the content of C=C bond, indicating that the DC is lower in the adhesive that penetrated into the demineralized zone. The amide I (C=O stretching vibration) mode is sensitive to the molecular conformation of the polypeptide chains.[21,22] The position and intensity of this band is typical of collagen fibril with triple-helical structure. In comparing this region in the spectra of unprotected collagen, there is a relative increase in the ratios of amide I/CH and amide I/amide III in the 90-day specimens. These spectral changes indicate that the ordered collagen structure has become disorganized.[21,23,24] The relative difference in intensity of these spectral features could be caused by a loosening of the collagen fibril structure from water absorption.[25]

These spectral results are in general agreement with high-resolution morphologic investigations, which reported degradation of denuded, acid-etched collagen fibrils during aqueous aging.[26,27] This study provides direct evidence of the breakdown of hydrolytically unstable adhesive monomers or oligomers at the hybrid layer/dentin interface in class II composite restorations, following 90 days of aqueous aging. The results also provide direct evidence of deterioration in the unprotected collagen at the gingival margin in the aged class II composite restorations. Two distinct advantages of micro-Raman spectroscopy are minimal sample preparation and the nondestructive nature of this technique. By combining this method of analysis with an excitation source that minimizes sample fluorescence, the a/d sample can be studied without altering or damaging the interface. Because the technique is nondestructive, the same sample can be evaluated both before and after storage. The sample is also available for analysis using complementary techniques, eg, scanning acoustic microscopy.

9.4 Case study 3: compare and contrast FTIR and Raman imaging analysis

FTIR IR imaging (FTIRI) represents the combination of spectroscopy with microscopy. This technique allows the collection of molecular information from samples, eg, materials, biologic tissues, and material/tissue interfaces, at the microscopic level. The FTIR images represent the inherent contrast associated with the unique chemical bonds of the components within the analyzed sample. A chemical image of each component is created by plotting the unique frequencies as a function of spatial position and spectral intensity. A color scheme can be applied to the intensity values to permit the creation of a "false-color composite" image.

In this case study, FTIRI was used to characterize the interface structure of adhesive bonded to dentin substrate. FTIR microspectroscopic and imaging analyses were completed using the Spectrum Spotlight FTIR imaging system (Perkin Elmer) with both single-point and imaging mode. The liquid nitrogen–cooled detector incorporates a narrow-band mercury-cadmium-telluride (MCT) array detector and single-point

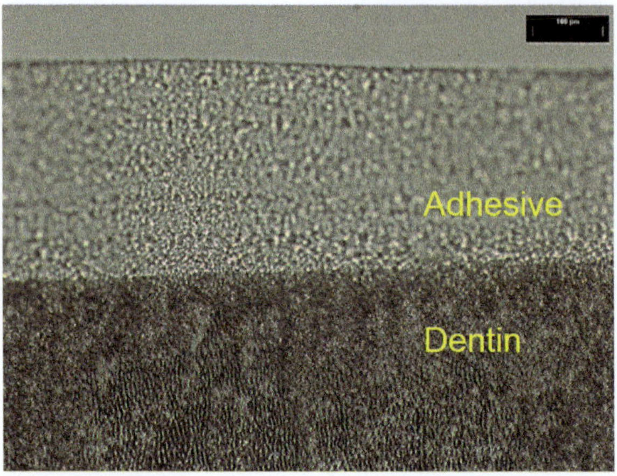

Figure 9.7 Visible image of the microtomed slice of the adhesive/dentin interface. The regions associated with the adhesive and dentin are indicated on the figure.

medium band MCT detector on a single substrate. It offers the wavelength range from 7800 to 720 cm^{-1}. This system provides 25 and 6.25 μm pixel resolution, and could generate chemical images of a size up to 1.64 cm^2. In the following case study, images were scanned between 4000 and 720 cm^{-1} at 4 cm^{-1} spectral resolution, with two scans per pixel. Image size was ~300 by ~300 μm, using 6.25 μm pixel resolution. Approximately 2600 spectra were acquired in less than 5 min. An atmosphere correction was applied to the raw image, subtracting the contribution of atmosphere absorbance, ie, water vapor and carbon dioxide. Images were created using Spectrum Spotlight software. The visible image of the microtomed a/d interface specimen that was analyzed using this technique is shown in Fig. 9.7. The two layers, ie, dentin and adhesive, are clearly visible, although lacking in detail.

The total absorbance image of the a/d interface specimen (Fig. 9.7) collected from a $200 \times 150\,\mu m^2$ area is shown in Fig. 9.8(a). Although there is no chemical information in the full absorbance image, it is a spatial representation of the energy impinging on the detectors. It is noted, however, that some additional features are observed, indicating stronger absorbance (less energy impinging the detectors) in the bottom half of the image. Inspection of Fig. 9.8(b)–(d) reveals clear delineation between layers. Images of three spectral parameters (1721, 1658, and 1027 cm^{-1}) provide information about the spatial distribution of the adhesive, collagen, and mineral components across the a/d interface. Investigation of all the images indicates that the interface is not a thin slice through the images. Its width appears to indicate an interaction between the adhesive and dentin layers, which is not obvious from the analysis of the visible image (Fig. 9.7). The interfacial width of the 1027 cm^{-1} image appears to be bigger than that of the 1721 cm^{-1} image. This indicates that the width of demineralized dentin layer is much deeper than the zone that was infiltrated by the adhesive. These FTIRI results are consistent with our previous micro-Raman spectroscopic investigation. The micro-Raman results showed a gradient of adhesive penetration into the demineralized dentin layer.[14,15]

Since these images contain thousands of very high-quality spectra at a pixel resolution of 6.25 μm, the relative composition and other chemical information can be determined

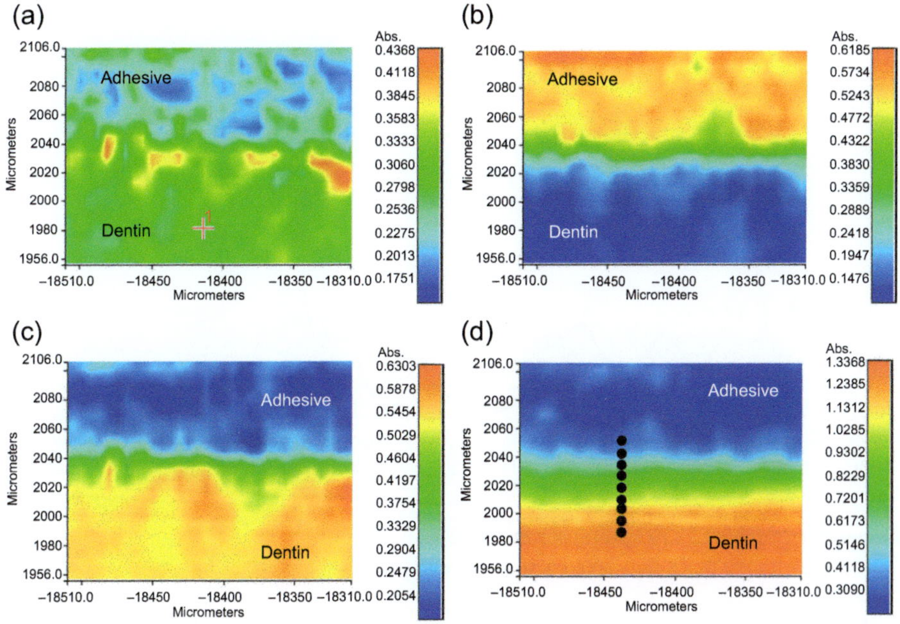

Figure 9.8 FTIR spectroscopic image of the adhesive/dentin interface. (a) Total absorbance image, (b) 1721 cm^{-1} image (carbonyl), (c) 1658 cm^{-1} image (amide I), and (d) 1027 cm^{-1} image (phosphate).

across the length and breadth of the a/d interface. As an example, a series of mapping spectra across the a/d interface (the position was represented by the dotted line in Fig. 9.8(d)) are shown in Fig. 9.9. The chemical characteristics of the two layers are apparent in the spectra. The three bottom spectra were acquired from pure adhesive, a methacrylate-based polymer. Vibrational bands associated with both adhesive and dentin components are noted in the fourth spectrum. The spectral intensity of the $\nu_1\nu_3 PO_4$ domain increases gradually as a function of depth. The high spectral intensity of the $\nu_1\nu_3 PO_4$ domain in the top spectrum indicates mineralized dentin. Spectral features associated with both adhesive (1721 cm^{-1}) and collagen (1658 cm^{-1}) appear in several spectra across the interface. This indicates that within the limits of resolution of this technique, the adhesive resin has penetrated into the dentin matrix, although the width of the interface layer could be overexaggerated due to the low spatial resolution of FTIR spectroscopy.

9.4.1 Raman microspectroscopic imaging

Case study #2 on a/d interfaces by Raman spectroscopy was performed using point-by-point mode across an individual line of the interface. Two-dimensional micro-Raman mapping/imaging can provide an important modality in studying the spatial relationships and distributions of the functional or chemical groups of heterogeneous specimens.

The Raman microspectroscopic images of SB a/d interface collected from a $20 \times 12\,\mu m^2$ area are shown in Fig. 9.10. The relative intensities of the spectral features associated with the mineral (P—O, 961 cm^{-1}) and adhesive resins, ie, 1453 cm^{-1} (CH_2)

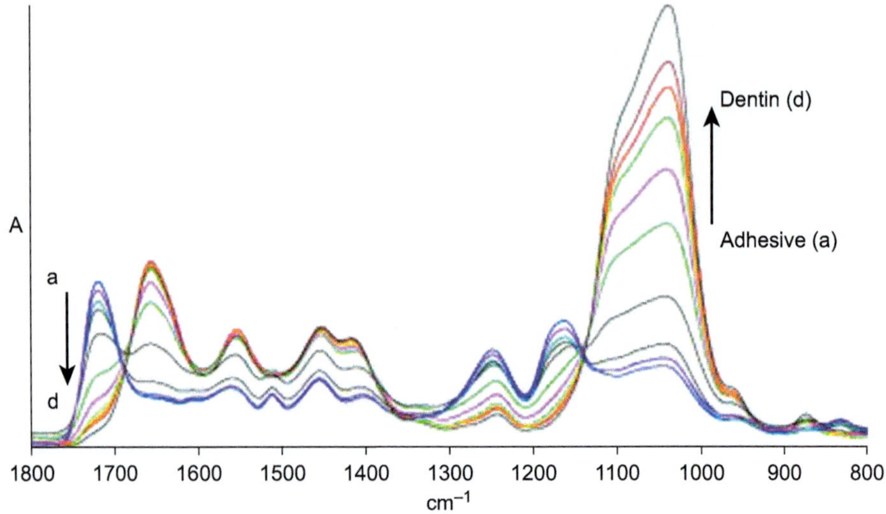

Figure 9.9 Mapping FTIR spectra across the adhesive/dentin interface. These spectra are associated with the black dots noted across the adhesive/dentin interface in Fig. 9.8(d).

or 1113 cm^{-1} (C—O—C) are represented by the color differences. Red represents the highest relative intensity, whereas black represents the lowest. Images of these three spectral parameters (961, 1113, and 1453 cm^{-1}) provide information about the spatial distribution of the mineral, 2,2-Bis[4-(2-hydroxy-3-methacryloxypropoxy) phenyl] propane (BisGMA) monomer, and adhesive components (both BisGMA and 2-hydroxyethyl methacrylate, eg, HEMA monomers) across the a/d interface. Investigation of all the images indicates that the interface is not a simple, uniform layer. Such survey maps of the molecular structure provide a reliable and powerful means of identifying dentin demineralization, the distribution of adhesive monomers, and flaws or defects in the pattern of adhesive infiltration of the demineralized dentin. As shown in Fig. 9.10(a), the image of mineral revealed a partially demineralized layer on the top of dentin substrate. Adhesive monomers readily infiltrated the dentin tubules and spread into the intertubular region (Fig. 9.10(b)). The diffusion of resin monomers (BisGMA and HEMA) differed substantially. In a comparison with HEMA, BisGMA monomer resisted diffusion into the demineralized dentin, especially, the intertubular area (Fig. 9.10(c)).

By combining Raman spectroscopy with microscopy, a comprehensive representation of the degree and depth of demineralization, distribution of adhesive resin monomers, and width of the interface can be obtained with spatial resolution at the microscopic level. A distinct advantage is that specimens can be analyzed directly, in air, at room temperature and pressure, wet or dry without destroying the specimen. In this study, the spectral data were recorded from samples that were wet throughout the analysis. Collecting spectral data from the demineralized dentin under wet conditions reduces the potential for collagen collapse as a result of drying/desiccation. Collagen collapse would lead to inaccurate characterization of the extent or degree of dentin demineralization. Water immersion also reduces the potential that the sample will be exposed to excess and potentially damaging heat during spectral imaging.

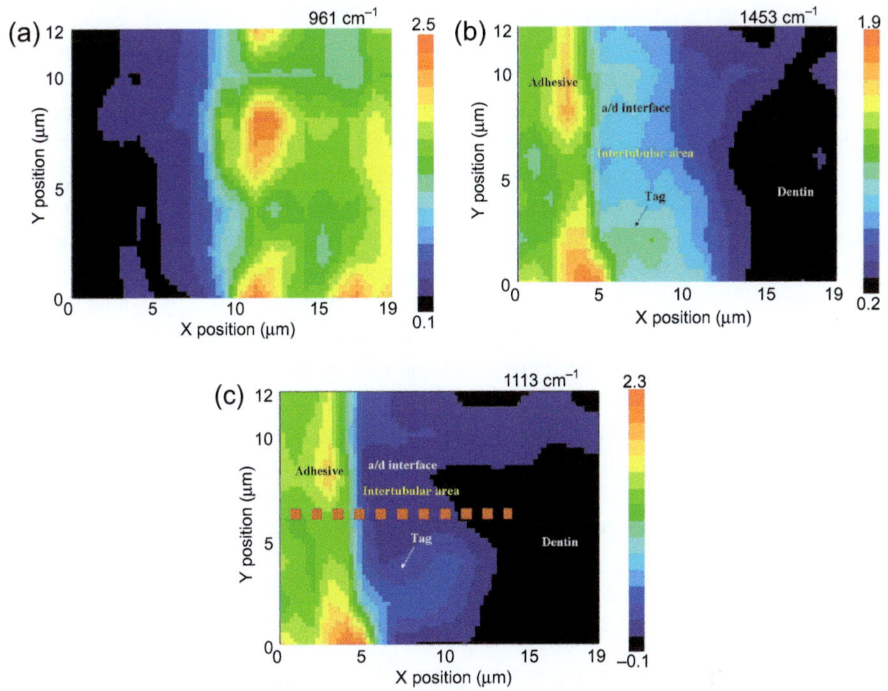

Figure 9.10 Micro-Raman spectroscopic images of the SB adhesive/dentin interface: (a) 961 cm^{-1} image (phosphate), (b) 1453 cm^{-1} image (CH_2), and (c) 1113 cm^{-1} image (C—O—C).

The Raman spectrum is similar to an IR spectrum in that it provides a “fingerprint” of the molecules present within the sample and can be used for qualitative identification and quantitative determination.[4,5] However, unlike IR spectroscopy, water does not present a strong Raman signal within the biological “fingerprint” region. Thus, specific functional groups of molecules can be identified in wet biological specimens with minor spectral interference from water. Additional differences between the two techniques are related to sample preparation. For example, a limitation of IR spectroscopy in transmission mode is the requirement for a finite thickness of the sample to control the absorption intensity of the molecular vibrations. Hygroscopic IR-transmitting materials must be used for many of the sample handling applications because a majority of the IR wavelengths are obscured by glass or quartz windows. In contrast, Raman spectroscopy has no restriction with respect to the sample size, shape, or thickness, and glass or quartz is a suitable sample-containment material for Raman samples.

Raman microspectroscopy is an exceptional tool for investigating the chemistry of material/tissue interfaces because it does not rely on homogenization, extraction, or dilution, but rather each structure is analyzed in situ. Investigation at this level of resolution is critical to our ability to isolate the factors that promote adhesive-phase separation, to identify those components that prevent such separation, and to understand how these components work synergistically to inhibit adhesive-phase separation at the interface of this material with "wet" demineralized dentin matrices. Such investigations are fundamental to the development of adhesives as well as other materials that will provide durable, long-term clinical function for our patients.

Spatial resolution is compromised in the IR microscope, since the fundamental resolution limit is about 10 μm (resolution depends on the wavelength). The shorter wavelengths examined using the visible excitation of Raman spectroscopy yield a diffraction-limited spatial resolution of 1 μm or less. Although FTIR microspectroscopic imaging does not have the high spatial resolution of micro-Raman spectroscopy, it offers the advantage that IR spectra, with acceptable signal-to-noise ratio, can be collected from a ~$400 \times 400\,\mu m^2$ area in minutes. FTIR microspectroscopy can be used to determine the relative composition, degree of cure, and homogeneity across the length and breadth of the a/d interface. Thus spectroscopic survey maps of the a/d interface can be collected in a very time- and labor-efficient manner. Regions of interest along the a/d interface can be identified quickly. Detailed analysis of these regions can then be completed at high spatial resolution using micro-Raman spectroscopy. IR spectra highlight the functional groups of a molecule, whereas Raman spectra offer more information about the skeletal movements of the molecule.

9.5 Case study 4: multivariate analysis of spectroscopic data to confirm phase partitioning in methacrylate-based dentin adhesive

It has been reported that our current dentin adhesives are sensitive to excess moisture, eg, water blisters in adhesives placed on overwet surfaces and phase separation with concomitant limited infiltration of the critical dimethacrylate component into the demineralized dentin matrix.[17,28–31] Large fluid shifts that occur during the bonding process (solvent evaporation and light curing), may allow dentinal fluid to mix with the hydrophilic comonomers, creating nanoleakage pathways within the adhesives.[32] We have investigated the ternary phase diagram for the BisGMA/HEMA/water system,[33] and determined the phase partition behavior of experimental adhesives containing more than two comonomers with different hydrophobicity. To determine quantitatively the components in the hydrophobic- and hydrophilic-rich phases when exposed to overwet environments, our group has used high-performance liquid chromatography (HPLC) to analyze the well-separated phases of model dentin adhesive.[33,34]

The HPLC technique is time consuming (chromatography typically takes 30–60 min) and labor intensive. Additionally, the increased requirements for sample handling during preparation can adversely affect the quality of the analysis. By contrast, FTIR spectroscopy is a very rapid chemical fingerprinting technique (typically 30 s or faster per sample) that can potentially resolve the problems and produce results in under a minute after minimal sample preparation.

Representative FTIR spectra collected from HEMA, BisGMA, and water are presented in Fig. 9.11. The assignments of the spectral features for monomers are 1690–1740 cm^{-1} (carbonyl C=O stretching), 1635–1645 (aliphatic C=C stretching),

1605–1609 (phenyl C=C), 1445–1457 cm^{-1} (CH_2CH_3), 1402–1406 CH_2 deformation, 1165–1180 cm^{-1} (C—O stretching), 830–836 cm^{-1} (C—C—O stretching), and 810 cm^{-1} (C=C twist). Assignments for water (H_2O) are O—H stretching, 3000–3700 cm^{-1}; O—H deformation/scissors, 1500–1700 cm^{-1}; and 650–900 water-hindered rotation. Overall, at the qualitative level, the spectra of HEMA and BisGMA look similar, and both overlap with the characteristic peaks of water. The obvious visible differences between BisGMA and HEMA appeared on the absorption bands related to the aromatic group.

When the absorption bands do not overlap, simple mathematical treatments, such as Beer–Lambert calibration of peak heights or area with respect to the concentration of a single analyte, are possible. However, intense water bands in the IR spectra obstruct the accuracy and sensitivity of quantitative analysis of multiple analytes. Because of the subtle differences highlighted earlier, it was not possible to use simple visual inspection to quantify the level of monomers and water. For this case, one of several multivariate methods such as partial least squares (PLS) and/or principal component regression (PCR) could be used in conjunction with the spectra to develop the multicomponent calibration models.

For the creation of a powerful model, a set of well-defined calibration samples is needed. In this case, calibration samples with a known composition were prepared by mixing the components in a well-defined ratio. Fig. 9.12 plots the water–HEMA–BisGMA ternary phase diagram, and all the standards shown in the single-phase region are used for calibration. There are two groups of standards, shown in Fig. 9.11, which are used for hydrophobic-rich model and hydrophilic-rich model separately.

The software used for the principal component analysis was Spectrum QUANT+ expert Version 4.60 (Perkin Elmer). Calibration models were developed from spectra in absorbance units using PLS and PCR methods with the first-derivative transformed spectra. The optimum number of factors for calibration was selected on the basis of the predicted residual sum of squares, which should be minimized, along with the regression percentage variance. The developed calibration models were first cross-validated

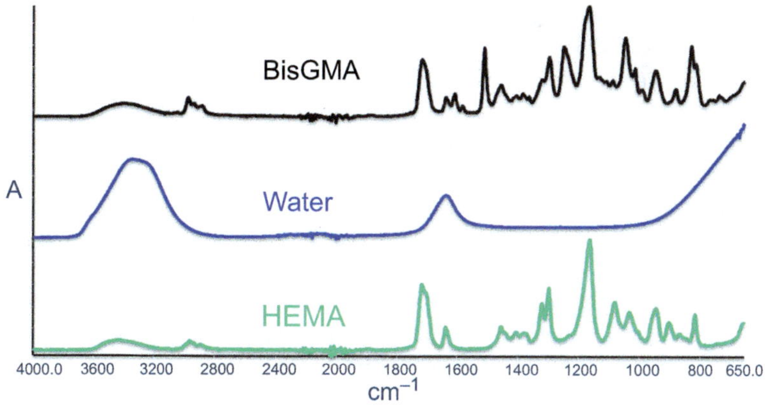

Figure 9.11 ATR-FTIR spectra of BisGMA (in black), HEMA (in green) and water (in blue). The spectra of both BisGMA and HEMA overlap with the characteristic peaks of water.

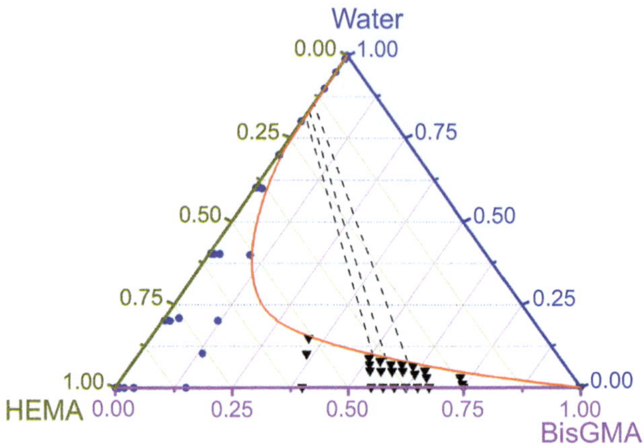

Figure 9.12 Standards in water–HEMA–BisGMA ternary phase diagram used for the calibration model. The solid-phase boundary line is drawn as a binodal curve, separating the single- and two-phase regions. *Filled circles and triangles* represent the standard samples used for the three-component models of hydrophobic- and hydrophilic-rich phases, respectively. Dashed lines represent three representative experimental tie lines.[33,34]

in all cases to minimize the risk of overfitting and then used for testing or validation using the new data. The model prediction was tested by computing the standard error of prediction (SEP) and standard error of estimation (SEE); SEE can be described as the square root of the residual variance divided by the number of degrees of freedom, and SEP is the magnitude of the error expected when independent samples are predicted using the model. Table 9.1 shows the summary statistics for PCR, PLS1, and PLS2 using the same training set associated with hydrophobic-rich samples. In this case, the PLS1 and PLS2 algorithms outperformed PCR. In general, they resulted in a 3-factor (or less) model with high correlation coefficient. All samples were predicted with a similar level of accuracy, and the SEP values were about 0.002–0.004 with %variance over 99%. Fig. 9.13 is a representative calibration model, which was developed using a calibration set identical to that used for the PLS1 prediction models.

The concentrations of HEMA, BisGMA, and water in the samples predicted by PLS methods compare favorably with data from the HPLC method, as presented in Table 9.2. Therefore, the technique is highly plausible as an alternative to the standard procedure for routine analysis of adhesive-phase compositions. Compared with HPLC, the disadvantage of FTIR chemometrics is the detection limit associated with spectroscopic analysis. The amount of BisGMA in the hydrophilic-rich-phase sample is very small (converted to weight percentage, the amount is less than 0.1 mass%), which is lower than the detection limit of FTIR chemometrics (about 0.2 mass%). However, the quantification of this minor component in the hydrophilic-rich samples is not critical for our research objective since this low concentration of BisGMA could not contribute significantly to the cross-link density of the polymer network (unpublished data). The results support previous conclusions from our group that water-

Table 9.1 Regression summary of different algorithms for 3-component hydrophobic-rich phase model

Property	No. of LVs	% Variance	SEE	SEP	Mean value
PCR					
Water	1	99.3	0.00253	0.00262	0.0362
BisGMA	5	99.8	0.00244	0.00253	0.586
HEMA	6	99.8	0.00225	0.00327	0.378
PLS1					
Water	1	99.3	0.00252	0.00263	0.0362
BisGMA	2	99.4	0.00360	0.00378	0.586
HEMA	3	99.2	0.00400	0.00464	0.378
PLS2					
Water	1	99.3	0.00253	0.00262	0.0362
BisGMA	2	99.4	0.00362	0.00379	0.586
HEMA	2	98.9	0.00461	0.00481	0.378

Note *LV*, latent variable.

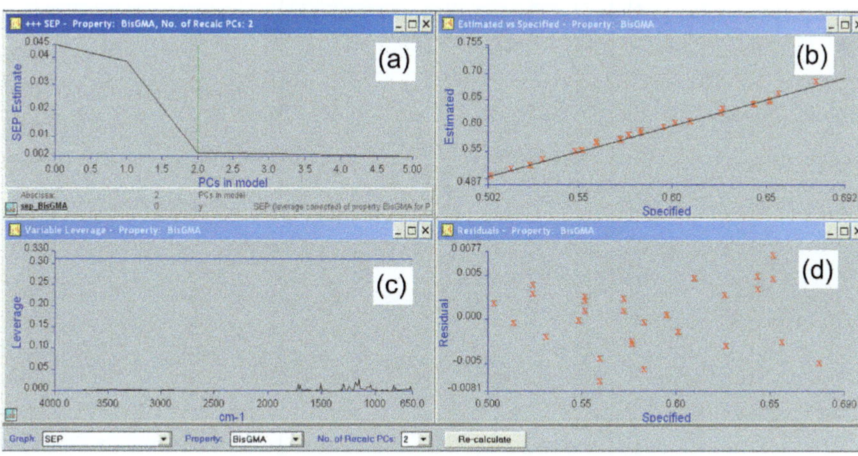

Figure 9.13 Representative calibration model. (a) Standard error of prediction graph, which gives a measure of the SEP associated with the model for a given number of principal components (PCs). The graph enables the selection of a different number of PCs to use to model the property (here, BisGMA) and a recalculation of the data. (b) Plot of estimated versus reference values. (c) Leverage graph displaying a cutoff line determined by the software, using parameters set by the operator. All standards that give results above the cutoff line are standard outliers. No significant outliers were found for any of the residual leverage plots. (d) Residual graph showing a random distribution of residuals about the 0 point of the *y*-axis. Any structure that is evident may indicate a problem with the model.

Table 9.2 Comparison of results obtained from HPLC versus FTIR chemometrics

Initial water content	Method	Hydrophilic-rich phase composition ($n=3$) at (mass%)			Hydrophobic-rich phase composition ($n=3$) at (mass%)		
		BisGMA	HEMA	Water	BisGMA	HEMA	Water
16.0%	HPLC	0.054 (0.002)	18.3 (0.8)	81.6 (0.6)	50.8 (0.5)	39.7 (0.4)	9.5 (0.3)
	FTIR	N/A[a]	18.0 (0.1)	82.0 (0.1)	50.9 (0.1)	39.9 (0.2)	9.4 (0.1)
33.0%	HPLC	0.030 (0.002)	16.8 (0.7)	83.1 (0.8)	53.9 (0.3)	37.4 (0.3)	8.6 (0.2)
	FTIR	N/A	16.5 (0.1)	83.5 (0.1)	53.9 (0.2)	37.5 (0.1)	8.5 (0.1)
50.0%	HPLC	0.014 (0.001)	14.7 (1.2)	85.3 (1.1)	58.9 (0.4)	33.1 (0.3)	7.9 (0.2)
	FTIR	N/A	14.5 (0.2)	85.5 (0.2)	58.8 (0.2)	33.2 (0.1)	7.9 (0.1)

[a]Note: BisGMA amount in aqueous phase is very small (<0.06%), which is lower than the detection limit of FTIR chemometrics (about 0.2%).
N/A, not available.

compatible cross-linkable comonomers must be included in adhesive formulations to address the defects that form in adhesives exposed to the wet, oral environment.[12,33–36]

When combined with appropriate multivariate statistical methods such as PLS regression or PCR, FTIR spectroscopy is an ideal solution for the quantitative analysis of the phase compositions. Multivariate statistics are useful in spectral analysis because it facilitates the simultaneous inclusion of multiple spectral intensities, which greatly improves the precision and predictive ability of the analysis.[37]

We have demonstrated that in tertiary mixtures of dental monomer(s) and water, FTIR spectroscopy in combination with multivariate analysis, such as PLS, provides an accurate, simple, and rapid technique for the quantitative assessment of separated phase composition. The sophisticated statistical approaches use the full or partial spectral region rather than unique and isolated analytical bands. We regard FTIR spectroscopy, in combination with multivariate analysis, as a suitable alternative to HPLC for the detection and quantification of phase compositions in phase-separated dentin adhesives.

9.6 Summary

In summary, the results presented in this chapter demonstrate the advantages of using molecular microanalysis to identify those factors that inhibit the development of an ideal bond at the adhesive interface with “wet” dentin. They demonstrate the utility of FTIR and Raman microspectroscopies in characterizing the fundamental phenomena underlying reactions at the material/tissue interfaces. We use the vibrational spectroscopic results in conjunction with chemometrics and morphologic analyses to explain the fundamental phenomena controlling reactions at the interface between biologic tissues and synthetic materials. These structure/property measurements have been utilized by our group in mathematical models to simulate the behavior of the a/d interface under occlusal function and loading conditions. The knowledge gained from these analyses is applied to the development of new materials and techniques for craniofacial and dental applications.

References

1. Pellitier MJ. *Analytical applications of Raman spectroscopy*. Ann Arbor, MI: Blackwell Science Ltd.; 1999. p. 1–52.
2. Nafie LA. Theory of Raman scattering. In: Lewis IR, Edwards HGM, editors. *Handbook of Raman spectroscopy*. New York: Marcel Dekker, Inc.; 2001. p. 1–10.
3. Larsen RA. Raman spectroscopy of polymers. In: Craver CD, Carraher CE, editors. *Applied polymer science 21st century*. New York: Elsevier; 2000. p. 759–85.
4. Chase B. A new generation of Raman instrumentation. *Appl Spectrosc* 1994;**48**:14A–8A.
5. Turrell G, Corset J. *Raman microscopy-developments and applications*. New York: Academic Press; 1996. p. 1–12.
6. Stansbury JW, Dickens SH. Determination of double bond conversion in dental resins by near infrared spectroscopy. *Dent Mater* January 2001;**17**(1):71–9.
7. Young JS, Bowman CN. Effect of polymerization temperature and cross-linker concentration on reaction diffusion controlled termination. *Macromolecules* 1999;**32**(19):6073–81.

8. Scherzer T, Decker U. Real-time FTIR-ATR spectroscopy to study the kinetics of ultrafast photopolymerization reactions induced by monochromatic UV light. *Vib Spectrosc* 1999;**19**(2):385–98.
9. Scherzer T, Decker U. The effect of temperature on the kinetics of diacrylate photopolymerizations studied by real-time FTIR spectroscopy. *Polymer* 2000;**41**(21):7681–90.
10. Dickens SH, Stansbury JW, Choi KM, Floyd CJE. Photopolymerization kinetics of methacrylate dental resins. *Macromolecules* 2003;**36**:6043–53.
11. Sano H, Yoshikawa T, Pereira PNR, Kanemura N, Morigami M, Tagami J, et al. Long-term durability of dentin bonds made with a self-etching primer, in vivo. *J Dent Res* 1999;**78**(4):906–11.
12. Spencer P, Ye Q, Park J, Topp EM, Misra A, Marangos O, et al. Adhesive/Dentin interface: the weak link in the composite restoration. *Ann Biomed Eng* 2010;**38**(6):1989–2003.
13. Hashimoto M, Ohno H, Kaga M, Endo K, Sano H, Oguchi H. In vivo degradation of resin-dentin bonds in humans over 1 to 3 years. *J Dent Res* 2000;**79**:1385–91.
14. Wang Y, Spencer P. Quantifying adhesive penetration in adhesive/dentin interface using confocal Raman microspectroscopy. *J Biomed Mater Res* 2002;**59**:46–55.
15. Wang Y, Spencer P. Hybridization efficiency of the adhesive dentin interface with wet bonding. *J Dent Res* 2003;**82**:141–5.
16. Spencer P, Swafford JR. Unprotected protein at the dentin-adhesive interface. *Quintessence Int* 1999;**30**(7):501–7.
17. Spencer P, Wang Y, Walker MP, Wieliczka DM, Swafford JR. Interfacial chemistry of the dentin/adhesive bond. *J Dent Res* 2000;**79**(7):1458–63.
18. Sano H, Takatsu T, Ciucchi B, H JA, Matthews WG, Pashley DH. Nanoleakage: leakage within the hybrid layer. *Oper Dent* 1995;**20**:18–25.
19. Bean TA, Zhuang WC, Tong PY, Eick JD, Yourtee DM. Effect of esterase on methacylates and methacrylate polymers in an enzyme simulator for biodurability and biocompatibility testing. *J Biomed Mater Res* 1994;**28**:59–63.
20. Cannon JM, Kostoryz E, Russo KA, Smith RE, Yourtee DM. Bisphenol A and its biomaterial monomer derivatives alteration of in vitro cytochrome P450 metabolism in rat, minipig, and human. *Biomacromolecules* 2000;**1**(4):656–64.
21. Goheen SC, Lis LJ, Kauffman JW. Raman spectroscopy of intact feline corneal collagen. *Biochim Biophys Acta* 1978;**536**:197–204.
22. Frushour BG, Koenig JL. Raman scattering of collagen, gelatin, and elastin. *Biopolymers* 1975;**14**:379–91.
23. Renugopalakrishnan V, Carreira LA, Collette TW, Dobbs JC, Chandraksasan G, Lord RC. Non-uniform triple helical structure in chick skin type I collagen on thermal denaturation: Raman spectroscopic study. *Z Naturforsch* 1998;**53**(5–6):383–8.
24. Sane SU, Cramer SM, Przybycien TM. A holistic approach to protein secondary structure characterization using amide I band Raman spectroscopy. *Anal Biochem* 1999;**269**:255–72.
25. Farrell RA, McCauley RL. On corneal transparency and its loss with swelling. *J Opt Soc Am* 1976;**66**:343–5.
26. Pashley DH, Tay FR, Yiu C, Hashimoto M, Breschi L, Carvalho RM, et al. Collagen degradation by host-derived enzymes during aging. *J Dent Res* 2004;**83**(3):216–21.
27. Armstrong SR, Vargas MA, Chung I, Pashley DH, Campbell JA, Laffoon JE, et al. Resin-dentin interfacial ultrastructure and microtensile dentin bond strength after five-year water storage. *Oper Dent* 2004;**29**(6):705–12.
28. Tay FR, Pashley DH, Yoshiyama M. Two modes of nanoleakage expression in single-step adhesives. *J Dent Res* 2002;**81**(7):472–6.

29. Spencer P, Wang Y. Adhesive phase separation at the dentin interface under wet bonding conditions. *J Biomed Mater Res* 2002;**62**(3):447–56.
30. Ye Q, Park JG, Topp E, Wang Y, Misra A, Spencer P. In vitro performance of nano-heterogeneous dentin adhesive. *J Dent Res* 2008;**87**(9):829–33.
31. Ye Q, Wang Y, Spencer P. Nanophase separation of polymers exposed to simulated bonding conditions. *J Biomed Mater Res B Appl Biomater* 2009;**88**(2):339–48.
32. Hashimoto M, Ito S, Tay FR, Svizero NR, Sano H, Kaga M, et al. Fluid movement across the resin-dentin interface during and after bonding. *J Dent Res* 2004;**83**(11):843–8.
33. Ye Q, Park J, Laurence JS, Parthasarathy R, Misra A, Spencer P. Ternary phase diagram of model dentin adhesive exposed to over-wet environments. *J Dent Res* 2011;**90**(12):1434–8.
34. Ye Q, Park J, Parthasarathy R, Pamatmat F, Misra A, Laurence JS, et al. Quantitative analysis of aqueous phase composition of model dentin adhesives experiencing phase separation. *J Biomed Mater Res B Appl Biomater* 2012;**100**(4):1086–92.
35. Park J, Ye Q, Topp EM, Misra A, Kieweg SL, Spencer P. Effect of photoinitiator system and water content on dynamic mechanical properties of a light-cured bisGMA/HEMA dental resin. *J Biomed Mater Res A* 2010;**93**(4):1245–51.
36. Singh V, Misra A, Parthasarathy R, Ye Q, Park J, Spencer P. Mechanical properties of methacrylate-based model dentin adhesives: effect of loading rate and moisture exposure. *J Biomed Mater Res B Appl Biomater* 2013;**101**(8).
37. Geladi P, Kowalski BR. Partial least-squares regression - a tutorial. *Anal Chim Acta* 1986;**185**:1–17.

Material-tissue interfacial phenomena: challenges in mathematical modeling

10

A. Misra[1], V. Singh[1], R. Parthasarathy[2]
[1]University of Kansas, Lawrence, KS, United States; [2]Tennessee State University, Nashville, TN, United States

10.1 Introduction

Adhesive biopolymers comprising hydrophobic/hydrophilic monomer pairs are the primary bonding agent for attaching composite restorative material to the tooth structure in restorative dentistry. These adhesive biopolymers form an interfacial construct when they are applied to the prepared tooth substrate. The life of composite tooth restoration primarily depends on the durability/strength of this dentin–adhesive (d-a) interface.[1–4] The d-a interface can be described as a transition zone between adhesive and dentin in a composite tooth restoration. Dentin is first etched using acidic agents, and adhesive is applied to the etched surface; subsequently, a relatively hydrophobic composite is attached to the adhesive. This d-a interface is a complex system of different material components and their varying mechanical properties. As previously reported, the properties of these material components greatly affect the overall mechanical behavior of the d-a interface.[1–3]

From the viewpoint of spatial scales, the d-a interface can be broadly considered at:

1. The macroscale defined at the millimeter level spanning 0.1–10 mm. At this scale, the d-a interface appears as a thin layer between the composite and dentin whose structure is difficult to describe or model for analysis.
2. The microscale defined at the micrometer level spanning 0.1–100 μm. At this scale, the d-a interface can be descried as a complex structure composed of composite, adhesive, adhesive–collagen composite, exposed collagen, and partially demineralized dentin. The analysis at this scale is influenced by complex and ill-defined structure property of components, including the heterogeneity and/or phase separation in adhesive, interdigitated polymerized adhesive and collagen composite, defects due to leached mineral in partially demineralized dentin, and presence of pore fluid.
3. The atomic scales defined at the nanometer level spanning 0.1–100 nm. The structure at this scale is largely unknown but can be surmised to consist of a variety of covalent, ionic, and hydrogen bonds among the multiatomic components of the adhesive polymeric network, the polymeric collagen network, and any remnant apatitic mineralite.

From the viewpoint of temporal scales, the polymeric composition of the d-a interface and the dynamic external loading produced at the occlusal surfaces indicate that the behavior of these interfaces is both rate and time dependent. Thus the durability

Material-Tissue Interfacial Phenomena. http://dx.doi.org/10.1016/B978-0-08-100330-5.00010-8

and long-term performance of the d-a interfaces depends on the rate dependence (viscoelastic-damage-plastic) behavior as well as the time-related biochemomechanical transformations of the various material components. Clearly, the characterization and modeling of this interfacial construct poses significant challenges associated with the spatial and temporal scales. This chapter describes findings from efforts made to understand the spatial scales issues using macro- and microscale elastic models and the temporal issues using microscale viscoelastic-damage-plastic models.

10.2 Macro- and microscale stress analysis of d-a interface

Owing to the nature of contacts between the maxillary and mandibular teeth during mastication, both axial and horizontal loads are produced on the occlusal surfaces. Although the overall chewing action may appear to produce compressive load on the tooth, the d-a interface will be subjected to multiaxial loading including tensile and shear loads, as schematically illustrated in Fig. 10.1.

10.2.1 Macroscale behavior

From the macroscale viewpoint, the stress transfer, particularly at the d-a interface in a restored tooth structure, can be illustrated with a global finite element (FE) model of mandibular right second permanent molar, as illustrated in Fig. 10.2.[3] Quarter geometry was considered to reduce the computational time. The three-dimensional (3D) global model considered the material component properties as follows: composite (E=30 GPa, ν=0.30), enamel (E=70 GPa, ν=0.20), and dentin (E=28 GPa, ν=0.25). Calculations were performed for several different properties of the d-a interface. The results given here are for two cases of d-a interface properties: case 1 for E=5 GPa, ν=0.4, and case 2 for E=25 GPa, ν=0.4. The model consists of 716,550 solid parabolic tetrahedral elements, of which 141,310 elements are within the 100-μm thick d-a interfacial region. Discretization refinement was performed to obtain converged results. The bottom

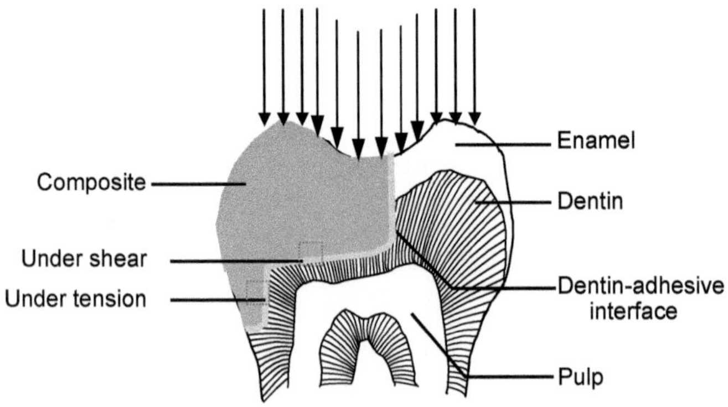

Figure 10.1 Schematic depicting the loading conditions at the d-a interface.

boundary nodes of the 3D tooth were constrained in the vertical direction. The nodes on the surface in the *z-x* plane and surfaces in the *y-z* planes were constrained in *x*- and *y*-axis, respectively. To simulate the physiological patterns of contact during chewing nonhomogeneous morsels that contain a combination of hard gum and bone,[5] a compressive traction force of 1 N/mm^2 is applied at 45 degree to the occlusal surface of the crown. The mesh discretization and the boundary conditions are given in Fig. 10.2.

The load transfer in the restored tooth can be visualized by considering the stress distributions at the horizontal and vertical sections of the 3D FE model, as shown in Fig. 10.3.

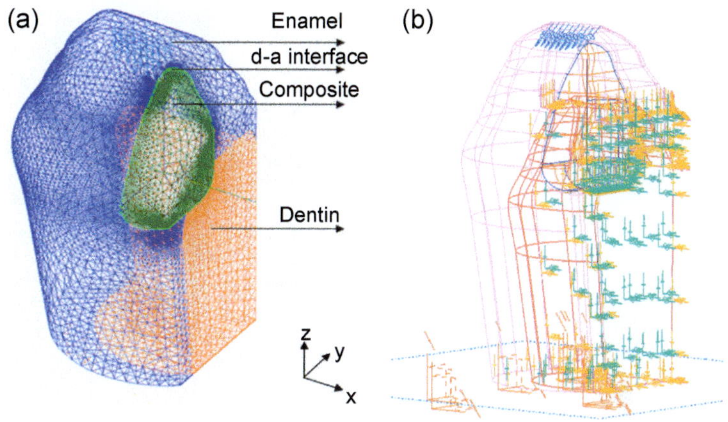

Figure 10.2 Macroscale analysis of the stress transfer in a restored molar including the loading conditions at the d-a interface: (a) FE model, and (b) boundary conditions.

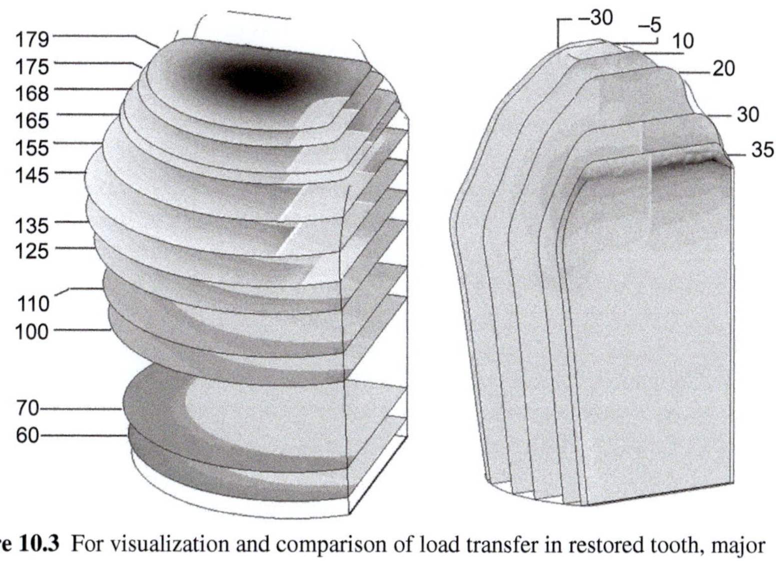

Figure 10.3 For visualization and comparison of load transfer in restored tooth, major principal stress distributions obtained from the FE model were plotted on horizontal and vertical sections.

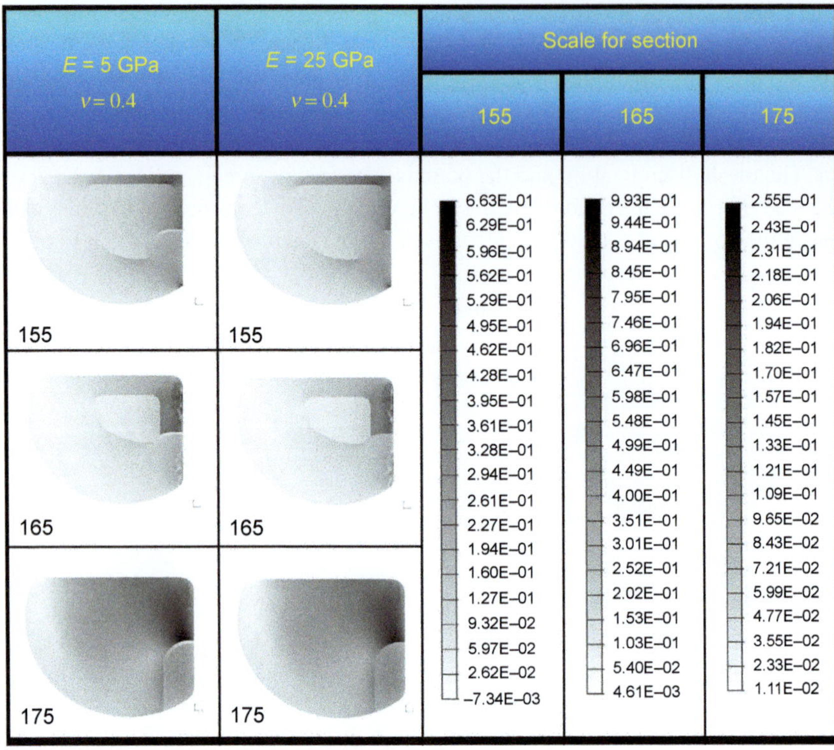

Figure 10.4 Major principal stress distributions in selected horizontal sections.

A larger number of sections were examined, and the stress distribution at three sections are given in Figs. 10.4 and 10.5. The following general observations may be made from these stress distributions: (1) the d-a interface is subjected to multiaxial stresses including compressive, tensile, and shear stresses; (2) the stress transfer through the d-a interface at the cavity wall for interface with low elastic moduli is minimal and the interface serves as a discontinuity; and (3) high stress concentrations in enamel and dentin proximal to cavity are only partially mitigated by the composite restoration, and as the stiffness of the interface layer increases, the stress concentration in the underlying tooth structure diminishes.

The results of the global model indicate that the stress conditions of the d-a interface are (1) complex, (2) depend on the occlusal loading conditions, and (3) vary from location to location along the d-a interface. Qualitatively, similar d-a interface stress distributions will be obtained for variations of the global model, although the quantitative details may be different. It is noteworthy that concurrent local–global modeling in which highly refined local model can be coupled to a global FE model would be too computationally intensive to provide practical, accurate results that capture all the physiologic loading conditions (such as soft versus hard morsels) as well as accurately represent the microstructural features of the tooth and, more importantly, the d-a interface. In view of these challenges, it is expedient to consider a detailed microscale analysis independent of the macroscale analysis as illustrated in Fig. 10.6. The stress analysis at the macroscales can provide an assessment

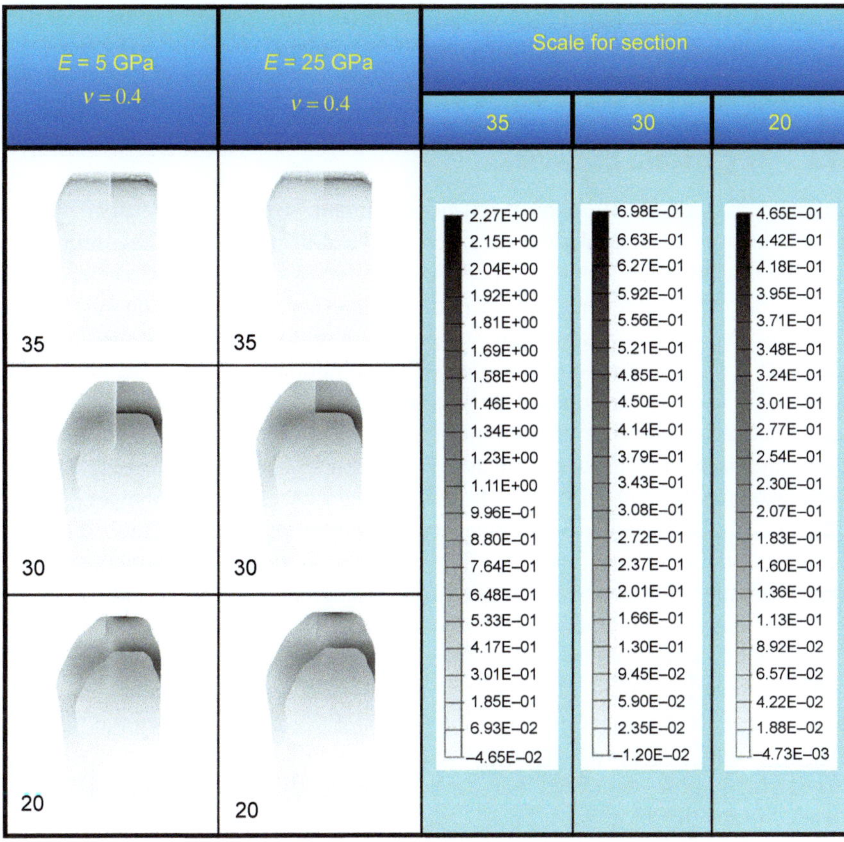

Figure 10.5 Major principal stress distributions in selected horizontal sections.

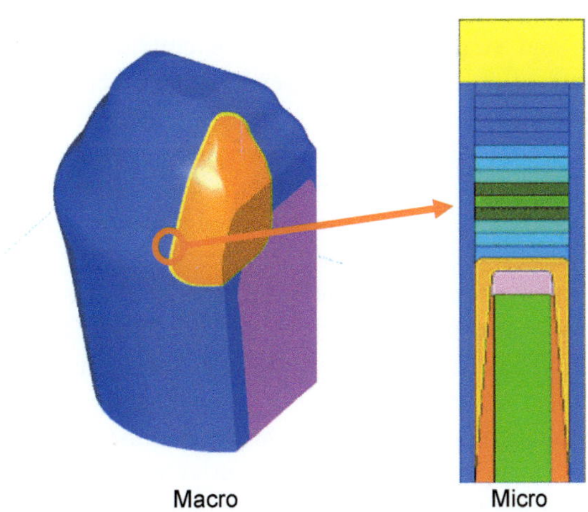

Figure 10.6 Load transfer at the d-a interface at the macro- and microscale.

of stresses at the d-a interface due to loading at the occlusal surfaces. On the other hand, the stress analysis at the microscales can give insights into the stress concentration location and the weak link within the d-a interface.

10.2.2 Microscale behavior

Based on microscale structure–property measurements, we have previously developed an idealized microstructural representation of the d-a interface.[1,2] This representation of the d-a interface was developed by considering the combined chemomechano-optical information generated from micro-Raman spectroscopy, scanning acoustic microscopy, and optical microscopic imaging.[6–8] Fig. 10.7 illustrates the conceived idealization as well as the two-dimensional (2D) computation unit cell. In our previous work, both 2D and 3D computational unit cells have been utilized to investigate a range of issues related to the role of d-a interface structure/properties on load transfer.[1–3] These computational cells have been analyzed for traction and displacement boundary conditions, since these provide an overall upper- and lower-bound behavior.[9] To capture the mechanical response of a-d interface, we have applied quasiperiodic boundary conditions on the computational cell. The imposition of quasiperiodic boundary conditions on nonperiodic meshes needs careful consideration.[10] The periodic boundary implies that shape and orientation of two opposite edges remains identical during the deformation and stress vectors acting on those sides should be equal and opposite.[11] The 2D computational unit cell along with the boundary conditions and applied load is given in Fig. 10.8. On the upper and lower edges of unit cell, periodic boundary conditions are applied. However, on the bottom edge of the d-a interface, all the nodes are fixed except those associated with the adhesive tag, because adhesive tag is freely suspended in the dentin tubules. These models have been used to perform parametric studies of adhesive infiltration, effect of interface geometry, varying degree of demineralization of intertubular and peritubular dentin during etching, the hybrid layer thickness, and anisotropy of hybrid layer.

Stress analysis using the microscale FE models of the d-a interface indicate that under both stress- and strain-controlled loading conditions, stress distribution is effected by the combination of material properties of the hybrid layer and the physical characteristics of the d-a interface. This analysis has shown that different material components of the d-a interface suffer different maximum stresses. As a result, the overall failure and fatigue life of the d-a interface is governed by the failure and fatigue life of the material component with the lowest strength and shortest fatigue life under a given loading condition. The fatigue life of the d-a interface predicted using these results was found to be a function of the boundary conditions, the properties of the adhesive, and the microstructure of the d-a interface. In fact, the fatigue life prediction curve in terms of the stress level and number of loading cycles does not follow a single function. Instead, different regions of this curve are governed by the different material components of the d-a interface. The results also show that d-a interfaces with thin hybrid layer that possesses uniform material properties experience less stress concentrations and show longer fatigue life when compared with the d-a interface with a graded hybrid layer (GHL).

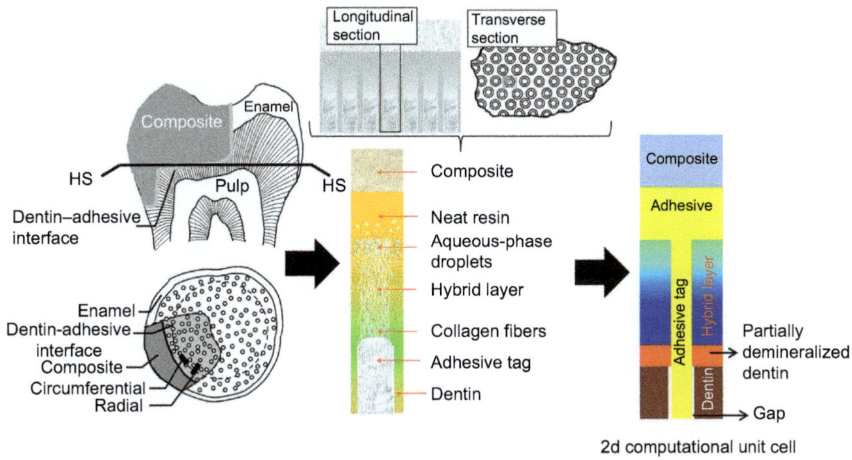

Figure 10.7 Schematic of the d-a interface and 2D rectangular idealized computational unit cell or representative volume element.

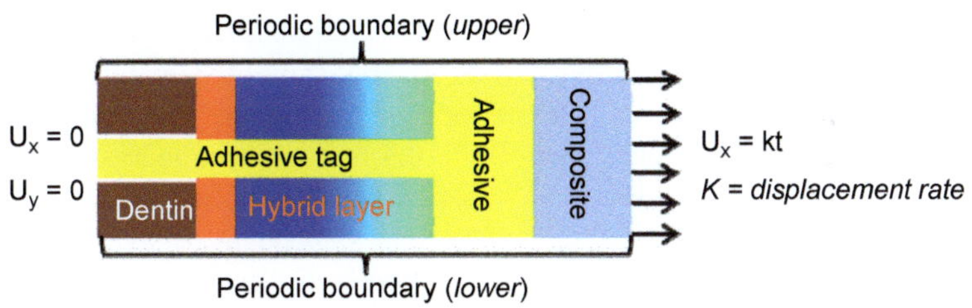

Figure 10.8 The 2D finite element model showing boundary conditions and load applied.

10.3 Rate-dependent microscale stress analysis of d-a interface

The properties of dentin adhesive and hybrid layer (collagen–adhesive composite) depends on the loading rate and moisture content.[12,13] The finite element models of d-a interface (such as[2,3]) have, typically, ignored rate-dependent behavior and assumed dentin adhesive and hybrid layer to be linear elastic. Here we present some results using a finite element model of d-a interface where the material components such as dentin adhesive, hybrid layer, and composite have nonlinear rate-dependent behavior and include deformation-induced damage. The constitutive equation used to describe mechanical response of dentin adhesive and hybrid layer is developed using the micromechanical approach (described in detail in[14–17]).

To study the stress distribution in the d-a interface, the developed computational cell of d-a interface was subjected to monotonic loading at different rates in an in-house developed finite element program into which the constitutive relationship mentioned previously has been implemented. The top surface of the idealized unit cell was subject to monotonically increased displacement at three different loading rates of 0.004 μm/s, 0.002 μm/s, and 0.0002 μm/s to show the effect of loading rate on the overall behavior of d-a interface. These simplified boundary conditions are chosen to study the behavior of the d-a interface under ideal conditions, which provides upper limit for the durability of the d-a interface. However, under clinical conditions, boundary and loading conditions are complex as shown by Singh et al. in 3D FE analysis of a restored tooth.[1,3] In the current model, there are 11,735 three-node triangular elements and 12,036 nodes.

The dentin adhesive in the composite tooth restoration appears predominantly in the following two places: (1) forms a layer under the dental composite and (2) as adhesive tags formed by the flow of adhesive into the dentinal tubules (tubules were opened as a result of acid etching). The thicknesses of the restorative dental composite, the adhesive layer, and the partially demineralized dentin, dentin and exposed collagen are 5, 5, 2.0, 5.0, and 3.0 μm, respectively. In the current study to show the effect of geometry on the overall response of d-a interface, the following variants of the d-a interface are studied: (1) uniform hybrid layer (UHL), in which mechanical properties of hybrid layer are assumed to be constant along the depth of the d-a interface; (2) GHL, in which the properties decrease linearly along the depth of the d-a interface; and (3) GHL with defect, which is case 2 with circular defect in the adhesive tag.

The results of finite element simulation of the d-a interface under different loading and geometry are shown in Figs. 10.9–10.12. Fig. 10.9 shows the evolution of overall stress in the computational cell of d-a interface as it is loaded under monotonically increasing displacement. It is clear from Fig. 10.9 that with the increase in loading rate, the stress–strain response of the d-a interface becomes stiffer and stronger. This increasing stiffness is expected because of the rate-dependent behavior of material components such as adhesive, composite, and hybrid layers. In particular, the strength of the d-a interface with UHL decreased from ~64 MPa at a relatively fast strain rate of $15e^{-5}$/s to ~11.5 MPa at slower rate of $7.5e^{-6}$/s, which is 20 times lower. It is worthwhile to note that not only the maximum stress increases with increase of loading rate but also the strain corresponding to maximum stress increases. Furthermore, if the

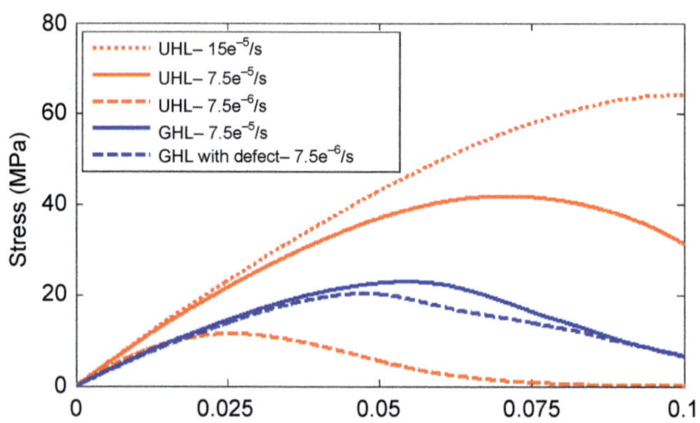

Figure 10.9 Overall stress–strain behavior of the d-a interface at different loading rate and geometry.

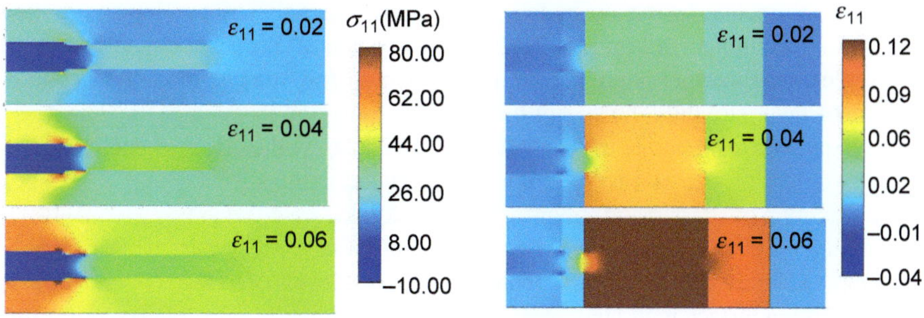

Figure 10.10 Stress–strain distribution in the d-a interface with uniform hybrid layer at different strain levels.

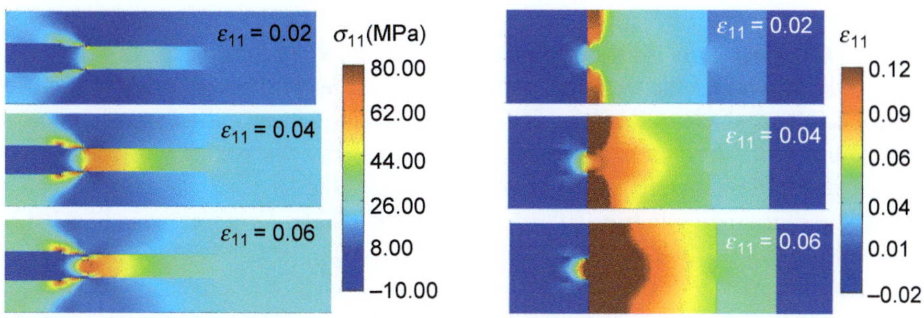

Figure 10.11 Stress–strain distribution in the d-a interface with graded hybrid layer at different strain levels.

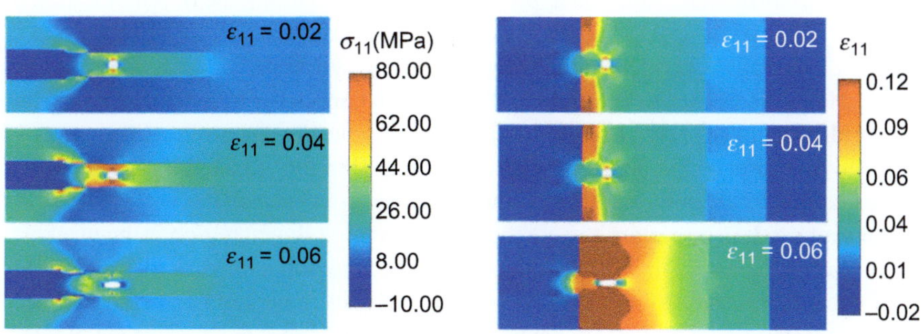

Figure 10.12 Stress–strain distribution in the d-a interface with graded hybrid layer and microdefect in adhesive at different strain levels.

loading rate is kept constant and the geometry of the d-a interface is changed, then the strength/durability of the d-a interface also changes. As seen from Fig. 10.9 at a strain rate of $7.5e^{-5}$/s, the peak strength of the d-a interface with UHL, GHL, and GHL with defect is found to be ~42, ~23, and ~20.5 MPa, respectively.

It is important to note that the dentin adhesive will often undergo some degree of phase separation when formed in the presence of water. This phase separation results in nanoscale defects. In the presented model, defects smaller than 250 nm are considered to be homogenized into the representative material properties specified at the microscales. On the other hand, defects larger than 250 nm may be modeled as part of the d-a interface. Not only the size of the defect but also the location of the defect will affect the overall response of the d-a interface. To illustrate the effect of such a defect, a circular defect of size radius 500 nm was introduced in the adhesive tag.

The evolution of stresses and strains in the d-a interface are given in Figs. 10.10–10.12, respectively, for UHL, GHL, and GHL-with-defect interface under a strain rate of $7.5e^{-5}$. The stress and strain contours are presented at the strain levels of 0.02, 0.04, and 0.06. In the case of d-a interface with UHL at 0.02 strain level, higher stress is observed in adhesive tags; these adhesive tags are formed when dentin adhesive flows into the hollow dentin tubules. However, hybrid layer experiences smaller and uniform stress, due to the presence of constant material properties along the depth of the hybrid layer. At the strain level of 0.04, adhesive tag experiences even larger stress; however, when the strain level reaches 0.06, stress in the adhesive tag decreases, as shown in Fig. 10.10. This decrease in the stress in adhesive tag with increase in strain indicates that this material component has reached its peak stress level and is exhibiting strain-induced softening, which indicates failure. If the loading is continued further, stress in adhesive tag will continue to decrease and will ultimately lead to rupture of adhesive tag.

Stress and strain distribution in the d-a interface with GHL is presented in Fig. 1011. In d-a interface with GHL, adhesive flows into the demineralized dentin from top to bottom and forms a collagen–adhesive composite of gradually decreasing properties. This process results in a layer of uninfiltrated demineralized dentin sometimes termed as exposed collagen. This exposed collagen is absent in the d-a interface with UHL. From Fig. 10.11 we observe that stress in adhesive tag increases gradually from top to bottom, whereas in UHL, stress is approximately uniform along the depth of adhesive tag at any given strain level. The increase in stress along the depth of adhesive tag is caused by the depth-dependent material properties of hybrid layer. Material properties of hybrid layer decreases from top to bottom, which causes the transfer of stress from the hybrid layer to adhesive tag. In contrast, if we consider the strain distribution in Fig. 10.11 we observe that larger strains are observed in the exposed collagen, which is expected due to the soft nature of collagen, and can experience larger deformations without rupture. It is important to note that the exposed collagen region is the weakest, and one would expect the failure to concentrate in this region. However, the redistribution of stresses indicates that stiff and less ductile phases may control the failure limit. Also, we observe that, similar to d-a interface with UHL, stress in adhesive tag in GHL decreases beyond a certain strain level, indicating failure, ie, reduction in the capacity of d-a interface to sustain load. Other material components of the d-a interface such as composite, adhesive, and dentin experience approximately uniform stress distribution. Finally, the presence of defect disrupts the stress and strain distribution as seen from Fig. 10.12. This microscale defect causes a localized failure in the adhesive tags; once the tag is failed, stress is transferred to the neighboring hybrid layer as seen in the stress distribution at strain level of 0.06 in Fig. 10.12. The presence of defects causes initial failure in tag, and thereafter failure propagates through hybrid layer, ultimately causing the fracture of the d-a interface.

10.4 Concluding remarks

This d-a interface is a complex system of different material components and their varying mechanical properties. The overall mechanical behavior of the d-a interface is greatly influenced by the properties of these material components. Mathematical modeling can provide an alternative noninvasive approach to understand the behavior of the interface and its impact on the durability of composite tooth restorations. This chapter has described some of the challenges associated with the development of such models as well as approaches to interpret the results. Feasible computational modeling approaches to address the issues related to spatial scales by using independent macro- and microscale models as well as temporal issues by developing rate-dependent models have been discussed. Nevertheless, for developing a comprehensive understanding of how composite tooth restorations perform in function, the current modeling efforts, which are typically based on classical elastic continuum mechanics, are inadequate, although they provide a fundamental point of departure for more refined modeling, such as the micromechanically based models that have the capability of connecting the microscale mechanisms to the macroscale phenomena.[16,18,19] An implementation of the micromechanical model for illustrating the rate effects on d-a interface behavior was described in this chapter.

References

1. Misra A, Spencer P, Marangos O, Wang Y, Katz JL. Micromechanical analysis of dentin/adhesive interface by the finite element method. *J Biomed Mater Res Part B Appl Biomater* 2004;**70B**:56–65.
2. Misra A, Spencer P, Marangos O, Wang Y, Katz JL. Parametric study of the effect of phase anisotropy on the micromechanical behavior of dentin-adhesive interface. *J R Soc Interface* 2005;**2**:145–57.
3. Singh V, Misra A, Marangos O, Park J, Ye Q, Kieweg SL, et al. Fatigue life prediction of dentin–adhesive interface using micromechanical stress analysis. *Dent Mater* 2011;**27**(9):e187–95.
4. Spencer P, Ye Q, Park J, Topp EM, Misra A, Marangos O, et al. Adhesive/Dentin interface: the weak link in the composite restoration. *Ann Biomed Eng* 2010;**38**(6):1989–2003.
5. Dejak B, Mlotkowski A, Romanowicz M. Finite element analysis of stresses in molars during clenching and mastication. *J Prosthet Dent* 2003;**90**(6):591–7.
6. Wang Y, Spencer P. Quantifying adhesive penetration in adhesive/dentin interface using confocal Raman microspectroscopy. *J Biomed Mater Res* 2002;**59**(1):46–55.
7. Wieliczka DM, Kruger MB, Spencer P. Raman imaging of dental adhesive diffusion. *Appl Spectrosc* 1997;**51**:1593–6.
8. Wieliczka DM, Spencer P, Kruger MB. Raman mapping of the dentin/adhesive interface. *Appl Spectrosc* 1996;**50**:1500–4.
9. Nemat-Nasser S, Hori M. *Micromechanics: overall properties of heterogeneous materials.* Elsevier; 1999.
10. Nguyen VD, Bechet E, Geuzaine C, Noels L. Imposing periodic boundary condition on arbitrary meshes by polynomial interpolation. *Comput Mater Sci* 2012;**55**:390–406.

11. Kouznetsova V, Brekelmans WAM, Baaijens FPT. An approach to micro-macro modeling of heterogeneous materials. *Comput Mech* 2001;**27**(1):37–48.
12. Singh V, Misra A, Marangos O, Park J, Ye Q, Kieweg SL, et al. Viscoelastic and fatigue properties of model methacrylate-based dentin adhesives. *J Biomed Mater Res B Appl Biomater* 2010;**95**(2):283–90.
13. Singh V, Misra A, Parthasarathy R, Ye Q, Park J, Spencer P. Mechanical properties of methacrylate-based model dentin adhesives: effect of loading rate and moisture exposure. *J Biomed Mater Res B Appl Biomater* 2013;**101**(8):1437–43.
14. Misra A, Parthasarathy R, Singh V, Spencer P. Micro-poromechanics model of fluid-saturated chemically active fibrous media. *Z Angew Math Mech* 2015;**95**(2):215–34.
15. Misra A, Singh V. Micromechanical model for viscoelastic materials undergoing damage. *Continuum Mech Thermodyn* 2013;**25**(2–4):343–58.
16. Misra A, Singh V. Thermomechanics-based nonlinear rate-dependent coupled damage-plasticity granular micromechanics model. *Continuum Mech Thermodyn* 2014;**27**(4–5):787–817.
17. Misra A, Singh V. Nonlinear granular micromechanics model for multi-axial rate-dependent behavior. *Int J Solids Struct* 2014;**51**(13):2272–82.
18. Misra A, Poorsolhjouy P. Granular micromechanics model for damage and plasticity of cementitious materials based upon thermomechanics. *Math Mech Solids* 2015. http://dx.doi.org/10.1177/1081286515576821. [published online].
19. Yang Y, Ching W-Y, Misra A. Higher-order continuum theory applied to fracture simulation of nano-scale intergranular glassy film. *J Nanomech Micromech* 2011;**1**(2):60–71.

Part Four

Lessons learned: next generation reconstructions and future opportunities

Dentinoenamel junction: motif for interfacial mechanics of dissimilar materials

11

A. Misra[1], O. Marangos[2], P. Spencer[1]
[1]University of Kansas, Lawrence, KS, United States; [2]Cyprus University of Technology, Limassol, Cyprus

11.1 Introduction

When dissimilar materials, whose properties possess wide variations, are combined in engineering practice, the interfacial regions are invariably defective and, typically, the location where failure initiates. On the other hand, interfaces found in natural material systems exhibit superior performance and seem to have overcome the difficulties that plague engineering interfaces/joints. Human teeth are a well-documented example of a natural system in which two materials with vastly different properties are combined effectively. The dentinoenamel junction (DEJ) represents a biological interface that successfully joins stiff, brittle enamel to compliant, relatively ductile dentin. The DEJ has been widely cited as an example of a material system in which structural hierarchy contributes significantly to the longevity and performance of the tooth under function.[1–6] The durability of the tooth has been attributed to the inability of cracks in the enamel to propagate through the DEJ to the subjacent dentin.[5,7,8] The DEJ region is a hierarchy of microstructures whose composition is derived from building blocks consisting of apatitic mineralite, collagen, and water (for example, see Fig. 11.1 for structural hierarchy of dentin). Highly cross-linked collagen forms the DEJ matrix, which is infiltrated with variable amounts of mineralite, glycosaminoglycans, and water. Although a number of morphological features and their sizes have been identified, a definitive structural description of this region has been elusive given the complex arrangements of the various components. As a result qualitative descriptions abound with respect to why cracks in the enamel do not propagate as monolithic cracks into the dentin.[2,5–11] It is unclear how and why the microscale composition, structure, and mechanical properties of the DEJ lead to a robust interface between the stiff enamel and the 2–4 times less stiff dentin.

11.2 DEJ literature review

The DEJ is described as the region spanning inner enamel to mantle dentin and a number of high-resolution techniques have been applied to study the DEJ. These studies have provided valuable insight to the structure and composition of the DEJ and its

Material-Tissue Interfacial Phenomena. http://dx.doi.org/10.1016/B978-0-08-100330-5.00011-X

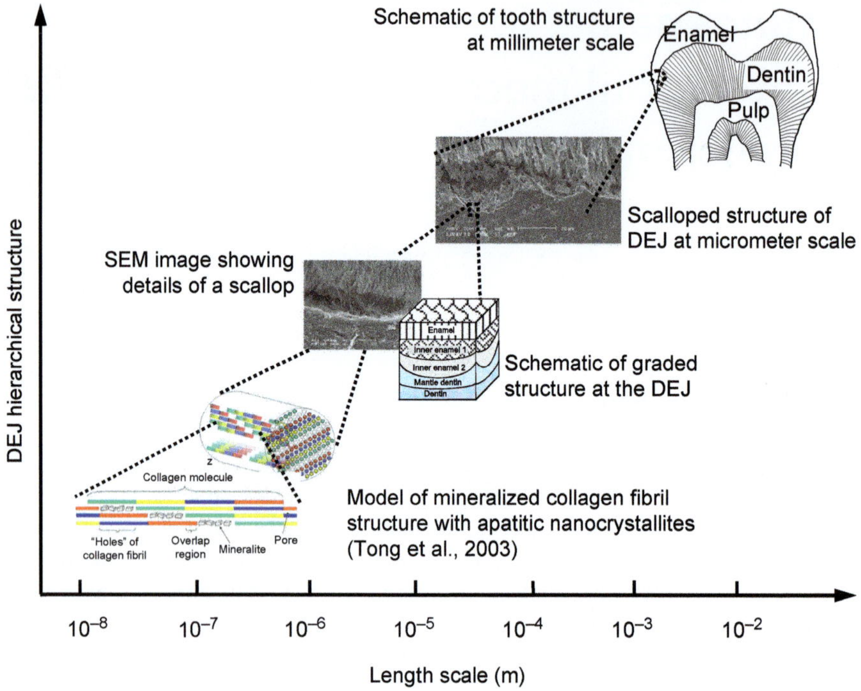

Figure 11.1 A schematic depiction of dentin-enamel junction hierarchical structure from molecular organization to the whole tooth.
Modified from Misra A, Marangos O, Parthasarathy R, Spencer P. Micro-scale analysis of compositional and mechanical properties of dentin using homotopic measurements. *Biomed Imagine Comput Model Biomech* 2013;**4**:131–41.

vicinity.[2,4,12–16] Mechanical and fracture behavior of the DEJ have also been measured using a variety of characterization techniques.[1,3,4,7–9,17,18]

11.2.1 Mechanical properties: indentation and fracture

Hardness measurements across the DEJ have been performed under a wide load range using Vickers indentation method.[1,5] Hardness and elastic modulus measurements have also been performed using Atomic Force Microscope (AFM)-based indentation or nanoindentation and modulus mapping.[4,17,18] These indentation measurements indicate the hardness and modulus transition from a high value in the bulk enamel to a low value in the bulk dentin. The thickness over which this transition occurs is a function of the indenter load and size, which is not unexpected, as this zone is known to possess an abrupt variation of composition and structure, as seen from Fig. 11.1. Clearly, a relatively small indenter load and size will interrogate a small region within this zone and provide the local-scale properties. On the other hand, a large indenter load and/or size will interact with a larger area and, therefore, provide an averaged property over a larger scale. Therefore, it is not surprising that DEJ width has been reported to vary from more than ~100 μm down to ~2–3 μm based on measurements with techniques of varying resolution.[1,4,17,18]

Fracture toughness of the DEJ has been studied by investigating fracture propagation across the DEJ.[5,8,9] The intent of these investigations has been to simulate the propagation of a fracture that emanates from the enamel, likely due to separation along enamel rods. The fact that oftentimes these fractures get arrested in the vicinity of the DEJ has fascinated researchers. In an article in *Nature*, Imbeni et al.[5] have investigated the fracture arrest/deflection process by following the propagation of fractures formed at the corners of Vickers indents. The fracture deflection was explained on the basis of linear elastic fracture mechanics concept for bimaterial interfaces. They also examined the fracture zones and found that as the fracture propagates into dentin, a diffused microfracture zone held together by bridging fibers forms ahead of the fracture tip. Further studies have indicated a different mechanism for the resilience of this junction whereby the existing cracklike defects are inhibited from propagating due to stress shielding from neighboring similar cracks in the enamel.[6] Fractography of fractured microbeams subjected to bending have been used to explain the failure propagation in DEJ.[19] The presence of microscale roughness in the form of scallops at the DEJ has also been hypothesized to contribute to the robustness of this interface.[11] These studies treat enamel and dentin as conventional homogeneous isotropic elastic media without any considerations of the nanoscale/microscale structure and component properties. The findings suggest that perhaps higher order micromorphic theories or multiscalar approaches are needed to correctly describe the fracture arrest mechanism. There are four aspects that make fracture and indentation studies of DEJ difficult to interpret in a quantitative manner: (1) microstructure, (2) heterogeneity, (3) nonlinearity, and (4) scale dependence. Fracture and failure mechanics of materials that combine structure, heterogeneity, nonlinearity, and scale dependence are in their infancy and are active areas of research within computational mechanics and physics communities.[20] This is specifically true when we seek understanding/solutions from the nanoscales.

11.2.2 Morphology and composition

The DEJ region is a conglomerate of microstructures and composition derived from building blocks consisting of apatitic mineralite, collagen, and water. Although a number of morphological features and their sizes have been identified, a definitive structural description of this region has not been established. A key structural feature at the DEJ appears to be the scallop whose characteristic size varies from 10 to 100 μm. The presence, shape, and size of scallops at the DEJ has been studied by Whittaker,[13] who has also provided a review of early work beginning from the description of Tomes.[21] Scallops vary in size and depth from cuspal to cervical locations, as described in 1997 by Doukoudakis et al.[22] The functional significance of the scallops from biomechanical viewpoint has been investigated in 2007 by Shimizu and Macho.[11] Their finding suggests that the scalloped structure can significantly affect the stress distributions at the DEJ. Based on high-resolution electron microscopy investigations, the morphology of inner enamel in the vicinity of the DEJ has been classified into three zones.[14,23] The innermost zone has been described as consisting of 5- to 10-μm-thick hypomineralized zone of disoriented crystallites that transitions through a 10- to 20-μm-thick intermediate zone to the outer enamel. Mantle dentin that underlies the optical DEJ is

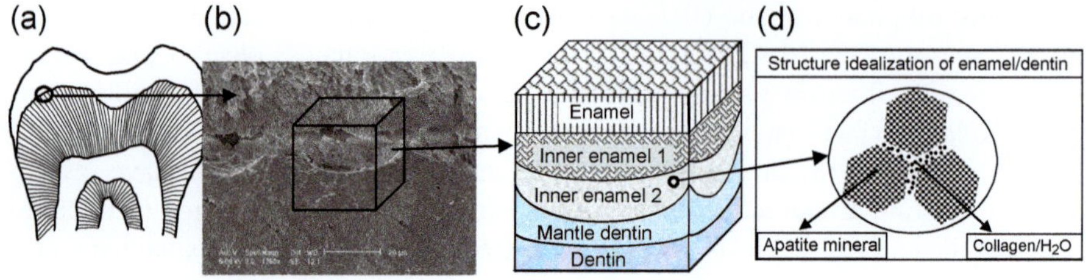

Figure 11.2 (a) Schematic cross-section through a molar; (b) scanning electron micrograph of dentin-enamel junction (DEJ) showing ~20-μm interdigitated (scalloped) geometry; (c) idealized DEJ geometry at ~10–100 μm^3; and (d) the building blocks that compose enamel, dentin and the DEJ.

characterized by the absence of dentinal tubules and has been described to be somewhat less mineralized than primary dentin. The relative proportions of mineral and organic components in the DEJ region have also been investigated.[2,4,15,16,24] Although qualitatively there is agreement about the general features of this region, there is also a considerable degree of conflicting information regarding the composition and structure, particularly with regard to the arrangement of crystallites in the inner enamel and the structure of mantle dentin. Clearly, the structural features, such as scallops, the orientation of crystallites in the inner enamel region, the morphology in the vicinity of mantle dentin, and the composition of this region are significant from the viewpoint of how mechanical loading is resisted within this region. The current empirical information is woefully insufficient for unraveling DEJ mechanics. Moreover, because of the lack of advanced mathematical models, our understanding of these interfaces is incomplete. Based on the current information, the microstructure of the DEJ can be depicted as shown in Fig. 11.2.

11.3 Homotopic experimental characterization of DEJ

Advances in nondestructive high-resolution techniques have enabled location-dependent measurement of biomaterial physical, chemical, and mechanical properties at the micro- and nanometer scales. Data interpretations from these measurements have to be performed carefully to extract meaningful information. Two aspects become significant when such techniques are used in a complementary manner.[25–27] First, it becomes necessary that the measurements with complementary techniques be performed at the same location for their proper interpretation or cross-correlations, such that "data fusion" considers the same material volume. Second, appropriate mathematical models must be applied to interpret the data in terms of material properties since the high-resolution techniques seldom measure the properties directly.

The mechanical and compositional properties of the DEJ region vary with location and scale. Furthermore, the mechanical behavior is expected to be characterized by anisotropy. Therefore, the properties should be characterized at different precise scales to completely understand how these properties vary both across and along the

DEJ. Such a characterization is necessary if we are to develop mathematical models to understand how small features affect the overall mechanics of the tooth structure. The concept of *homotopic* measurements (Greek *homos* meaning identical and *topos* meaning place) describes the methodology in which a set of material properties are measured at the same location of the same sample using different methods and different scales.[25–27] Here we describe homotopic measurements using optical microscope, optical profilometry, scanning acoustic microscopy (SAM) and micro-Raman spectroscopy (μRS). The micromechanical elastic properties were determined by SAM. The same area was mapped by μRS to obtain quantitative homotopic characterization of the mechanical properties and composition at a similar spatial scale.

11.3.1 Sample preparation

Extracted unerupted third molars collected under approved institutional review board protocol were used for the experimental work. The teeth samples were placed in separate vials containing phosphate-buffered saline solution with 0.002% sodium azide and stored at 4°C. Only tooth samples that are not fractured were used for this study. The specimen preparation proceeded as follows. The cervical third, right below the neck of the tooth, was sectioned perpendicular to its long axis by means of a H_2O-cooled low-speed diamond saw (Buehler, Lake Bluff, IL). The crown was vertically sectioned at ~1-mm increments using a H_2O-cooled low-speed diamond saw resulting in at least five ~1-mm-thick longitudinal slabs parallel to the buccolingual plane shown in Fig. 11.3. To remove surface irregularities such as saw marks and the smear layer caused by the diamond saw, the longitudinal 1-mm sections were polished by successively increasing the grit size. Whenever the samples were not used, they were placed in vials containing phosphate-buffered saline solution with 0.002% sodium

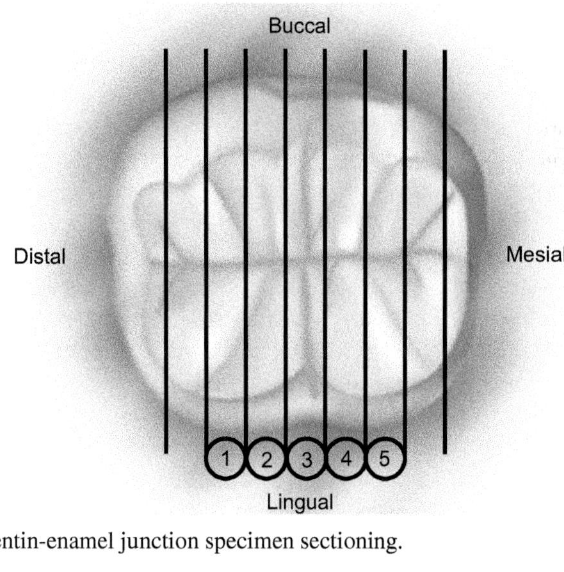

Figure 11.3 Dentin-enamel junction specimen sectioning.

azide and stored at 4°C. The mesial surface of a prepared slab was first analyzed by SAM. The same surface was then analyzed by μRS.

Prior to analyses, the topography of the DEJ specimens was analyzed by profilometry. Knowledge of topography is important as surface techniques can be affected by topography. Assumptions of the theoretical models used to analyze surface technique data assume that the surface roughness is small when compared with measurement scales. Although in principle it is possible to model surface topography, the resultant methods for property interpretation become immensely complicated. The profilometric analyses assists in ensuring (1) that the average height of the surface topography of the prepared specimen is much smaller (at least 100 times) when compared with the smallest ultrasound wavelength (~3 μm) and (2) that the near-surface integrity at the vicinity of the DEJ is maintained and the DEJ region is free from defects, such as microcracks, saw-cut marks, interfacial separation, and/or undercut between surfaces. Hand polishing using 600 to 1200 grit paper produced uniform and smooth surfaces for SAM analysis of the DEJ. The surface prepared as described has an average surface roughness in the range of ~0.02 μm. We also find that the SAM results are not affected provided the polishing is done by applying a light pressure and the surfaces are sonicated and rinsed clean promptly after polishing.

11.3.2 SAM analysis

SAM offers a versatile nondestructive method for determining the elastic moduli at different scales. The traditional SAM, based on the reflection coefficient and V(z) curve measurements (see Ref.[28]) using spherical lens is, however, not ideally suited for anisotropy measurements of elastic constants. The acoustic field generated by a spherical lens is symmetric. When the symmetric field interacts with the unknown substrate placed perpendicular to the lens axis, both the reflected wave and the Rayleigh wave contribution to the returned signal are averaged over all directions. Thus the directional properties due to material anisotropy are smeared out. For our measurements, the DEJ slab was placed in a distilled (deionized) temperature-controlled H_2O bath and positioned relative to the acoustic lens using a positioning system schematically depicted in Fig. 11.4. The positioning setup permits 3-axis translational motion, X-Y motion for interrogating different regions of the specimen and Z-positioning to enable focusing and defocusing on the specimen. The positioning system also includes a tilt stage to allow for θ-rotation of the specimen relative to the transducer axis.

Since SAM can function as a conventional microscope, it can be used to identify morphological features based on the contrast in acoustic properties of a specimen. Therefore, a surface scan (C-scan) was first performed to locate the DEJ contour for the sample. The peak signal amplitude was recorded at each location, and a gray scale image generated as shown in Fig. 11.5. Enamel being stiffer reflects a larger portion of the signal and therefore appears as smaller grayscale value than dentin in the image. The grayscale contrast of the two distinct regions delineates the DEJ contour. It is very important for these measurements that the transducer axis be

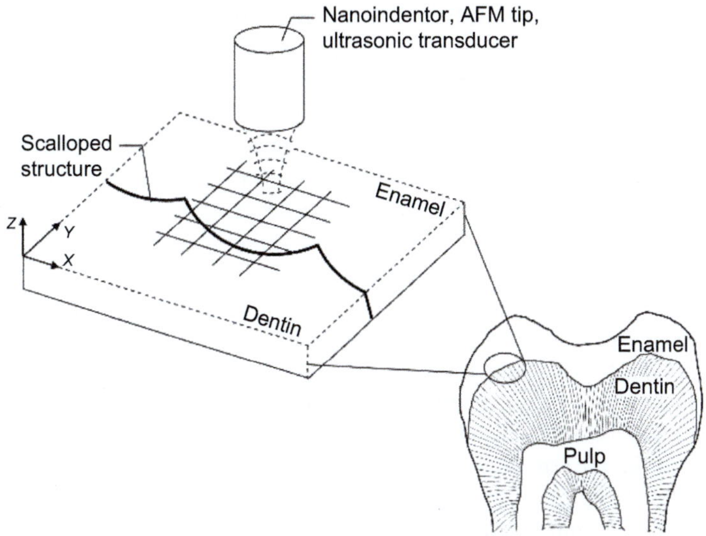

Figure 11.4 Schematic of experimental protocol over the dentin-enamel junction region.

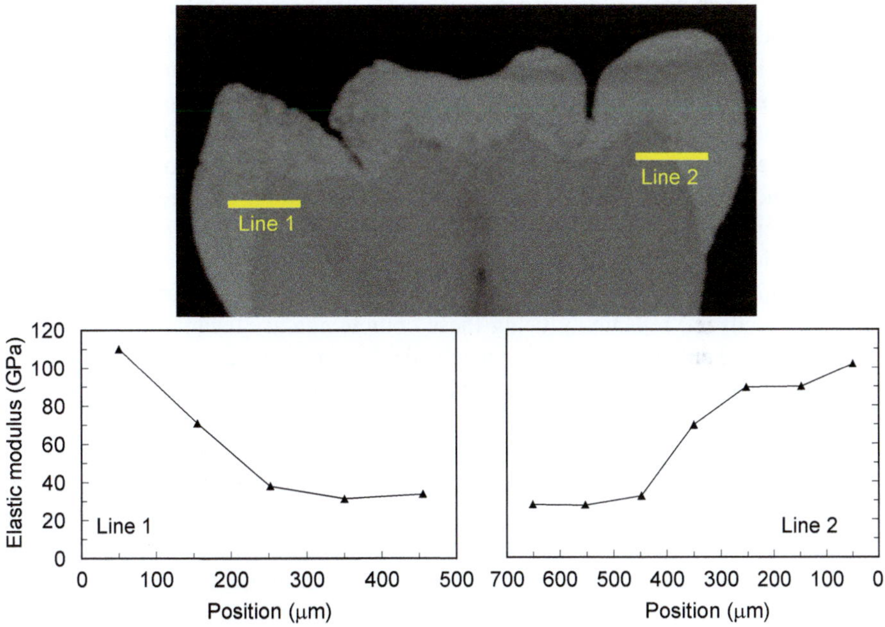

Figure 11.5 C-scan scanning acoustic microscopy image of a tooth section using 30-MHz focused transducer. Also shown are the elastic moduli determined along two lines crossing the dentin-enamel junction as shown in the C-scan.

perpendicular to the sample surface. For this purpose, the θ-tilt stage was tilted at 0.1 degrees increments, while the ultrasonic transducer was focused at the sample surface. At each increment, the peak signal amplitude was recorded. The θ-position that gave the highest signal amplitude was set as the sample tilt position for further measurements. Fig. 11.5 demonstrates the capabilities of SAM in determining the micromechanical properties of the DEJ region. In this case, the measurements were performed at the mesoscale (~100 μm) resolution using a 30-MHz focused transducer. Fig. 11.5 also shows the elastic modulus variation across the DEJ at two different locations. Each point on the curves for lines 1 and 2, represents the modulus of a ~100-μm spot of the tooth section. The moduli obtained across the DEJ are similar to those obtained by previous investigators using indentation techniques. The clear advantage of characterization using SAM is that it is nondestructive. Therefore, the same sample can be imaged at a higher resolution with a higher frequency transducer. SAM offers us the only viable way to obtain such multiscalar data. Once the location of the DEJ on the sample was defined, a small area (~100 × 100 μm) was chosen for further evaluations with a focus on the acquisition of A-scan data from various locations within this area. A schematic of the acquisition protocol is shown in Fig. 11.4.

11.3.3 μRS analysis

The DEJ region is primarily composed of apatitic mineralite, collagen, and water, with a higher organic content than either enamel or dentin.[15,29] However, what is unknown in sufficient detail is how the relative composition varies in the DEJ region and how this composition is correlated with the micromechanical properties at the different scales. μRS can be used to characterize the spatial distributions of organic compounds and inorganic compounds with a spatial resolution of about 1 μm. Importantly, for biological samples, it is a nondestructive technique and the analysis is not affected by the presence of water. Combining μRS and SAM provides the means to relate chemical composition to the micromechanical properties at the DEJ. Since both techniques are nondestructive, the same sample and the same area on the sample can be analyzed repeatedly using these complementary techniques. Moreover, these data can be enhanced by further mechanical behavior measurements with AFM and nanoindentation. The sample was placed directly on glass microscope slides and covered with H_2O and imaged using a 60X H_2O immersion lens. Spectra was acquired at various locations within the selected DEJ region at a spatial resolution of ~1 μm using a computer-controlled *x*-*y*-*z* stage with a minimum step width of 50 nm. Spectra will be obtained at a wave number resolution of ~6 cm^{-1} over the spectral region of 400–1800 cm^{-1} with an integration time of 120 s. The experimental apparatus used to collect the Raman spectra was a LabRam model (Horiba Jobin Yvon Inc., Edison, NJ) model. The optical microscope allows for visual identification of the position at which the Raman spectrum was obtained. Instrument fluctuation was evaluated by comparing spectra from standards such as silicon, and each spectrum was frequency calibrated and corrected for chromatic variations in the spectrometer system detection.

11.3.4 Composite data

A composite image of the DEJ region obtained by applying complementary imaging techniques to the same sample is shown in Fig. 11.6. As a first step, the prepared sample was analyzed using an optical profilometer (Wyko NT1100, Veeco). The average roughness in the area of interest was determined to be less than 0.02 μm. More importantly, the profilometry clearly showed defects such as remnants of saw marks and uneven height locations on the DEJ. These features normally cannot be detected through optical microscopy; however, they can introduce artifacts during mapping with the analytical techniques. Using profilometry, we were able to identify several ~100 × 100 μm locations along the DEJ that were appropriate for our analysis with SAM and μRS. A DEJ area close to the cuspal region, shown in Fig. 11.6, was chosen for further studies. A C-scan image of the area was acquired using SAM (C-SAM Gen 5, Sonoscan) with a 230-MHz transducer with 4-μm lateral resolution at a grid spacing of 4 μm. This system allows us to store A-scan signals at all the grid locations for future analyses. Since SAM measurements are nondestructive and the sample is in an aqueous environment, it is preserved in its near-natural state. Thus, the same area of the sample could be imaged with μRS (LabRam ARAMIS, Horiba Jobin Yvon) using a He–Ne laser (632.8 nm) and 60X water immersion lens. The spectra were acquired at a grid spacing of 4 μm to match the SAM image. The acquired μRS spectra were then analyzed to develop normalized intensity maps of spectral features associated with the mineral (PO_4, 960 cm^{-1}) and collagen (amide I, ~1660 cm^{-1} and C–H stretching 2940 cm^{-1}). The intensity maps are shown in Fig. 11.7 along with the SAM C-scan. In Fig. 11.8, we show the A-scan signals and Raman spectra from three arbitrarily chosen spots within our 100 × 100-μm region. These figures illustrate one of the distinct advantages of using SAM to determine the micromechanical properties, ie, the same small region of a single sample can be analyzed using complementary techniques. Thus, the structure as determined by measurement of the molecular features can be related directly to the acoustic impedance within the same small region of the sample. These complementary techniques allow us to relate differences in the micromechanical behavior—specifically the acoustic impedance—to the molecular structure within

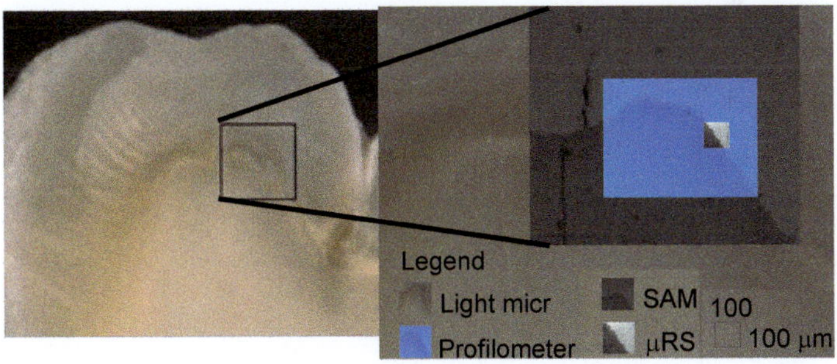

Figure 11.6 Composite image of data superposition from scanning acoustic microscopy and micro-Raman spectroscope at 4-μm grid spacing using homotopic measurement of the dentin-enamel junction region. Also shown are the profilometer data of the same region. The data are overlain on the optical image of the sample to indicate location.

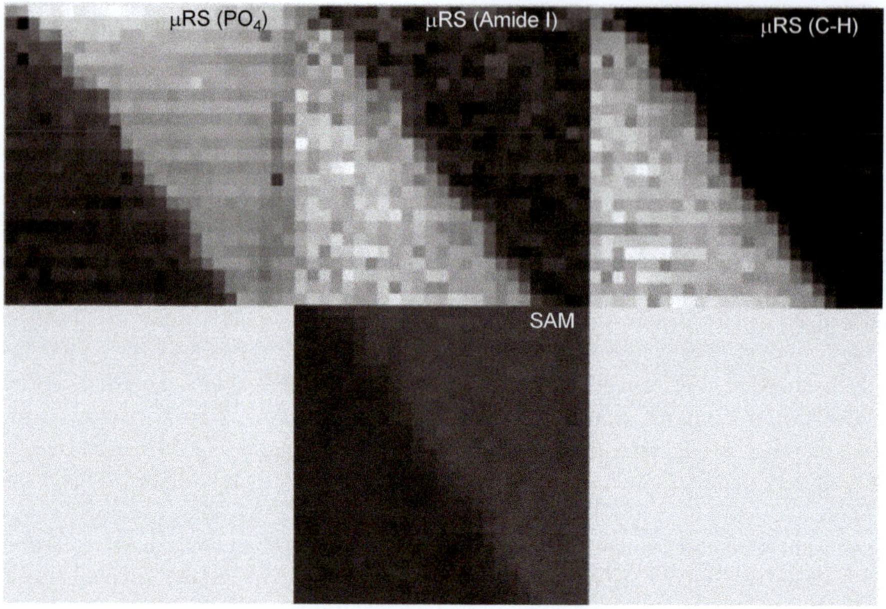

Figure 11.7 Maps of same 100 × 100 μm dentin-enamel junction area, as in Fig. 11.6, at 4 μm grid spacing. Top row: micro-Raman spectroscope maps of normalized intensity. Bottom map is scanning acoustic microscopy C-scan using a 230 MHz transducer.

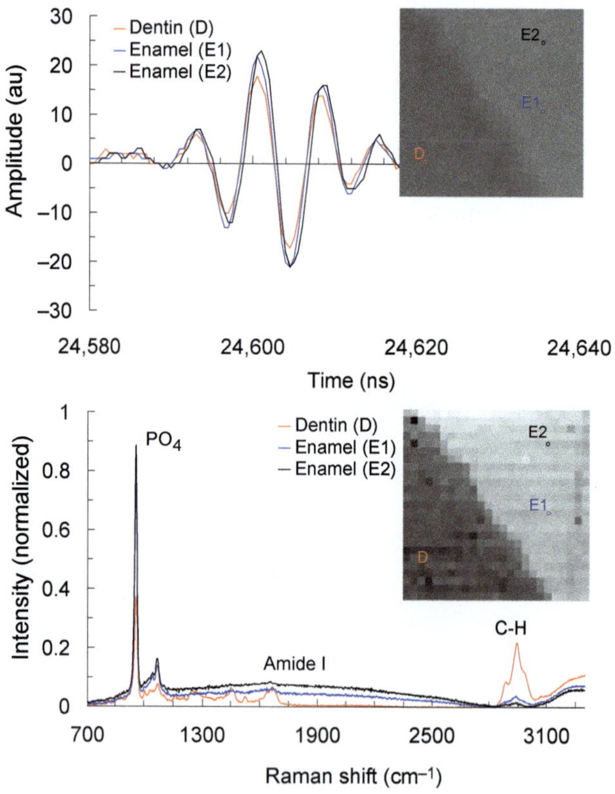

Figure 11.8 Scanning acoustic microscopy A-scan signals and Raman spectra from same spots.

the region analyzed. These measurements amply demonstrate the homotopic nature of the acquired data and point to the ability to perform a wide range of property correlations with the data set.

11.4 FE modeling of the DEJ region

To begin developing an understanding of how micromorphology and micromechanical properties influence the DEJ behavior, we have created two-dimensional finite element (FE) models as shown in Fig. 11.9. The FE model represents a 70×70-μm cross-section through a single scallop. The model was divided into five layers with an enamel layer at the top, two layers of inner enamel, a mantle dentin layer, and a dentin layer at the bottom. The micromorphology is based on the discussion in Section 2. An important feature of the DEJ micromorphology is the scalloped structure. These microscallops range in size from 25 to 100 μm both within a tooth and between different teeth.[29] Moreover, the scalloped structure exhibits pseudoperiodicity, that is, the scallops repeat themselves, although with variation in size. As a first step, our FE model was chosen to be of an average scallop size in the cuspal region.

Furthermore, we take advantage of the pseudoperiodicity by limiting the FE model to a single scallop and applying periodic boundary conditions to the sides. In this way, the 70×70-μm computational cell serves as a representative volume element (RVE) of the DEJ in the proximity of the scallop of assumed size and structure. We note that the structure changes in size, composition, and micromechanical properties as we traverse along the DEJ. Consequently, similar RVE will need to be created for cervical and cuspal regions of a tooth. For this preliminary study, plane stress elements were chosen and element

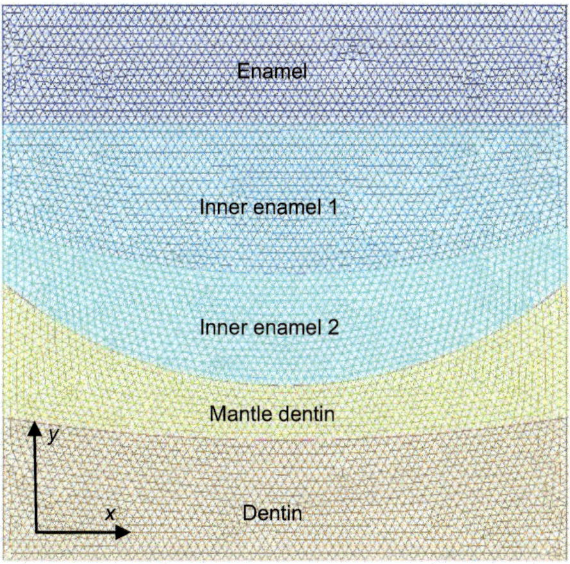

Figure 11.9 FE model of section through a dentin-enamel junction scallop. This computational cell serves as a representative volume element.

sizes were taken to be 0.1 μm. The elastic properties of the various layers were assigned as shown in Table 11.1. The enamel layer was given a transverse isotropic property based on measurements presented by He et al.[30] The properties of the two inner enamel layers were inferred using the morphological and compositional data provided by Kodaka et al.[15,23] According to Kodaka et al.,[15] the apatitic mineralites are highly randomly oriented in the inner enamel in the 10- to 15-μm zone above the interface identified as the "DEJ." Since the apatitic mineralites are highly oriented into rodlike motifs in the outer enamel, we assume that a gradual randomization must occur from the highly ordered rodlike enamel to completely randomized inner enamel. Kodaka et al.[15] also reported a gradual decrease in the mineral content from the outer enamel toward the DEJ. Thus the elastic moduli of inner enamel layer 1 are inferred to be slightly lower in magnitude to those of the enamel but slightly more isotropic, whereas those of the inner enamel layer 2 were assumed to be lower in magnitude than those of the enamel layer 1 and isotropic.

Four realizations of the aforementioned model were created to investigate the effect of the scalloped shape and anisotropy of the enamel layers on the overall modulus of the DEJ RVE. For model 1, we ignored the scalloped microstructure and assumed a 2-layer planar structure formed by joining enamel and dentin (similar to the layered microstructure assumed by Imbeni et al.[5]). Planar structure, albeit with graded isotropic properties, was assumed by Huang et al.[31] In contrast, for model 2 we considered a 2-layered scalloped structure. Thus by comparing models 1 and 2, we can assess the effect of scallops on the overall RVE properties. For models 3 and 4, we assumed a multiple-layer graded scalloped structure shown in Fig. 11.1. For model 3, we assumed all layers to have isotropic properties, whereas for model 4, the layer properties were assigned as shown in Table 11.1. Models 3 and 4 were designed to study the effect of anisotropy on the overall RVE properties.

To obtain the overall properties of the RVE, we performed calculations using the FE model for two uniaxial tension tests along the x- and y-directions and a simple shear loading test. As a result we are able to compute the overall elastic constants of the RVE assuming a transverse isotropic symmetry shown by Eq. (11.1):

$$\{\sigma\} = [C_{ij}]\{\varepsilon\}, \qquad where \qquad [C_{ij}] = \begin{bmatrix} C_{11} & C_{12} & C_{13} & 0 & 0 & 0 \\ C_{12} & C_{11} & C_{13} & 0 & 0 & 0 \\ C_{13} & C_{13} & C_{33} & 0 & 0 & 0 \\ 0 & 0 & 0 & C_{44} & 0 & 0 \\ 0 & 0 & 0 & 0 & C_{44} & 0 \\ 0 & 0 & 0 & 0 & 0 & (C_{11}-C_{12})/2 \end{bmatrix} \tag{11.1}$$

In Eq. (11.1), $\{\sigma\}$ is the six-component stress vector and $\{\varepsilon\}$ is the six-component strain vector. For uniaxial tensile tests, we apply the displacement boundary conditions as $u_i = \varepsilon_{ij}x_j$, where only one strain component is specified to be nonzero. Thus, for the y-direction or vertical uniaxial tensile loading, y-displacement of the

Table 11.1 Layer elastic moduli in gigapascals

Layer	Anisotropy	E_y	$E_x=E_z$	$\nu_{yx}=\nu_{yz}\nu_{xz}$	G_{yx}
Enamel	Transverse	100	80	0.3	38.5
Inner enamel 1	Transverse	95	85	0.3	36.5
Inner enamel 2	Isotropic	60	60	0.3	23.1
Mantle dentin	Isotropic	20	20	0.3	7.7
Dentin	Isotropic	30	30	0.3	11.5

Table 11.2 Effective elastic moduli of the four models

Models (GPa)	1	2	3	4
C_{11}	69.8	72.9	59.5	60.7
C_{13}	30.2	31.8	25.6	26.3
C_{33}	68.9	72.3	59.8	60.6
C_{44}	26.0	26.4	21.4	22.7

boundary nodes are specified as $u_y=y\varepsilon_{11}$, where $\varepsilon_{11}\neq 0$, whereas the other five components are identically zero. Similar boundary conditions are applied for the uniaxial tensile loading in the x-direction and the shear loading in the x-direction. As a result, we obtain the stress distribution within the FE model under these boundary displacements. The stresses can be volume or surface averaged in order to obtain the overall stress vector of the RVE.[32] Thus by performing two uniaxial tensile tests with FE models, we can get three independent equations from Eq. (11.1) to compute the longitudinal elastic constants C_{11}, C_{13}, and C_{33}. Similarly, by performing simple shear tests we can get the shear elastic constant C_{44}. The resultant overall properties of the RVE are tabulated in Table 11.2.

We find that the magnitudes of the moduli significantly depend upon the microstructure and the layer properties. The longitudinal elastic constants for model 2 with scalloped structure are found to be higher when compared with model 1 with planar structure, everything else remaining the same. Remarkably, the shear modulus C_{44} is found to be the same for the two models. These calculations show that the scallops have a tendency to stiffen the DEJ in the longitudinal direction, but not in the shear direction. The anisotropy of the four models are quite similar; however, models 3 and 4 are considerably softer when compared with models 1 and 2 due to the presence of a soft inner enamel and mantle dentin layers. These limited calculations tend to indicate that the anisotropy of the phases alone does not seem to affect the overall properties significantly as seen from the comparison of moduli for models 3 and 4. However, the stresses within the RVE are significantly affected by both the scalloped structure and anisotropy of the phases. Calculations with three-dimensional (3D) models based on realistic micromorphological and mechanical properties are needed to clarify the effects of scalloped structures and anisotropy of the phases on the overall elastic property of the RVE.

The calculations performed with the FE model can also be used to understand how the stresses transfer within the DEJ region. The stress distributions within the DEJ region can point to the potential microscale failure initiation locations and mechanisms. The local stress distribution within the RVE has significant variations depending on the presence of scalloped or planar microstructure and layer anisotropy. In Fig. 11.10, we have plotted the major principal stress distributions within models 1 and 2 under uniaxial tensile loading in the y-direction and simple shear loading in the x-direction. As seen, in the case of model 1 with planar microstructure, the stress distribution is uniform within the RVE under tensile loading, which is in marked contrast to the stress distribution within the RVE of model 2 with scalloped structure. Clearly, the scallops have a major role to play in how the occlusal loading is transmitted as stress within the tooth structure. Such analyses at the local scales have been rarely performed to clarify the role of the DEJ microstructure.[33] To our knowledge, investigations of the effect of these small features at larger scales, such as a whole tooth model, have been rare.

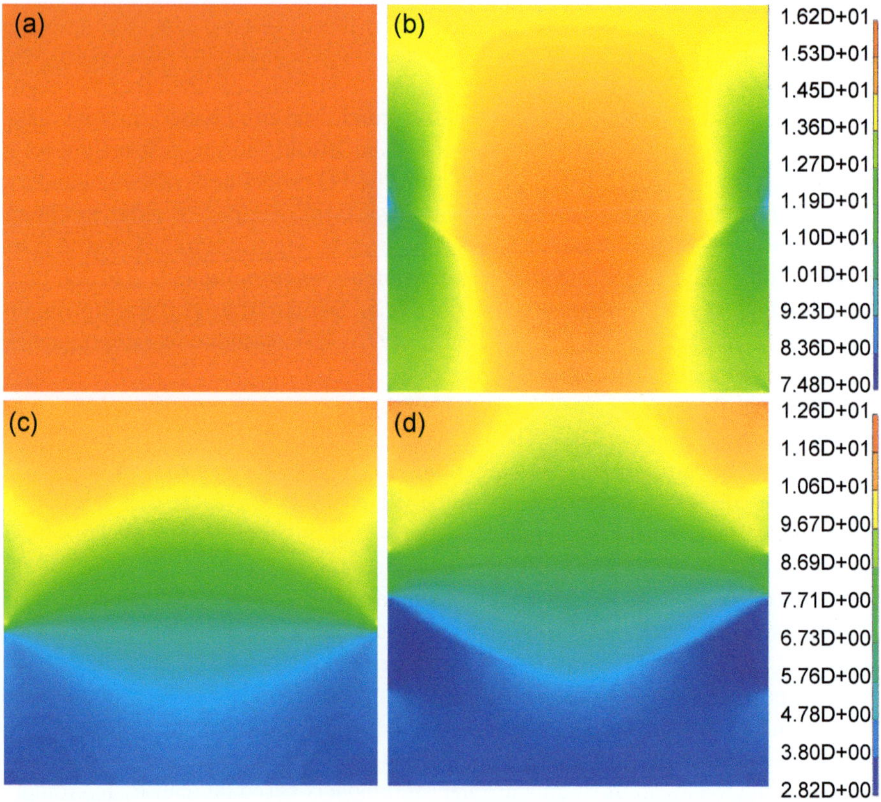

Figure 11.10 Major principal stress distribution in models 1 (a, c) and 2 (b, d) under tensile (a, b) and simple shear (c, d) loading (stress units: megapascals).

11.5 Discussion and conclusion

Although there is a considerable amount of literature devoted to DEJ, there remain significant gaps that impede a complete understanding of the mechanical behavior of the DEJ in function. A systematic multiscale measurement of mechanical behavior and composition using complementary techniques has not been made. High-resolution techniques than can provide information of the 3D structure and mechanical behavior at spatial scales that spans the nano- to micrometer scales do not directly provide material properties. Since the measurement techniques at these scales are imperfect, there is an urgent need for mathematical and computational model that can be used for realistic data interpretation.

At the nano- and microscales, there is a severe lack of reliable computational methods for simulating mechanical behavior including failure and fracture processes in textured or granular materials. Both the traditional continuum approaches for fracture modeling and the discrete approach such as molecular dynamics or discrete element have severe limitations. In the first case, the ability to describe effects of granularity or treatment of nonlinear fracture process with many branched failure zones or pathways is replete with ad hoc assumptions. In the case of discrete approach, the artifacts associated with simulating quasistatic process with dynamic methods by mass scaling or specification of pseudodamping coefficients to control numerical calculations; the specification of local interaction laws between coarse-grained particles; the assumption of highly idealized, many times, unrealistic microstructure; and the sheer computational expense associated with performing parametric studies with these models make the method highly unattractive. Many attempts have been made at multiscale modeling in the past two decades; however, methods that connect different scales have to rely on microstructure descriptions that may not be readily available. Moreover, multiscale simulations of macroscale mechanical behavior are not feasible for materials that are suffused with complex structures and interfaces. Appropriate continuum models are needed that can greatly reduce the computational needs and provide accurate simulations. In summary, the identification of strategic elements that mitigate damage and crack propagation and provide a durable bridge between brittle and ductile materials as in the DEJ can benefit from further systematic and comprehensive investigations that combine experimental analysis and mathematical modeling.

References

1. White SN, Paine ML, Luo W, Sarikaya M, Fong H, Yu Z, et al. Dentino-enamel junction is a broad transitional zone uniting dissimilar bioceramic composites. *J Am Ceram Soc* 2000;**83**(1):238–40.
2. Goldberg M, Septier D, Bourd K, Hall R, Jeanny JC, Jonet L, et al. The dentino-enamel junction revisited. *Connect Tissue Res* 2002;**43**(2–3):482–9.
3. Marshall Jr GW, Balooch M, Gallagher RR, Gansky SA, Marshall SJ. Mechanical properties of the dentinoenamel junction: AFM studies of nanohardness, elastic modulus, and fracture. *J Biomed Mater Res* 2001;**54**:87–95.

4. Marshall SJ, Balooch M, Habelitz S, Balooch G, Gallagher R, Marshall GW. The dentin-enamel junction - a natural, multilevel interface. *J Eur Ceram Soc* 2003;**23**(15):2897–904.
5. Imbeni V, Kruzic JJ, Marshall GW, Marshall SJ, Ritchie RO. The dentin-enamel junction and the fracture of human teeth. *Nat Mater* 2005;**4**(3):229–32.
6. Chai H, Lee JJ, Constantino PJ, Lucas PW, Lawn BR. Remarkable resilience of teeth. *Proc Natl Acad Sci USA* 2009;**106**(18):7289–93.
7. Dong XD, Ruse ND. Fatigue crack propagation path across the dentinoenamel junction complex in human teeth. *J Biomed Mater Res A* 2003;**66**(1):103–9.
8. Lin CP, Douglas WH. Structure-property relations and crack resistance at the bovine dentin-enamel junction. *J Dent Res* 1994;**73**(5):1072–8.
9. Rasmussen ST. Fracture properties of human teeth in proximity to the dentinoenamel junction. *J Dent Res* 1984;**63**(11):1279–83.
10. Zaslansky P, Friesem AA, Weiner S. Structure and mechanical properties of the soft zone separating bulk dentin and enamel in crowns of human teeth: insight into tooth function. *J Struct Biol* 2006;**153**(2):188–99.
11. Shimizu D, Macho GA. Functional significance of the microstructural detail of the primate dentino-enamel junction: a possible example of exaptation. *J Hum Evol* 2007;**52**(1):103–11.
12. Hayashi Y. High resolution electron microscopy in the dentino-enamel junction. *J Electron Microsc* 1992;**41**(5):387–91.
13. Whittaker DK. The enamel–dentine junction of human and *Macaca irus* teeth: a light and electron microscopic study. *J Anat* 1978;**125**(Pt 2):323–35.
14. Kodaka T, Kuroiwa M, Abe M. Fine structure of the inner enamel in human permanent teeth. *Scanning Microsc* 1990;**4**(4):975–85.
15. Lin CP, Douglas WH, Erlandsen SL. Scanning electron microscopy of type I collagen at the dentin-enamel junction of human teeth. *J Histochem Cytochem* 1993;**41**(3):381–8.
16. Gallagher RR, Demos SG, Balooch M, Marshall Jr GW, Marshall SJ. Optical spectroscopy and imaging of the dentin-enamel junction in human third molars. *J Biomed Mater Res A* 2003;**64**(2):372–7.
17. Fong H, Sarikaya M, White SN, Snead ML. Nano-mechanical properties across dentin-enamel junction of adult human incisors. *Mat Res Soc Symp Proc* 2000;**599**:85–90.
18. Balooch G, Marshall GW, Marshall SJ, Warren OL, Asif SA, Balooch M. Evaluation of a new modulus mapping technique to investigate microstructural features of human teeth. *J Biomech* 2004;**37**(8):1223–32.
19. Chan Y, Ngan A, King N. Nano-scale structure and mechanical properties of the human dentine–enamel junction. *J Mech Behav Biomed Mater* 2011;**4**(5):785–95.
20. NSF. *Simulation-based engineering science, revolutionizing engineering science through simulation.* National Science Foundation Blue Ribbon Panel Report. 2006.
21. Tomes CS. *A manual of dental anatomy*. London: Churchill; 1898.
22. Doukoudakis S, Kranias N, Spanou M, Stavridakis M. Morphologic characteristics of dentin at the dentinoenamel junction as viewed by scanning electron microscopy. *J Esthet Dent* 1997;**9**(2):94–9.
23. Kodaka T, Debari K, Kuroiwa M. Mineral content of the innermost enamel in erupted human teeth. *J Electron Microsc* 1991;**40**(1):19–23.
24. Tesch W, Eidelman N, Roschger P, Goldenberg F, Klaushofer K, Fratzl P. Graded microstructure and mechanical properties of human crown dentin. *Calcif Tissues Int* 2001;**69**(3):147–57.
25. Marangos O, Misra A, Spencer P, Bohaty B, Katz JL. Physico-mechanical properties determination using microscale homotopic measurements: application to sound and caries-affected primary tooth dentin. *Acta Biomater* 2009;**5**(4):1338–48.

26. Marangos O, Misra A, Spencer P, Katz JL. Scanning acoustic microscopy investigation of frequency-dependent reflectance of acid-etched human dentin using homotopic measurements. *IEEE Trans Ultrason Ferroelectr Freq Control* 2011;**58**(3):585–95.
27. Misra A, Marangos O, Parthasarathy R, Spencer P. Micro-scale analysis of compositional and mechanical properties of dentin using homotopic measurements. *Biomed Imagine Comput Model Biomech* 2013;**4**:131–41.
28. Briggs GAD. *Acoustic microscopy*. Oxford: Clarendon Press; 1992.
29. Ten Cate AR. *Oral histology*. St. Louis: Mosby; 1994. p. 174.
30. Khuri-Yakub B, Chou C. *Acoustic microscope lenses with shear wave transducers*. IEEE; 1986. p. 741–4.
31. Miyasaka K, Nakabayashi N. Combination of EDTA conditioner and phenyl-P/HEMA self-etching primer for bonding to dentin. *Dent Mater* 1999;**15**:153–7.
32. Tittmann BR, Miyasaka C, Maev RG. Technique of visualization of anisotropy of biomedical tissue by shear wave acoustics elastography. *IEEE Ultrason Symp Abstr* 2007:579.
33. Raum K, Brien W. Pulse-echo field distribution measurement technique for high-frequency ultrasound sources. Ultrasonics, ferroelectrics, and frequency control. *IEEE Trans* 1997;**44**(4):810–5.

Chimeric biomolecules: biomolecular recognition–based self-organization at the bio-material interfaces

12

E. Yuca[1,2], F.S. Utku[3], P. Spencer[1], C. Tamerler[1]
[1]University of Kansas, Lawrence, KS, United States; [2]Yildiz Technical University, Istanbul, Turkey; [3]Yeditepe University, Istanbul, Turkey

12.1 Introduction

Molecular recognition plays a critical role in biological interactions. Hierarchical composite structures are a result of molecular recognition in which biomolecules, mainly proteins, play a crucial role. In Nature, biomolecules control nucleation, growth, and assembly of biological tissues at nano-, meso-, and macroscales. The peptide-based molecular recognition is the key to our approach in generating self-assembling interfaces and controlling interactions with the surrounding environment (Tamerler et al., 2010; Sarikaya et al., 2003).

Proteins play a critical role in maintaining the specific interactions in the organism; formation of controlled structures at all scales in the system depends on biomolecule–material interactions (Sarikaya et al., 2003, 2004; Tamerler et al., 2007, 2010; Lowenstam and Weiner, 1989; Meyers et al., 2009; Berman et al., 1988; Paine and Snead, 1997). During the past decade, several innovative surface engineering approaches, which are based on our understanding of the complex hierarchical design and diverse functionality of bone and dental tissues, have been developed (Fratzl and Weinkamer, 2007; Aizenberg et al., 2005; Sarikaya et al., 2003). The surface engineering approaches include various deposition-based methods, eg, mineral coatings (Narayanan et al., 2007; Zhang et al., 2009; Leeuwenburgh et al., 2006; Shirkhanzadeh, 1998; Munch et al., 2008; Deville et al., 2006a; Lowenstam, 1981; Addadi and Weiner, 1992; Niemeyer, 2001; Woesz et al., 2006; Gungormus et al., 2012; Utku et al., 2008). Among these approaches, solid-binding peptides, ie, peptides that have affinity and selectivity for the inorganic surfaces, have attracted increasing interest. These solid-binding peptides offer the potential of predictable and controlled interactions at the bio-material interfaces. Solid-binding peptides have been identified using combinatorial biology–based approaches, ie, phage and cell surface display techniques (Sarikaya et al., 2003, 2004; Kriplani and Kay, 2005; Sarikaya, 1999; Sarikaya and Tamerler, 2009; Naik et al., 2002a; Thai et al., 2004; Sano et al., 2005; Gungormus et al., 2008; Whaley et al., 2000).

Material-Tissue Interfacial Phenomena. http://dx.doi.org/10.1016/B978-0-08-100330-5.00012-1

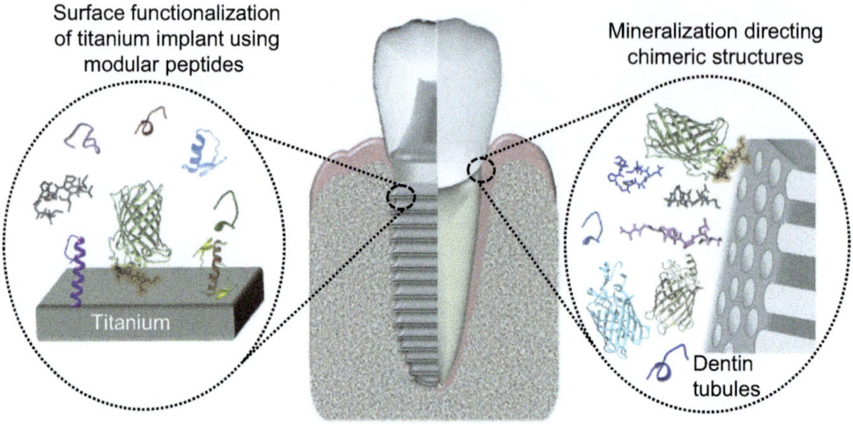

Figure 12.1 Schematic representation of solid-binding peptide–based biomimetic approach. Engineered peptides can be exploited in association with various peptide or protein fusion partners to build multifunctional units to control and monitor the interactions at the bio-material interfaces.

With the modularity of the peptides, our group has focused on designing chimeric molecular constructs that contain both inorganic substrate-binding ability and additional functionalities, eg, bioactive or nonfouling properties and integration into existing proteins and enzyme constructs (Khatayevich et al., 2010; Yuca et al., 2011; Hnilova et al., 2012b; Yucesoy et al., 2015a; Yazici et al., 2013). These multifunctional units may be fine-tuned for a variety of directed self-assembly applications. Binding kinetics and thermodynamic parameters drive the fine-tuning of these multifunctional units. Such fine-tuning allows us to engineer the competitive binding ability of the solid-binding peptides over a wide range of biomolecular interactions toward creating a functional molecular interface (Tamerler et al., 2006; Seker et al., 2009; Evans et al., 2008; Yazici et al., 2013; Khatayevich et al., 2010; Shiba, 2010). Exploitation of solid-binding peptides with various peptide or protein fusion partners allows us to build multifunctional units that potentially lead to controlled interactions at the bio-material interfaces. The focus of this chapter is the design and development of these bioenabled peptide-based interactions. Several examples will be used to illustrate the bioenabled peptide-based interactions. The examples include applications for disease prevention, control or restoration of oral tissues, and biofunctionalization of dental implants (Fig. 12.1).

12.2 Controlled hierarchical interface of mineralized hard tissues

Biomineralization is the process by which organisms produce minerals with controlled hierarchical structures; the hierarchical organization leads to superior properties when compared with synthetic materials with similar phase compositions (Lowenstam, 1981; Addadi and Weiner, 1985). Deposition of minerals in living organisms leads to the formation of hard tissues such as bone and teeth, with hydroxyapatite (HA) as the principal mineral of these hard tissues. Differences in the organization of the HA crystals provide bone and teeth with unique mechanical properties (Fong et al., 2003).

Bone, a product of vertebrate biomineralization, is a hierarchically structured, graded composite material of high complexity (Reznikov et al., 2014; Weiner and Wagner, 1998; Fratzl et al., 2004). Bone consists of type I collagen, extracellular matrix (ECM) proteins and molecules, glycoaminoglycans, and noncollagenous proteins, carbonated HA, and water (Weiner and Traub, 1986; Cowin, 1999; Nomura et al., 1977; Robinson, 1952; Utku et al., 2008). Modeling of bone as a hierarchically organized material involves the complexity of a nine-level scheme (Reznikov et al., 2014). The collagen fibrils are organized in an ordered phase, with the mineralized collagen fibril oriented as unidirectional, limited alignment and fanning arrays, and in a disordered phase. The ground mass, which possibly consists of proteoglycans, exists as thin or extensive layers of nonoriented mineralized fibrils between the ordered collagen fibril arrays, filling the spaces between them and forming the osteocyte lacunae and canaliculi (Reznikov et al., 2014).

The complexity of mineralized hard tissues has made the development of hybrid materials with controlled structures and functions all the more interesting, yet difficult (Boonekamp et al., 1986; Kasaj et al., 2008; Lowenstam, 1981; Addadi and Weiner, 1985; Brown et al., 2000). A case in point is the bone-embedded titanium implants that are used in oral implantology and restorative dentistry. The use of these implants has brought about a fundamental change in oral health care, making commercially pure (cp) titanium (Ti) and Ti alloys good replacements for the roots of teeth.

Titanium implant materials that are used in orthopedic and dental applications provide the strength and toughness required of a load-bearing material. Ti alloys and cpTi, as inert materials with high toughness and strength, excellent corrosion resistance, low density, and elastic modulus (Geetha et al., 2009; Liu et al., 2004; Kokubo et al., 2004), have significant superiority over other metals and thus are widely used in hard tissue implants. The cpTi implants are available in four different grades, which vary based on the amount of interstitial elements such N, C, H, Fe, and O in the Ti lattice and, hence, in the mechanical strength of the Ti unit structure (Boyer et al., 1994). Grade 4 cpTi, which is commonly used in oral implantology, exhibits the highest mechanical strength (~550 MPa tensile strength, ~250 MPa Vickers hardness) compared with Grade 1 cpTi, which has the lowest yield strength (240 MPa tensile strength, ~120 MPa Vickers hardness), yet better formability (Boyer et al., 1994).

12.3 Functional integration of titanium-based implant materials

Despite the favorable aspects, the integration of titanium-based synthetic implant materials with bone needs improvement. In traditional materials science and engineering, metallic materials are produced using conventional methods, such as melting and solidification, thermomechanical treatments, solution/vacuum deposition, and crystal growth. Due to the differences in mechanical properties between the metal-based implant and the host tissue, the full, functional integration of implants has been a critical constraint in the design of implants with optimal osseointegrative properties (Maia et al., 2013; Cranford et al., 2013; Saiz et al., 2013; Dalby et al., 2007; Deville et al., 2006b).

The medical-grade cpTi and its alloys have been modified with a focus on the improvement of metal surface biocompatibility and long-term stability (Hanawa, 2009; Variola et al., 2011; Long and Rack, 1998). The modification of surface topography and chemistry, ie, roughening by means of grinding, micro-machining, sand/grit blasting, rough polishing, etching, or some combination thereof to a root mean square micrometer to nanometer roughness, has generally resulted in surfaces that are more favorable for cell adhesion and enhanced bioactivity (Le Guéhennec et al., 2007; Hanawa, 2009; Variola et al., 2011; Bagno and Di Bello, 2004; Sarikaya et al., 2004). Methods for the modification of chemical and phase composition and nanoscale features, ranging from physical deposition, sputtering of thin films, ion deposition, thermochemical surface treatments, porous surface generation, ceramic coating, atmospheric plasma and vacuum plasma spraying of Ca-P and TiO_2 coatings, and biological modifications, have been used to improve functional properties. These functional properties play decisive roles in molecular interactions, cellular response, bone regeneration, and osseointegration of the titanium-based implant materials (Bagno and Di Bello, 2004; Geetha et al., 2009; Fukumoto et al., 1999; Alves et al., 2005; Stojanovic et al., 2007; Yazici et al., 2013).

Chemical surface modification of titanium not only alters the surface roughness and composition but also enhances the wettability of the implant (Bagno and Di Bello, 2004). The major chemical methods used are hydrogen peroxide treatment, sol–gel treatment, chemical vapor deposition, acidic or alkaline treatment, and anodization. Treatment with strong acids is a routine process and removes the surface oxide and cleans and polishes the implant surface, giving a uniform roughness of 0.5–2 μm, while increasing the surface area and producing a macroporous surface (Luo et al., 2015; Kulkarni et al., 2015; Orsini et al., 2000). The extent of polishing is determined by the acid concentration, temperature, and treatment time. During the acid treatment, titanium is oxidized to a bivalent state; on the titania surface, oxygen ions are generated, which react with the Ti^{+2} cations to give TiO_2 (Kokubo et al., 2004; Le Guéhennec et al., 2007). In addition to acid etching, dual-acid polishing can be employed, using different mixtures of acids, eg, concentrated HNO_3 and HF or concentrated HCl and H_2SO_4, heated above 100°C (Le Guéhennec et al., 2007; Kulkarni et al., 2015; MacDonald et al., 2004). The dual-acid etching method has been shown to enhance several properties including the attachment of fibrin and osteogenic cells, production of ECM and direct bone formation on the implant surface (Orsini et al., 2000), adhesion of platelets, colonization of osteoblasts, and osseointegration with less bone resorption (Cochran et al., 1998; Trisi et al., 2002; Buser et al., 2004). The alkaline treatment with sodium or potassium hydroxide proceeding the acidic treatment leads to the formation of a bioactive, rough TiO_2 surface layer, increasing biocompatibility (Oh et al., 2005).

As a result of acidic or alkaline anodization of the titanium implant surface connected to the anode of an electrochemical cell, an oxide film is formed; this change in the

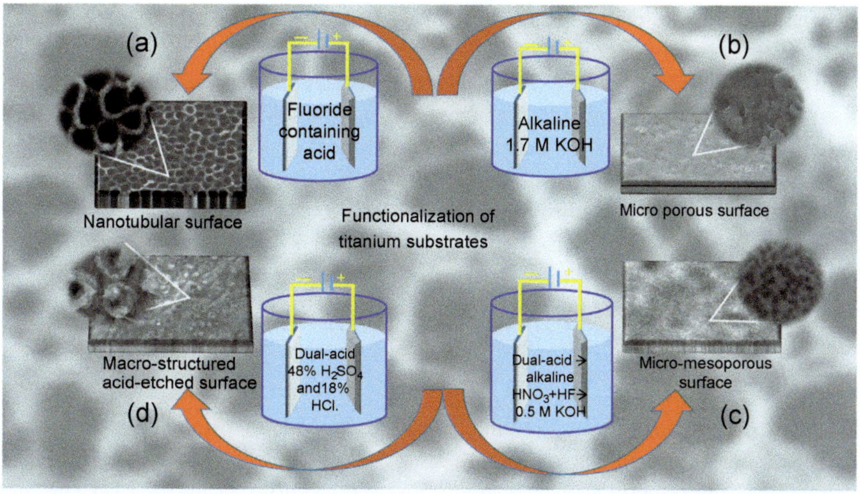

Figure 12.2 Electrochemical functionalization of titanium substrates: Surface functionalization using (a) fluoride-containing ethylene glycol, forming nanotubular structures; (b) alkaline solution, forming microporous surface; (c) dual-acid solution followed by alkaline solution, forming macro-mesoporous surface: and (d) dual-acid solution, forming macrostructured, acid-etched surface.

titanium implant surface leads to improved cellular adhesion and bonding (Fig. 12.2). The oxide layer thickness can be modulated by altering the electrochemical process parameters, such as current density, electrolyte solution concentration, composition, and temperature (Luo et al., 2015; Kulkarni et al., 2015; Orsini et al., 2000; Schliephake et al., 2009). In addition to the non–fluoride-containing electrolytes, ie, alkaline treatment with sodium or potassium hydroxide, anodization can be conducted using fluoride-containing electrolytes. In this case, the TiO_2 layer formed by the concurrent reactions taking place at various interfaces of titania reacts with fluoride ions to form soluble titanium fluorides. Nanotubular titania surfaces, produced by anodization in fluoride-containing electrolytes, provide a canaliculi-like tubular site for osteoblastic anchorage, associated with an advanced stage of cellular development (Fig. 12.2) (Chehroudi et al., 1992; Kunze et al., 2008; Kulkarni et al., 2015; Park et al., 2007). However, the bonding strength of titania nanotubes to the titanium base, may pose a risk in biomedical use, and thus can be improved by annealing at high temperature (Kar et al., 2006; Narayanan et al., 2008). Titania surfaces that can dissipate the bonding stress, ie, macro-mesoporous surfaces with a higher bonding strength may also be used (Fig. 12.2) (Narayanan et al., 2008; Jiang et al., 2013; Utku et al., 2014). Biomimetic replicas of biological materials with controlled and arranged surface porosity (Wegst et al., 2014), from the macroscale of Ti metal, down to the micronanoporous metal oxide level interdigitating with the bone tissue, further down to the nanocrystalline bioactive mineral layer enabling bone regeneration by the bone-forming cells of the body, have been developed (Jiang et al., 2013). The macro-mesoporous oxide layer with wider and nonuniformly shaped micron to submicron macroporosity, ranging between 0.050 and 1.0 μm in size, and inhomogeneously distributed mesopores, below 0.050 μm in size, within the macroporosity have been formed (Utku et al., 2015a; Jiang et al., 2013). Production of a hierarchically organized macro-mesoporosity with increased osteoblastic colonization and osseointegration (Le Guéhennec et al., 2007; Jiang et al., 2013) may thus overcome the mechanical concerns related to interfacial interactions at the implant–host level (Fratzl and Weinkamer, 2007; Aizenberg et al., 2005; Tamerler and Sarikaya, 2009a).

12.4 Osteointegration of biofunctionalized implant materials

The biological performance of titanium-based dental and orthopedic implants is evaluated by their osseointegration with host tissues through a functional interface; the functional interface is a result of the optimal conditions of implant surface morphology, composition, chemistry, topography, and roughness, without an intervening connective tissue (Albrektsson et al., 1983; Branemark, 1983; Zhou et al., 2015). With adequate mechanical interlocking between the implant and bone, the bone tissue grows into the surface porosity (Hulbert et al., 1973) of the roughened surfaces (Chehroudi et al., 1992; Kunze et al., 2008; Tomsia et al., 2011; Deporter, 2009), forming complex three-dimensional geometries confined to intact interfacial layers. This mechanical interlocking offers promise in terms of long-term mechanical stability and in vivo performance.

Comparing the mechanical properties of biological hard tissues with those of Ti implants, it is readily apparent that the mineral–protein composites, produced by organisms as controlled complex hierarchical structures at scales from nanometer and upward, display superior properties compared with the synthetic materials (Lowenstam, 1981; Addadi and Weiner, 1985). The mineral–protein composites of native structures are dynamic, complex, multifunctional, and self-healing hard tissues produced through the deposition of minerals on the splendid organic designs created by macromolecules. The mechanical properties of hard tissues are attained not only by the inclusion of minerals within the proteins, thus increasing both compressive and impact strength (Pokroy et al., 2009, 2006, 2004), but also by the generation of porosities and interfaces that sustain loads and prevent or deflect crack propagation.

The interface between the mineral-coated implant and the dental tissue requires the recruitment of desired cells, cell-to-cell communication at the interface of the surface and the biological host (Kitaori et al., 2009; Omar et al., 2010), as well as nanoscale in vivo biological effects, such as bonding on the atomic scale between the oxide and apatite nanocrystals (Palmquist et al., 2010). The mechanical compatibility between the tissue and implant surface has been explained by anisotropic stresses developed by cells (Bettinger et al., 2009), where surfaces with lower stiffness may promote cellular attachment due to higher compatibility in modulus between the substrate surface and the ECM (Discher et al., 2005; Bao and Suresh, 2003). Mammalian cells of various phenotypes and cell adhesion receptors (Yeung et al., 2005) display different cell morphologies and migration patterns (Lo et al., 2000) based on the wettability, roughness (Boyan et al., 2001), and stiffness of the substrate (Yeung et al., 2005). Therefore, studies have been conducted on the control of implant surface properties at the microscale (Frenkel et al., 2002; Jayaraman et al., 2004), and various molecular processes leading to adhesion and tissue integration of the implant materials at the nanoscale (Tomsia et al., 2011; Park et al., 2007; Variola et al., 2011).

12.5 Solid-binding peptides as molecular building blocks to control specific interactions at the materials interfaces

The growing complexity of mineralized hard tissues and the interfaces has brought about the challenge of developing hybrid materials with controlled structures and functions for biotechnology and medicine. One of the methods used by scientists, who undertake this challenge, is to use the traditional biomimetic approach, ie, to observe and imitate the biological mechanisms, to be inspired from nature, and thus design useful materials and systems generally using synthetic components and conventional methods (Mann, 1993; Seeman and Belcher, 2002). In addition to traditional biomimetics aspects emulating or duplicating biosystems, engineering of materials at the molecular level has been possible using the molecular biomimetics approach. Molecular biomimetics is a promising route for material assembly, fabrication, and application of technologically exquisite materials based on advances in molecular biology, molecular engineering, and physical sciences (Sarikaya, 1999; Sarikaya et al., 2003; Seeman and Belcher, 2002; Tamerler et al., 2010; Tamerler and Sarikaya, 2009a). Using molecular biomimetics, peptides can be selected and engineered to molecularly recognize the specific inorganic surface (Mayer and Sarikaya, 2002; Fong et al., 2003; Sarikaya et al., 2003, 2004; Tamerler, 2011; Tamerler and Sarikaya, 2009b). The potential use of peptides has been increasingly demonstrated in various scientific disciplines including surface functionalization (Sarikaya et al., 2003; Shiba, 2010; Khatayevich et al., 2010; Tamerler et al., 2010; Meyers et al., 2009), biomineralization (Gungormus et al., 2008; Sano et al., 2005), tissue engineering (Tamerler et al., 2010), and regenerative medicine (Kretsinger et al., 2005; Kashiwagi et al., 2009). The specificity and the recognition functions of genetically engineered peptide–based and protein-based materials have thus been exploited as building blocks in nanotechnology to generate bi-/multifunctional molecular structures and devices and for fabrication of novel practical systems (Woodbury et al., 1998; Brown, 2001; Sarikaya, 1999; Kacar et al., 2009a; Sarikaya et al., 2003, 2004; Tamerler and Sarikaya, 2009a).

Proteins participating in biomineralization influence nucleation, crystallography, polymorphism, and morphology of biogenic inorganics (Addadi and Weiner, 1985; Sarikaya, 1999; Mann, 1996). These proteins have been used in the design and engineering of functional materials using the biomimetic approach. Following the isolation, purification, and cloning steps (Cariolou and Morse, 1988; Glimcher and Nimni, 1992; Paine et al., 2003; Liou et al., 2000), biomineralizing peptides can be used in the synthesis of certain inorganics (Berman et al., 1988; Belcher et al., 1996; Cha et al., 1999). Hard tissues usually contain many proteins with a complex spatial and temporal distribution. The extraction and purification of these proteins can be difficult. Therefore, the combinatorial selection of peptides through display techniques is efficient for the selection of peptides that specifically bind to inorganic surfaces (Brown et al., 2000; Sarikaya et al., 2003). To overcome the clinical constraints of nonbiological conditions with demonstrated loss of biological activity (Cranford et al., 2013; Castner and Ratner, 2002; Tomsia et al., 2011), peptide- and protein-based chimeric structures have been constructed to provide bioinspired interfaces to implant surfaces (Evans et al., 2008; Huang et al., 2005; Levy and Onuchic, 2006; Wen et al., 2011). These peptide- and protein-based chimeric structures provide both molecular recognition and self-assembly and the ability to direct cell differentiation by inducing osteogenesis.

The utilization of combinatorial screening techniques has led to the development of a large number of novel peptides that can specifically bind to solid substrate with demonstrated binding kinetics and surface stability (Tamerler et al., 2003, 2010). Peptide sequences that are specific to a myriad of inorganic materials have been identified. The materials include noble metals, eg, gold (Brown et al., 2000; Hnilova et al., 2008; Huang et al., 2005), silver (Naik et al., 2002b; Nam et al., 2008; Hnilova et al., 2012b), and platinum (Seker et al., 2007a); oxides, eg, SiO_2 (Oren et al., 2007; Tamerler et al., 2007), ZnO (Thai et al., 2004), Cu_2O (Thai et al., 2004), and TiO_2 (Yazici et al., 2013; Dickerson et al., 2008; Sano et al., 2005; Sano and Shiba, 2003); minerals, eg, HA (Gungormus et al., 2008; Roy et al., 2008), calcite (Gaskin et al., 2000), and sapphire (Krauland et al., 2007); semiconductors, eg, GaAs (Whaley et al., 2000), ZnS, and CdS (Lee et al., 2002); as well as polymers (Sanghvi et al., 2005).

Polypeptide sequences that specifically bind to inorganics with unique physical properties are determined using the combinatorial selection protocols (Fig. 12.3). The oligonucleotides encoding random sequences of amino acids are inserted into phage genomes or into bacterial plasmids for the generation of phage and cell surface display libraries. The randomized amino acid sequences, which are incorporated with proteins, such as the coat protein of the phage or the outer membrane or flagellar protein of a bacterium, are expressed on the surface of the organism, eventually leading to the production of a different and random peptide by each organism (Brown et al., 2000; Whaley et al., 2000). The mixture of recombinant cells or phages is exposed to the target solid surface. Following the washing cycles to eliminate nonbinding phages or cells, the binders are eluted from the material surface. After this step, phages and cells are amplified and a round of biopanning is completed. To obtain strong binders, three to five rounds are repeated. After the biopanning rounds, clones carrying the peptides binding to the inorganic material are sequenced to obtain the DNA sequences (Tamerler and Sarikaya, 2008).

The binding characteristics of solid binders can be tested by microscopic or spectroscopic analyses such as fluorescence microscopy (FM), surface plasmon resonance spectroscopy, and quartz crystal microbalance (QCM). These techniques are used to determine the specificity and kinetics of the molecular binding of peptides to surfaces (Tamerler et al., 2006, 2007; Seker et al., 2007a,b). In addition to these methods, (Bailey et al., 2002), for the shorter peptide sequences, circular dichroism and nuclear magnetic resonance (NMR) spectroscopy is used (Kulp et al., 2004). Computational modeling

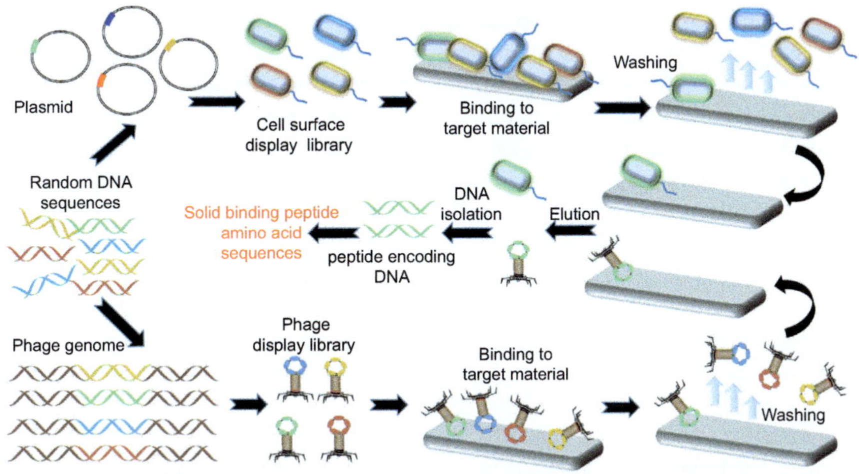

Figure 12.3 Combinaotorial biology–based display technologies: Phage display and cell surface display protocols adapted for selecting solid-binding peptides with binding affinity to a given inorganic surface.

is also applicable for molecular characterization to understand the conformation and mechanism of crystallographic surface recognition in the absence of the structural experimental data (Barth et al., 2005; Tomasio and Walsh, 2007; Oren et al., 2007). Supramolecular self-assembly and surface coverage of solid-binding peptides are visualized by atomic force microscopy giving quantitative data and nanostructural images (Tamerler and Sarikaya, 2007). Although the use of peptides as a technique for surface functionalization has become common (Hnilova et al., 2008; Kacar et al., 2009b), there is limited mechanistic understanding of molecular assembly, organization, and binding to solids (Evans, 2008; Sarikaya, 1999; Tamerler et al., 2010). Data obtained from techniques such as NMR spectroscopy (Kulp et al., 2004), computational modeling (Oren et al., 2007; Tomasio and Walsh, 2007), and experiments with geometrically constrained peptides (Dai et al., 2005) have led to some hypotheses regarding the mechanisms, eg, the secondary structures of the engineered peptides in solution can play an important role in their solid binding and selectivity (Wei et al., 2009).

12.6 Biofunctionalization of titanium dental implants materials using solid-binding peptides

Immobilization of bioactive molecules, such as ECM proteins or native matrix protein–derived peptides, on implant surfaces has been investigated as a means of controlling cell response on the implant surface. Immobilization of peptide on Ti surfaces using silane chemistry has been studied (Ruoslahti, 1996; Xiao et al., 1997). Fibronectin-derived peptide fragments, ie, Arg–Gly–Asp (RGD) and the Arg–Gly–Asp–Cys (RGDC) peptides, covalently attached to the Ti surface using 3-aminopropyltriethoxylsilane and *N*-succinimidyl-3-maleimidopropionate (Xiao et al., 1997; Morra, 2006) have been used widely, owing to the stimulation of cell adhesion through the activation of integrin receptors. These methods provide advanced biocompatibility to Ti implant surfaces. There are concerns regarding the effect of chemical modifications on the implant surface under physiological conditions (Love et al., 2005; Mrksich and Whitesides, 1996). Using the organic solvent–based chemical process, low coupling efficiencies with bioactive molecules and diminished activity and stability of the bioactive moiety have been observed. Therefore, despite the established biofunctional molecules, eg, RGD, polyethylene glycol (PEG), and bone morphogenetic protein (Bierbaum et al., 2003a,b; Ku et al., 2005; Martin et al., 2007; Darouiche et al., 2007; Balasundaram and Webster, 2007), using silane chemistry, control of inorganic surface properties to induce enhanced interaction at the bio-material interface has been challenging.

The proposed peptide-binding adsorption mechanism relies on the formation of a passivated oxide layer and charged group interactions contributed from amino acid residues. Characterized peptides have hydroxyl-containing residues with high cationic charge and exhibit histidine residues (Naik et al., 2002a; Fang et al., 2008). It seems that the binding affinity is controlled by a complex mechanism, where the amino acid content of the sequence and the net charge correlation properties specify peptide–surface interactions. In a study on Ti-binding peptides (TiBP), TiBP1 and TiBP2 have displayed a similar high affinity, despite their distinctive physicochemical properties, whereas TiBP60 has demonstrated the lowest affinity, despite exhibiting physicochemical properties similar to that of the higher affinity TiBP1 (Yazici et al., 2013). These differences are potentially related to the conformation of the molecular structure of the peptide on the given solid surface; conformation potentially dictates the specific molecular interactions with a surface. Similar relationships are observed in several material-specific polypeptides, which exhibit some degree of intrinsic disorder or unfolded structure (Gungormus et al., 2008; Hnilova et al., 2008; Amos and Evans, 2009; Delak et al., 2008; Evans et al., 2008). Folding tendency (Delak et al., 2009; Evans et al., 2008) is a molecular characteristic of the solid-binding protein sequences (Gungormus et al., 2008; Amos and Evans, 2009). Since TiBP60, TiBP1, and TiBP2 have slightly more compact structures, it can be proposed that the differences in folding may reflect the ability of each disordered TiBP sequence to adapt to Ti surfaces (Gungormus et al., 2008; Hnilova et al., 2008; Amos and Evans, 2009; Delak et al., 2008; Evans et al., 2008; Evans, 2008; Yazici et al., 2013).

Since Ti is the main metal used in dental implantology, several research groups have selected peptides that are specific to Ti/TiOx surfaces, various-sized particles of Ti oxide powders, bulk Ti oxide (anatase), amorphous TiO_2 plasma vapor deposited on a stainless-steel substrate, and even metallic Ti particles with native surface oxide using phage display techniques (Yazici et al., 2013; Sano and Shiba, 2003; Chen et al., 2006; Fang et al., 2008; Vreuls et al., 2010). The contribution of specific residues of TiBP to binding has been investigated by mutating the amino acids within the oligopeptide (Sano and Shiba, 2003). Peptides for Grade 4 cpTi have been selected using a FliTrx cell surface display library and characterized semiquantitatively for affinity to their respective Ti surfaces using FM. Quantitative characterization of peptide binding to the Grade 4 cpTi surface has been assessed using QCM, whereas the molecular conformation properties have been assayed using protein structure interrogation techniques and cytotoxicity was analyzed using osteoblastlike MC3T3-E1 cells (Anselme, 2000; Jaeger et al., 2007).

12.7 Self-organized chimeric peptides toward creating controllable biomaterial interfaces

Controlling the microscale properties of the implant surface, as well as nanoscale recognition, adhesion, and integration at the implant–tissue interface, metal implant surfaces with lower stiffness may promote cell attachment due to higher compatibility of the substrate surface with the modulus of the ECM (Discher et al., 2005; Bao and Suresh, 2003; Yeung et al., 2005). The organic interface that is produced as an integrated hybrid composite layer has potential use in a wide range of orthopedic and dental applications (Dietz et al., 2006). In a comparable application of bifunctional proteins, with the use of self-organized chimeric peptides, the cell-to-implant interactions have been directed by a simple one-step procedure. As an example, the conjugated integrin recognition peptide domain, Arg–Gly–Asp–Ser (RGDS) with TiBP1 and TiBP2, forming the TiBP–RGDS functionalized Grade 4 cpTi surface, ie, conjugating these peptides to integrin recognition peptide sequence RGDS, has resulted in a single molecule when coated on Ti surfaces in a single step, and it has enhanced the bioactivity of RGDS in the presence of preosseoblast and fibroblast cells (Fig. 12.4) (Anselme, 2000; Jaeger et al., 2007).

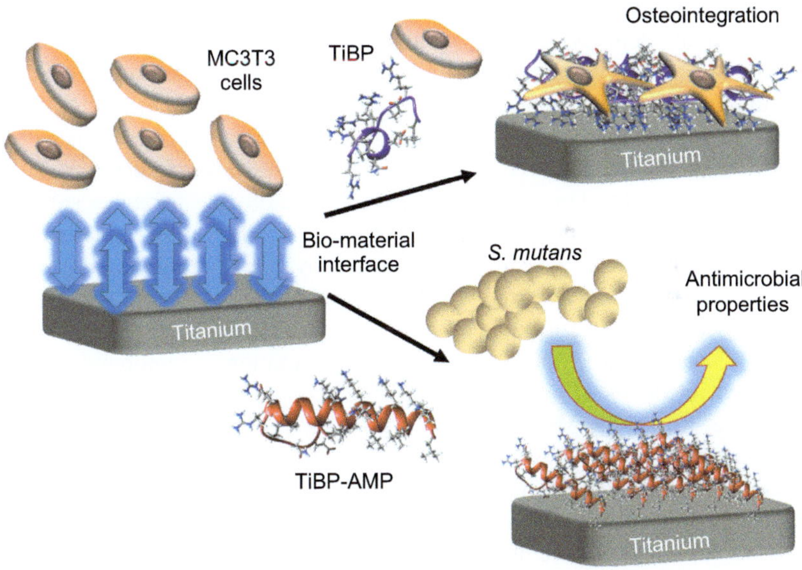

Figure 12.4 Titanium implant material surface is biologically functionalized by either titanium-binding peptides or titanium-binding peptide–based chimeric structures to present controllable interactions at the bio-material interfaces for developing biocompatible and antimicrobial implant materials.

In another example, an engineered peptide, peptide binding implant–bone-inducing protein (PBI-BIP), has been designed to incorporate implant binding as well as osteogenic activity, by guiding human stem cells to osteogenesis at the implant interface using molecular recognition and bioenabled self-assembly, thus avoiding the problems of chemical coupling to the implant interface and the loss of biological activity (Zhou et al., 2015). The chimeric peptide has been constructed from a PBI domain that has been proved to be effective for specific self-adherence onto a Ti/Ti alloy implant surface fused to a BIP that contains a biochemical signal that guides stem cells to differentiate by activating the Wnt signaling pathway for bone formation (Wen et al., 2011). The Wnt-induced cells have displayed enhanced mineral deposition in an ECM of their creation and an enhanced gene expression profile consistent with osteogenesis, thereby providing a bone-to-implant interface that promotes bone regeneration.

The modular peptide design has permitted the incorporation of other moieties for cell adhesion or antimicrobial activity to the PBI, demonstrating the potential for tuning the host cell response through an engineered chimeric molecule. An ideal bone replacement construct is expected to functionally replicate the lost tissue while becoming fully integrated with the host bone (Deville et al., 2006b), simultaneously promoting osteogenesis, antimicrobial function, and bioactivity at the bone–implant interface, and thus improving cell–implant interactions and reducing the recovery period (Wen et al., 2011).

Pathogens can adhere to virtually any surface through their various types of adherins and form a biofilm complex on the implant surface or at its periphery. The biofilm complex creates a barrier that decreases the penetration of antimicrobial agents and reduces the susceptibility of the biofilms members to drug delivery (Costerton et al., 1999; Antoci et al., 2008; Kazemzadeh-Narbat et al., 2010).

The potential toxicity of conventional antibiotics (Hetrick and Schoenfisch, 2006; Rathbone et al., 2011) and the development and spread of antibiotic-resistant pathogens such as the methicillin-resistant *Streptococcus aureus* remain a challenge to hospital-acquired infections (Campoccia et al., 2010; Kazemzadeh-Narbat et al., 2010). To render the implant surfaces nonadhesive and/or to introduce antimicrobial surfaces, PEG and its derivatives (Harbers et al., 2007; Shimotoyodome et al., 2007), coatings of albumin (An et al., 1996), covalently attached conventional antibiotics (Jose et al., 2005; Price et al., 1996; Russell et al., 1998; Wininger and Fass, 1996), chlorhexidine (Harris et al., 2006), silver, nitrogen oxide (Banerjee et al., 2011; Zhao et al., 2009), and quaternary ammonia compounds (Russell et al., 1998; Gottenbos et al., 2002) requiring complex covalent coupling strategies (Love et al., 2005; Mohorcic et al., 2010; Mrksich and Whitesides, 1996) have been used.

The slow release of derivatives of antimicrobial agents from preloaded implant devices may be linked to increased incidences of bacterial resistance and cytotoxicity (Harris et al., 2006). To reduce the number of complications leading to failure due to implant-associated bacterial infections (Uckay et al., 2013), bioactivation of implant surfaces with more biocompatible and nontoxic biomolecules, eg, antimicrobial peptides (AMPs) has emerged as a feasible approach to overcome infection-derived implant failure (Yucesoy et al., 2015a).

The short, cationic AMPs are evolutionary conserved constituents of the innate immune defense systems of organisms (Brogden, 2005; Giuliani et al., 2007; Zasloff, 2002), where the working mechanism of AMP may be to specifically target and disrupt the integrity of the negatively charged cell membrane of microorganisms. Although there is no consensus in the sequence and structure of AMPs, they usually have an amphipathic structure, which leads to an efficient ionic recognition between the cationic residues of peptide and the phospholipids of the bacterial membrane (Pasupuleti et al., 2012; Reddy et al., 2004) with highly sophisticated reaction mechanisms and considerably rapid rate action (Brogden, 2005; Jenssen et al., 2006) against a broad spectrum of gram-positive and gram-negative bacteria, fungi, and viruses. AMPs can work synergistically with conventional antibiotics and facilitate antibiotic penetration to the infection site, thus enabling more aggressive biofilm treatment (Brogden, 2005). It has also been demonstrated that the sequence and/or resulting structure of natural AMPs can be utilized as templates for the design of synthetic variants with enhanced effectiveness in antimicrobial activities (Fjell et al., 2009; Hilpert et al., 2006; Ingham and Moore, 2007), but without the cytotoxic consequences and collateral damage through vascular redistribution (Jiang et al., 2008).

The bifunctional chimeric peptides, composed of an AMP agent and an implant surface–binding peptide (Fig. 12.4), rely on the properties of the solid-binding peptides (Sarikaya et al., 2003) that selectively bind to the titanium surface and freely expose the AMP motif to combat invading bacteria. This interface on the implant surface is constructed by combining combinatorially selected solid-binding peptides and AMP sequences in different combinations through an intervening flexible linker (Appendini and Hotchkiss, 2001; Campoccia et al., 2013; Etienne et al., 2004; Kwakman et al., 2006; Zhou et al., 2015). Their antimicrobial efficacy has been tested either in solution or by immobilizing on the surface against *Streptococcus mutans*, *Streptococcus epidermidis*, and *Escherichia coli,* commonly found in oral implant and orthopedic infections (Campoccia et al., 2006; Socransky and Haffajee, 2002; Costa et al., 2011; Meyers et al., 2009; Yoshinari et al., 2010). The bifunctional chimeric peptides, containing other identified AMP sequences binding to a wide range of biomaterials other than titanium can be created by deploying different solid-binding sequences (Campoccia et al., 2013; Yazici et al., 2013; Yoshinari et al., 2010).

12.8 Calcium phosphate coating of titanium implants to increase biocompatibility

Another common method used to increase the biocompatibility of titanium implants is to coat them with calcium phosphate in the form of tricalcium phosphate (TCP) and/or HA (Heimann et al., 1998; Kurzweg et al., 1998; Bigi et al., 2008; Hanawa et al., 1997; Rautray et al., 2010; Ogawa et al., 2008). HA, being the principal inorganic component of the hard tissues of mammals, is widely utilized in hard tissue repair, replacement, and implant surface coating; as a gene/drug and cell delivery agent (Dash and Cudworth, 1998; Liu et al., 2005; Tan et al., 2007; Ma et al., 2008; Braux et al.,

2009); and as a regulator of cell bioactivity (Oh et al., 2005; Kasaj et al., 2008). Coating the implant surfaces with HA increases implant success, through the provision of biological activity and chemical integration. The microporous topography and surface chemistry of the scaffold renders the bone-forming cells the chemical base to attach, differentiate, and osteointegrate (Narayanan et al., 2008; Lin et al., 2003). The nanometer-sized HA crystals deposited on the microscale substrate have been shown to further contribute to surface topography and mechanics as the key factors in the cellular adhesion and integration of implants, indicating that the metal–tissue interface needs to be dealt with at the molecular scale (Ryu and Nam, 2000; Junker et al., 2009).

Presence of a biologically active oxide layer and a stable crystalline base for Ca-P deposition is of critical importance in shaping the cellular interaction between the host tissue and the implant, enabling transmission of forces and long-term implant success (Kokubo et al., 2004; Narayanan et al., 2008). A firm layer of nanocrystalline HA has been shown to establish approximately twice or three times more rapid response and several-fold increase in interfacial strength compared with uncoated surfaces (Narayanan et al., 2007; Zhang et al., 2009; Leeuwenburgh et al., 2006; Shirkhanzadeh, 1998). Insufficient and inhomogeneous surface coverage of the ceramic layer and the low bonding strength between the coating and the metal often result in cracking and spallation; these deficiencies have limited the broad use of HA-coated implants in clinical settings (Chang et al., 2001; Rakngarm and Mutoh, 2009; Ryu and Nam, 2000). With the aim of producing implants with bonding strength and shear strength higher than that of the human bone (with a bonding strength of ~18 MPa and a shear strength of ~44 MPa), the mechanical properties of HA-deposited implant surfaces have been improved by annealing under argon environment at 450°C (Kar et al., 2006).

HA can be deposited on implants using wet chemistry, high-temperature processes, and electrochemical techniques. Using wet chemistry, dense Ca-P coatings with good biological performance can be produced biomimetically by first immersing the surface to be coated in a fluid consisting of physiological anions and subsequently adding calcium. Using high-temperature processes such as the plasma spray method, producing thick, inhomogeneous coatings; the ion beam method, producing thin coatings; the laser method, producing thin coatings with diverse compositions, crystallinities, and high fatigue strength; radio frequency (RF) sputtering, producing thin, but dense and adhesive coatings; and hot isostatic pressing of uniform Ca-P granules, titanium surfaces can be coated with HA and HA phases (Cook et al., 1991). Ca-P coatings can be deposited on implant surfaces using electrophoresis, where negatively charged Ca-P particles migrate toward the cathode (Smith, 1993), and electrochemical deposition (ECD), where the cations are deposited on the cathodically polarized working electrode, followed by the electrostatic attraction of the anions.

Using the high-temperature processes at values greater than 900°C, biphasic HA containing both TCP and HA are deposited. After implantation, the difference in the solubility of the components of biphasic HA leads to loosening of the implant (Klein et al., 1991). The wet chemistry processes produce Ca-P compounds, which take a longer time to form. The ECD method, on the other hand, is faster and enables Ca-P coating of implant materials of any size and shape by controlling various factors that determine the chemistry of Ca-P coating, eg, current density, length of cathodic and anodic deposition cycles, temperature, and type of solution used (Cook et al., 1991; Kokubo et al., 2004; Angelescu et al., 2011; Narayanan et al., 2008; Shirkhanzadeh, 1998; Leeuwenburgh et al., 2006; Redepenning et al., 1996; Rossler et al., 2003). By modulating the ECD parameters, calcium phosphate compounds, ie, HA, monocalcium phosphate monohydrate, octacalcium phosphate, dicalcium phosphate dihydrate, monocalcium phosphate anhydrous, carboapatite, and dicalcium phosphate anhydrous, can be deposited (Albayrak et al., 2008; Lin et al., 2003; Kokubo et al., 2004). Compound deposition is determined as a function of (1) alkalization at the cathode and conversion of acid phosphates to phosphates in the presence of hydroxide ions or electron donators, determining the type of orthophosphate ion that reacts with calcium, and (2) the diffusion of phosphate ions as the rate-determining step in the deposition of calcium phosphates (Kokubo et al., 2004; Narayanan et al., 2008). The alkalinity of the micro-/nanoenvironment, the ionic strength, surface/diffusion control mechanisms, and temperature, affecting the reaction rates and the kinetics of adsorption and diffusion, govern the chemistry, particle size, and morphology of the Ca-P compound deposited (Nancollas and Wu, 2000; Wang and Nancollas, 2009; Brown and Fulmer, 1991).

HA deposition begins with the alkaline surface treatment, which enables the formation, polymerization, and condensation of sodium titanate and titanium hydroxide groups into negatively charged titanium oxide around pH 7.4 (Branemark, 1983; Hench and Wilson, 1993; Bavykin et al., 2006). These groups then interact with calcium ions to form positively charged amorphous calcium titanate, which reacts with the phosphate ions to form ACP, which then transforms into crystalline HA and grows by incorporation of calcium, phosphate, and hydroxide ions (Cook et al., 1991; Branemark, 1983). The ACP to HA conversion rate is highly temperature dependent, taking only 5 min at 60°C compared with 24 h at 25°C (Brown and Fulmer, 1991).

Crystal morphology and size have been affected by both the substrate type and temperature (Utku et al., 2014), with uniformly distributed crystals of acicular morphology and higher Ca/P ratios on nanotubular titania than on anodized titania, and with displayed temperature-dependent differences in crystal organization, shape, and size. The change in crystal morphology correlates with the change in Ca/P ratios of minerals formed with different monovalent, bivalent, and trivalent cations and anions incorporated into the crystal lattice. The Ca/P ratio of stoichiometric HA being 1.67, in biological HA, both cations and anions may be replaced by various ions, resulting in single or multiple substitutions or cosubstitutions. In the case of HA, Ca^{+2} may be substituted with K^{+}, Na^{+}, Mg^{+2}, Sr^{+2}, Ba^{+2}, Pb^{+2}, La^{+3}, and many rare earth elements; $PO_4{}^{-3}$ may be substituted with $CO_3{}^{-2}$; $VO_4{}^{-3}$, $AsO_4{}^{-3}$, and $SiO_4{}^{-4}$; and OH^{-} may be substituted with Cl^{-}, F^{-}, or $CO_3{}^{-2}$ (Kannan et al., 2008; Elliott, 1994; Brown and Constantz, 1994; Ślósarczyk et al., 2005). Typically, biological and synthetic HA contain carbonate ions, forming carbonated hydroxyapatite, ie, HA with a higher carbonate moiety (Elliott, 1994; Brown and Constantz, 1994; Rehman and Bonfield, 1997). The carbonate substitution may appear as Type A (replacing OH^{-}), Type B (replacing $PO_4{}^{-3}$), or Type AB (replacing both). Calcium-deficient hydroxyapatite (CDHA) may be formed in Type B substitution, where a decrease in anionic charge without a decrease in ionic content may result in cationic and anionic cosubstitutions to neutralize the mineral (Elliott, 1994; Brown and Constantz, 1994).

Micro- and nanofunctionalized surfaces have been electrochemically coated using modified saturated simulated body fluid (SBF) with Ca/P atomic ratios of 1.5, 1.67, and 2.5, at pH ranging from 4 to 7.2 (Kokubo et al., 2004; Shirkhanzadeh, 1998; Leeuwenburgh et al., 2006; Redepenning et al., 1996; Chehroudi et al., 1992; Raja et al., 2005; Oh et al., 2005; Kunze et al., 2008; Wang et al., 2009). Highly crystalline HA and CDHA derivatives are formed at pH above 7.2 and temperature above 60°C, whereas poorly crystalline HA and other Ca-P compounds (Utku et al., 2014) are formed at neutral to acidic pH (≤7.2) and temperature below 60°C. Even at the lower temperature, the nanotubular titania substrate, with a 100 times larger surface area than the unfunctionalized substrate, enables deposition of HA due to the generation and entrapment of hydroxide and phosphate ions formed by reduction of water and electron donation as a direct function of current density (Liu et al., 2001; Shirkhanzadeh, 1998). Despite these favorable aspects, unannealed Ca-P deposits on nanotubular substrates have displayed a lower shear strength than those on anodized surfaces (Utku et al., 2014).

The possibility of fine-tuning the nanotubular composite material under physiological conditions provides additional flexibility to design these scaffolds as potential biomaterials for future biomedical applications. Using a biomimetic HA coating approach that exploits peptides that can bind both to titanium and HA surfaces, the titanium implant surface has been homogeneously coated with HA, without any display of immediate cytotoxicity (Kelly et al., 2015).

12.9 Peptides to tune calcium phosphate recognition and mineralization

The three different layers of mammalian tooth, ie, enamel, dentin, and cementum, have been formed using proteins and peptides that associate with HA as the main constituent and take part in their formation (Lowenstam and Weiner, 1989). A natural exemplary biological material for the protein-based molecular recognition, transition, and control is enamel, the hardest tissue in the body. Consisting of thousands of 30-nm-diameter, micrometer-long HA crystallites, enamel integrates with dentin, the softer adjacent tissue, and protects the underlying dental tissues by absorbing energy during cutting and mastication and preventing premature fracture or failure (Zaslansky et al., 2006). Hierarchically ordered woven structure of mammalian tooth enamel is controlled by more than 40 different proteins that have been known to take part in its formation. The overall architecture, the nano- and microstructural characteristics, and the amount of HA crystallites determine the distinguishing characteristics of dental bioceramics and hard tissues, the enamel, cementum, and dentin.

The tissue-specific ECM proteins found within each of these tissues during its development (Lowenstam and Weiner, 1989; Mann, 2001; Begue-Kirn et al., 1998; Dsouza et al., 1997; Gajjeraman et al., 2007) act as regulators of nucleation and growth of biological apatite (Lowenstam and Weiner, 1989; Mann, 2001; Cölfen and Antonietti, 2008), offering great potential in the repair of mineralized dental tissues damaged due to caries, trauma, or periodontal disease (Taubman et al., 2005; Goldberg et al., 2001). Studies on the effects of these proteins on the biofabrication of dental tissues have contributed to progress in the regeneration or restoration of hard tissues (Fong et al., 2003; Tamerler et al., 2007, 2010).

Amelogenin, expressed during tooth enamel formation, exerts control over the dimension and directionality of HA crystals formed within the assembled protein matrix (Bartlett et al., 2006; Du et al., 2005; Snead et al., 2006). Certain regions of amelogenin amino acid sequence, proposed to interact with calcium phosphate minerals, provide knowledge on the mapping of putative crystal interaction or mineral nucleation domains (Fan et al., 2011; Iijima and Moradian-Oldak, 2004; Delak et al., 2009). Since the use of native or recombinant dental ECM proteins as therapeutic agents to repair damage caused by disease has been limited due to technical challenges in the identification, extraction, and purification of these proteins, research has focused on peptide mimicry or identifying functional domains within these naturally occurring proteins (Capriotti et al., 2007; Goldberg et al., 2001; Gu et al., 2011; Kim et al., 2010; Taller et al., 2007; Wazen et al., 2007; Zhang et al., 2007; Pampena et al., 2004; Tye et al., 2003).

By exploiting small peptide domains of native proteins, the structure–function relationships of proteins in the facilitation of biomineralization can be further investigated, and these peptides can be utilized to engineer mineral formation (Gungormus et al., 2012; Oren et al., 2007). A novel approach for identifying peptide sequences from native proteins has been described to repair dental tissues by controlling HA biomineralization (Gungormus et al., 2012). Amelogenin has been demonstrated to contain similarity regions, ie, domains with similar amino acid sequences, with a set of previously selected HA-binding peptides (HABPs) (Gungormus et al., 2008). The peptide regions function to direct the cell-free remineralization of the tooth root, resulting in a cementomimetic (cementum-like) material, contributing to cell-based regeneration of periodontal tissue in peptide-assisted biomineralization. The mineralized tissue covering the tooth root and anchoring it to the bone, a 22-amino acid long peptide, referred to as amelogenin-derived peptide 5 (ADP5), has been shown to facilitate cell-free formation on demineralized human root dentin of a cementomimetic HA mineral layer. This cementomimetic HA mineral layer supported attachment of periodontal ligament cells in vitro with the potential clinical application to repair diseased root surfaces to promote the regeneration of periodontal tissues (Gungormus et al., 2012).

A biomimetic process using primers containing phosphoprotein analogs for remineralizing mineral depleted resin–dentin interfaces has been applied to acid-etched dentin prior to the use of ion-releasing resin-based system, displaying that this biomimetic approach provides a suitable bonding treatment for remineralization of resin–dentin interface (Sauro et al., 2015). In another study, it has been shown that self-assembled oligopeptide amphiphile can be used for biomimetic mineralization on the enamel surface (Li et al., 2014a). Dentin matrix protein one derived peptides containing collagen-binding domains and calcium-binding domains have also been used for induction of biomimetic mineralization of demineralized enamel (Padovano et al.,

2015). Similarly, combinatorially selected solid-binding peptide-based mineralization approaches can be a potential molecular tool for resin–dentin interface or enamel surface biomineralization.

Binding and molecular structural properties of phage display–selected HABPs have indicated (Gungormus et al., 2008) a high-affinity HA-binding heptapeptide, CMLPHHGAC, with demonstrated mineral-forming capabilities, slowing the rate of initial mineralization, increasing the rate of transformation from amorphous to the crystalline phase, and forming larger particles when compared with weak binder sequences (CNPGFAQAC). The peptide-assisted mineral formation that mimics biomineralization, where the protein control over the formation of biomineral brings new insights into the evolution of protein–mineral interactions, demonstrates that strong binding affinity of a peptide to an inorganic solid is not necessarily an indication of its mineral-forming capability (Gungormus et al., 2008). A 27-residue peptide designed to contain a heptapeptide (MLPHHGA) at the C-terminal has been shown to direct the formation of HA, with the peptide folding and assembling to form a hydrogel network (Gungormus et al., 2010).

12.10 Chimeric genetically fused protein as a modular biomolecular device at the interface: from monitoring to biomolecular mediation of mineral layer

Solid-binding peptides have also been fused to proteins (Dai et al., 2005) and other peptides (Slocik and Naik, 2006; Yucesoy et al., 2015a), conjugated to functional small molecules or attached to quantum dots (Zin et al., 2005, 2007; Ma et al., 2007) to develop molecular building blocks or multifunctional molecular entities for various applications. These applications have included efficient immobilization of enzymes, conjugation of nanoentities, nanoparticle synthesis with controlled size (Kramer et al., 2004; Krauland et al., 2007; Kacar et al., 2009b), selective immobilization of fluorescent proteins (Yokoo et al., 2010), and for direct assembly or the in situ synthesis of other functional inorganic nanostructures (Brown, 2001; Pender et al., 2006; Sano et al., 2006; Slocik and Naik, 2006).

Probes that combine fluorescent properties and molecular recognition have been used to visualize biological events at many levels from molecules to an organism (Finney, 2006; Giepmans et al., 2006). Stability and cofactor-independent chromophore formation makes green fluorescent protein (GFP) suitable for use in living systems (Zimmer, 2002) in the detection of promoter activity, protein localization, motility, and interactions with other proteins in living cells or various cellular parameters in living animals (Hoffman, 2002; Wiedenmann et al., 2009; Chudakov et al., 2005). GFP is also suitable for tracking HA formation, via efficient labeling in biomedical applications, eg, gene/drug delivery and bone and teeth formation/remodeling, and in nanotechnological implementations, eg, nanoparticle composites. The gold standards for in vitro staining (ex vivo labeling) of HA, such as alizarin red S (Lipman, 1935) and von Kossa staining (Meloan and Puchtler, 1985) have been complemented with fluorescent labeling methods, ie, synthesis of HA particles doped with fluorescent ions (De Araujo et al., 2007; Yang et al., 2008) and HA quantum dot composites (Guo et al., 2008; Hsieh et al., 2009) or modification of the HA surface using chemical coupling agents such as bisphosphonates (Zaheer et al., 2001; Zhang et al., 2008).

Various bi-/multifunctional fusion protein construction strategies have been exploited, and a variety of solid-binding peptide–based fusion proteins have been produced. Solid-binding peptides have been fused to functional proteins, such as maltose-binding protein (Hnilova et al., 2012a), a GFP derivative (GFPuv) (Yuca et al., 2011), red fluorescent protein (Zhang et al., 2015), DNA-binding protein (Dai et al., 2005), alkaline phosphatase (Kacar et al., 2009b), L-lactate dehydrogenase (Cetinel et al., 2013) and formate dehydrogenase (Yucesoy et al., 2015b). Solid-binding peptides can be genetically fused to the C- (Yuca et al., 2011) and N-termini (Cetinel et al., 2013) or within the permissive sites of the functional protein (Dai et al., 2005), followed by the cloning of the fusion protein encoding the DNA fragment into an expression plasmid vector system. Following the cloning, fusion proteins are expressed in one of the appropriate host microorganisms such as bacteria and yeast, and then purified using various affinity chromatography techniques (Hnilova et al., 2012b; Yuca et al., 2011; Cetinel et al., 2013).

To produce the bifunctional GFPuv-HABP1 fusion protein, the nucleotide sequence encoding HABP1 was genetically linked to the N-terminus of the open reading frame of GFPuv encoding DNA and the fusion DNA fragment was cloned into pQE1 expression vector encoding N-terminal 6xhistidine-tag. Following expression in *E. coli*, the immobilized metal affinity chromatography technique was applied taking advantage of the 6xhistidine-tag. The excitation and emission wavelengths and fluorescence intensity of the fusion protein GFPuv-HABP1 were compared with a those of the negative control GFPuv, showing that GFPuv-HABP1 and GFPuv proteins have equivalent excitation and emission wavelengths with similar intensities and that HABP1 conserves its HA-binding ability without interfering with the GFPuv fluorescence property (Fig. 12.5) (Yuca et al., 2011).

The genetically engineered fusion protein, that is, GFPuv-HABP, has been demonstrated as a bifunctional molecular probe to label biological tissues or monitor HA mineralization (Yuca et al., 2011; Guo et al., 2008; Hsieh et al., 2009). The application of GFPuv-HABP system has been characterized using FM and spectroscopy as well as QCM. The utility of GFPuv-HABP fusion protein has been assessed for both timewise mineralization monitoring and visualization of mineralized tissues, showing formation of a uniform protein layer on the substrate surface coated with HA with the protein organized onto the HA substrate, where the fluorescence intensity per surface coverage of mineral is correlated with the amount of HA surface coating. Following the mineralization reactions, calcium phosphate layers were formed on glass cover slides, and samples were examined by optical microscopy and fluorescent microscopy (Fig. 12.6). GFPuv-HABP was also used for efficient fluorescence labeling of mineralized regions on the extracted human incisors. Single-rooted teeth were collected and kept in 70% ethanol. Following the sterilization and ultrosonication, cylindrical pieces were cut from the acellular afibrillar cementum (AAFC), close to the cementoenamel junction. The AAFC has a mineralized matrix but lacks collagen fibers and cementocytes. The teeth samples were incubated with GFPuv-HABP and negative controls. The samples were

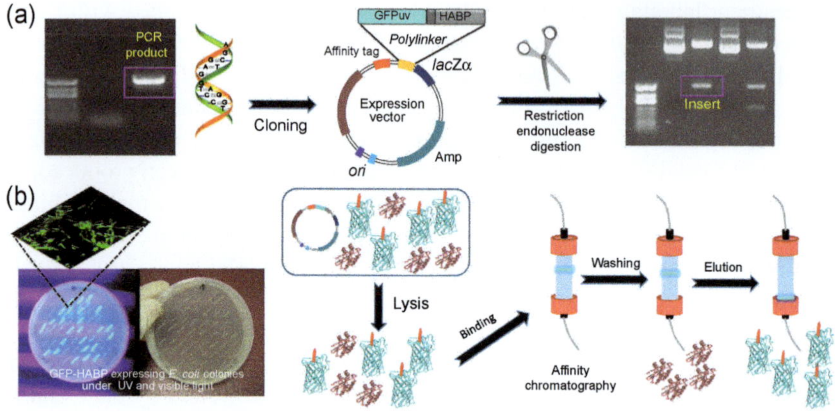

Figure 12.5 Solid-binding peptide–based fusion protein construction. (a) The solid-binding peptide is fused to functional proteins, such as GFPuv. To produce the bifunctional GFPuv-HABP1 fusion protein, nucleotide sequence encoding HABP1 is genetically linked to the N-terminus of the open reading frame of GFPuv encoding DNA and the fusion DNA fragment is cloned into the expression vector encoding the N-terminal 6xhistidine-tag. (b) Following transformation and expression in *Escherichia coli*, an immobilized metal affinity chromatography technique is applied taking to advantage of the 6xhistidine-tag. *GFP*, green fluorescent protein; *HABP*, hydroxyapatite-binding protein.

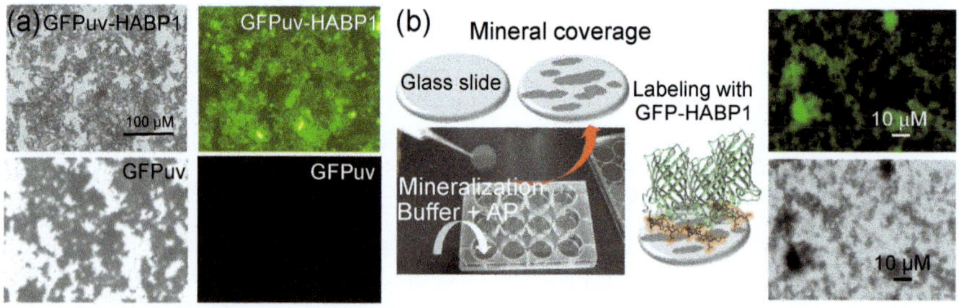

Figure 12.6 Genetically engineered GFPuv-HABP demonstrated as a bifunctional molecular probe to monitor HA mineralization. (a) The application of GFPuv-HABP system has been characterized using fluorescence microscopy. (b) Following the mineralization reactions, calcium phosphate layers were formed on glass cover slides and samples were examined by optical microscopy and fluorescent microscopy. *GFP*, green fluorescent protein; *HA*, hydroxyapatite; *HABP*, hydroxyapatite-binding protein.

rinsed after a 2-h incubation at room temperature. The FM images demonstrated that the GFPuv-HABP protein can recognize biologically mineralized tissues specifically. A simple and versatile application of solid-binding peptides conjugated with fluorescence protein as heterofunctional bioimaging molecular probes that target mineralization has been demonstrated. This bifunctional molecular probe can be employed to a wide range of biomimetic processing and cell-free tissue engineering (Yuca et al., 2011).

Chimeric biomolecules–assisted formation of hybrid composite interface on metal oxide substrate offers a wide range of opportunities to design and fabricate novel

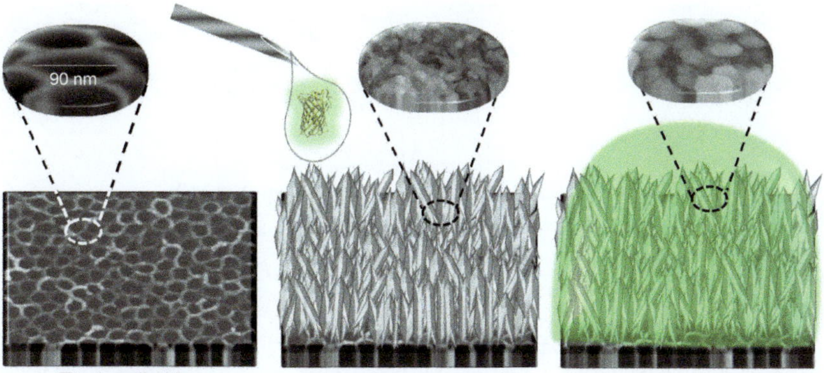

Figure 12.7 Hydroxyapatite deposition on nanotubular titania and coating with a layer of bifunctional GFPuv-HABP protein. GFPuv-HABP simultaneously provide two functionalities, with one domain binding to the HA surface through an HA-binding domain, whereas the other domain displays fluorescence property. *GFP*, green fluorescent protein; *HA*, hydroxyapatite; *HABP*, hydroxyapatite-binding protein.

interfaces. The bifunctional fusion protein, GFPuv-HABP, has been utilized to form a biomolecular-mediated mineralization layer on the implant surface by codepositing the protein with the HA precursors on nanotubular titania using the cathodic ECD at physiological pH and temperature (Narayanan et al., 2007; Shirkhanzadeh, 1998; Rossler et al., 2003; Kar et al., 2006; Utku et al., 2014, 2015b) (Fig. 12.7). Using the molecular probing system, either bound or codeposited, a firmly attached organic layer has been obtained at the interface of the synthetically produced metal oxide–mineral composite, thus approximating the modulus of the organic layer to that of the ECM. Ordered titanium dioxide nanotubular surfaces formed by anodization were coated with HA at physiological pH and temperature using SBF and pulsed electrochemical cathodization. The HA deposit interdigitated into the nanotubes, producing a metal oxide–mineral composite. The bifunctional GFPuv-HABP protein was then self-assembled on the HA, forming a biomodulated interface. Additionally, a protein-mediated HA composite layer was developed on the nanotubular titania surface, where the GFPuv-HABP was codeposited with the precursor ions of HA mineral onto the titania nanotube forming a biomodulated interface. Biomediated assembly resulted in the formation of a hybrid composite as an integrated interface on the nanotubular surface (Fig. 12.8).

12.11 Future prospects

Realizing controllable interactions at the bio-nano-material interfaces are vital in developing next-generation engineered implant materials. Our examples covered titanium-based implants as one of the key reconstructions in dentistry. Next-generation dental implants include advanced biointerfaces that allow manipulation with the

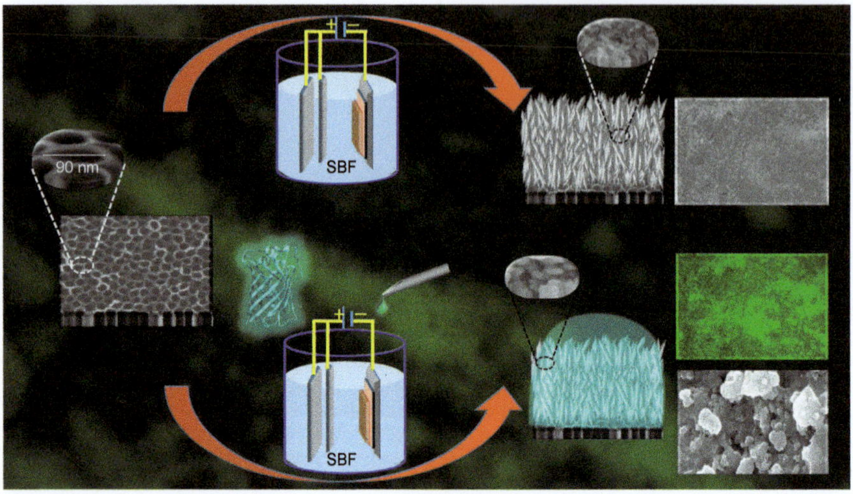

Figure 12.8 HA coating of nanotubular titania using electrochemistry. Nanotubes with 90 nm diameter are cathodically coated with HA in a modified SBF and with HA and GFPuv-HABP in modified SBF. The HA coating is displayed using optical microscope, showing the HA crystals; fluorescence microscope, displaying the codeposition of the fluorescently labeled peptide; and Field Emission-Scanning Electron Microscope (FE-SEM), showing the protein layer codeposited with the mineral. *HA*, hydroxyapatite; *SBF*, simulated body fluid.

biological molecules as one of the keys to provide and enhance favorable interactions with the surrounding biological species. Biomolecular-assisted fabrication of hybrid composite interface offers a wide range of opportunities for addressing the clinical challenges associated with dental implants. Realizing these opportunities will require a deeper understanding of the relationships between the host defense and regeneration as well as access to the interface for diagnostic and monitoring purposes. The next generation of oral implant systems may be constructed as complex three-dimensional geometries with time and functionally programmed properties, pharmacological modulation, as well as incorporation of cellular components and organic macromolecules. Potentially, these elements will act synergistically to provide an organic coating on dental implants that has a modulus approximating that of the ECM.

In addition to dental implants, biomolecular-assisted fabrication has the potential to address disease development and chemomechanical failure at the interface between restorative materials and tooth structure. For example, resin-based composite is rapidly becoming the most popular material for direct restorative dentistry, but composite restorations fail prematurely and patients at highest risk for decay are particularly susceptible to early failure (Derouen et al., 2006; Van de Sande et al., 2013). The primary reason for failure is recurrent decay (Opdam et al., 2010), and 80–90% of recurrent decay is located at the gingival margin of Class II and V composite restorations (Li et al., 2014b). Many clinical decisions to replace the composite restoration, even when caries has not yet developed, are based on defective margins; faulty margins frequently represent a breakdown of the bond between the composite and tooth (Gordan et al., 2009).

The viscous composite is not bonded directly to the tooth—a low viscosity adhesive must be used to connect the composite to the tooth (enamel and dentin). At the vulnerable gingival margin, the adhesive is the barrier between the restored tooth and the oral environment (Spencer et al., 2010). The lack of adhesives that form a durable seal at the composite/tooth interface is a major problem with the use of composites in direct restorative dentistry (Spencer et al., 2010).

One approach to this problem involves a threefold strategy that (1) exploits peptide engineering to disinfect the cavity and remineralize the deficient dentin matrices; (2) engineers resins to resist chemical and enzymatic hydrolysis, and (3) employs iterative feedback between the synthesis, characterization, and modeling to predict properties and promote targeted optimization. Targeted peptides will serve as the anchoring molecules to control the localization of silver nanoparticles for disinfection of the cavity, and HABP will promote remineralization of defective dentin matrices. Anchoring peptides to the adhesive and dentin will concentrate the antimicrobial and remineralization activities at the surface of the substrate. The targeted peptides are used to address acute attacks on the bond, whereas chronic deterioration is addressed by engineering new polymers that are resistant to chemical and enzymatic hydrolysis. The modeling will use the acquired physical, chemical, and mechanical data to predict the behavior of the new adhesives under conditions relevant to oral function. Iterative feedback between synthesis, characterization, and modeling will provide a rational approach to the design and development of robust dentin adhesives. The optimal adhesive is produced by balancing the desired properties with the need for enhanced intraoral stability and function. These novel adhesives are engineered to provide a durable, integrated bond at the composite/tooth interface.

Acknowledgments

Authors gratefully acknowledge the funding from the Research grants AR062249-03 from the National Institute of Arthritis and Musculoskeletal and Skin Diseases (NIAMS), and R01DE025476- 01 from the National Institute of Dental and Craniofacial Research (NIDCR), National Institutes of Health–United State, Bethesda, MD 20892 through University of Kansas.

References

Addadi, L., Weiner, S., 1985. Interactions between acidic proteins and crystals – stereochemical requirements in biomineralization. Proceedings of the National Academy of Sciences of the United States of America 82, 4110–4114.

Addadi, L., Weiner, S., 1992. Control and design principles in biological mineralization. Angewandte Chemie: International Edition in English 31, 153–169.

Aizenberg, J., Weaver, J.C., Thanawala, M.S., Sundar, V.C., Morse, D.E., Fratzl, P., 2005. Skeleton of *Euplectella* sp.: structural hierarchy from the nanoscale to the macroscale. Science 309, 275–278.

Albayrak, O., El-Atwani, O., Altintas, S., 2008. Hydroxyapatite coating on titanium substrate by electrophoretic deposition method: effects of titanium dioxide inner layer on adhesion strength and hydroxyapatite decomposition. Surface and Coatings Technology 202, 2482–2487.

Albrektsson, T., Branemark, P.I., Hansson, H.A., Kasemo, B., Larsson, K., Lundstrom, I., Mcqueen, D.H., Skalak, R., 1983. The interface zone of inorganic implants in vivo – titanium implants in bone. Annals of Biomedical Engineering 11, 1–27.

Alves, C., Neto, C., Morais, G.H.S., Da Silva, C.F., Hajek, V., 2005. Nitriding of titanium disks and industrial dental implants using hollow cathode discharge. Surface & Coatings Technology 194, 196–202.

Amos, F.F., Evans, J.S., 2009. AP7, a partially disordered pseudo C-RING protein, is capable of forming stabilized aragonite in vitro. Biochemistry 48, 1332–1339.

An, Y.H., Stuart, G.W., Mcdowell, S.J., Mcdaniel, S.E., Kang, Q., Friedman, R.J., 1996. Prevention of bacterial adherence to implant surfaces with a crosslinked albumin coating in vitro. Journal of Orthopaedic Research 14, 846–849.

Angelescu, N., Ungureanu, D.N., Catangiu, A., Bratu, V., Anghelina, F.V., 2011. Synthesis and characterization of hydroxyapatite powders obtained by wet chemical method. Metalurgia International 16, 125–128.

Anselme, K., 2000. Osteoblast adhesion on biomaterials. Biomaterials 21, 667–681.

Antoci Jr., V., Adams, C.S., Parvizi, J., Davidson, H.M., Composto, R.J., Freeman, T.A., Wickstrom, E., Ducheyne, P., Jungkind, D., Shapiro, I.M., Hickok, N.J., 2008. The inhibition of *Staphylococcus epidermidis* biofilm formation by vancomycin-modified titanium alloy and implications for the treatment of periprosthetic infection. Biomaterials 29, 4684–4690.

Appendini, P., Hotchkiss, J.H., 2001. Surface modification of poly(styrene) by the attachment of an antimicrobial peptide. Journal of Applied Polymer Science 81, 609–616.

Bagno, A., Di Bello, C., 2004. Surface treatments and roughness properties of Ti-based biomaterials. Journal of Materials Science: Materials in Medicine 15, 935–949.

Bailey, L.E., Kambhampati, D., Kanazawa, K.K., Knoll, W., Frank C.W., 2002. Using surface plasmon resonance and the quartz crystal microbalance to monitor in situ the interfacial behavior of thin organic films, *Langmuir* 18, 479–489.

Balasundaram, G., Webster, T.J., 2007. Increased osteoblast adhesion on nanograined Ti modified with KRSR. Journal of Biomedical Materials Research Part A 80A, 602–611.

Banerjee, I., Pangule, R.C., Kane, R.S., 2011. Antifouling coatings: recent developments in the design of surfaces that prevent fouling by proteins, bacteria, and marine organisms. Advanced Materials 23, 690–718.

Bao, G., Suresh, S., 2003. Cell and molecular mechanics of biological materials. Nature Materials 2, 715–725.

Barth, J.V., Costantini, G., Kern, K., 2005. Engineering atomic and molecular nanostructures at surfaces. Nature 437, 671–679.

Bartlett, J.D., Ganss, B., Goldberg, M., Moradian-Oldak, J., Paine, M.L., Snead, M.L., Wen, X., White, S.N., Zhou, Y.L., 2006. Protein–protein interactions of the developing enamel matrix. In: Schatten, G.P. (Ed.)Schatten, G.P. (Ed.), Current Topics in Developmental Biology, vol. 74.

Bavykin, D.V., Friedrich, J.M., Walsh, F.C., 2006. Protonated titanates and TiO_2 nanostructured materials: synthesis, properties, and applications. Advanced Materials 18, 2807–2824.

Begue-Kirn, C., Krebsbach, P.H., Bartlett, J.D., Butler, W.T., 1998. Dentin sialoprotein, dentin phosphoprotein, enamelysin and ameloblastin: tooth-specific molecules that are distinctively expressed during murine dental differentiation. European Journal of Oral Sciences 106, 963–970.

Belcher, A.M., Wu, X.H., Christensen, R.J., Hansma, P.K., Stucky, G.D., Morse, D.E., 1996. Control of crystal phase switching and orientation by soluble mollusc-shell proteins. Nature 381, 56–58.

Berman, A., Addadi, L., Weiner, S., 1988. Interactions of sea-urchin skeleton macromolecules with growing calcite crystals – a study of intracrystalline proteins. Nature 331, 546–548.

Bettinger, C.J., Langer, R., Borenstein, J.T., 2009. Engineering substrate topography at the micro- and nanoscale to control cell function. Angewandte Chemie: International Edition 48, 5406–5415.

Bierbaum, S., Beutner, R., Hanke, T., Scharnweber, D., Hempel, U., Worch, H., 2003a. Modification of Ti6Al4V surfaces using collagen I, III, and fibronectin. I. Biochemical and morphological characteristics of the adsorbed matrix. Journal of Biomedical Materials Research Part A 67A, 421–430.

Bierbaum, S., Hempel, U., Geissler, U., Hanke, T., Scharnweber, D., Wenzel, K.W., Worch, H., 2003b. Modification of Ti6Al4V surfaces using collagen I, III, and fibronectin. II. Influence on osteoblast responses. Journal of Biomedical Materials Research Part A 67A, 431–438.

Bigi, A., Fini, M., Bracci, B., Boanini, E., Torricelli, P., Giavaresi, G., Aldini, N.N., Facchini, A., Sbaiz, F., Giardino, R., 2008. The response of bone to nanocrystalline hydroxyapatite-coated Ti13Nb11Zr alloy in an animal model. Biomaterials 29, 1730–1736.

Boonekamp, P.M., Vanderweepals, L.J.A., Vanwijkvanlennep, M.M.L., Thesing, C.W., Bijvoet, O.L.M., 1986. Two modes of action of bisphosphonates on osteoclastic resorption of mineralized matrix. Bone and Mineral 1, 27–39.

Boyan, B.D., Lohmann, C.H., Dean, D.D., Sylvia, V.L., Cochran, D.L., Schwartz, Z., 2001. Mechanisms involved in osteoblast response to implant surface morphology. Annual Review of Materials Research 31, 357–371.

Boyer, R., Welsch, G., Collings, E.W., 1994. Materials Properties Handbook – Titanium Alloys. ASM International, Materials Park, OH, USA.

Branemark, P.I., 1983. Osseointegration and its experimental background. Journal of Prosthetic Dentistry 50, 399–410.

Braux, J., Guillaume, C., Jallot, E., Nedelec, J.M., Laurent-Maquin, D., Laquerriere, P., 2009. Effect of strontium treatment on human primary osteoblasts. Hydroxyapatite: a drug delivery system? International Journal of Artificial Organs 32, 458.

Brogden, K.A., 2005. Antimicrobial peptides: pore formers or metabolic inhibitors in bacteria? Nature Reviews Microbiology 3, 238–250.

Brown, P.W., Fulmer, M., 1991. Kinetics of hydroxyapatite formation at low temperature. Journal of the American Ceramic Society 74, 934–940.

Brown, S., Sarikaya, M., Johnson, E., 2000. A genetic analysis of crystal growth. Journal of Molecular Biology 299, 725–735.

Brown, P.W., Constantz, B., 1994. Hydroxyapatite and Related Materials. CRC Press, Boca Raton.

Brown, S., 2001. Protein-mediated particle assembly. Nano Letters 1, 391–394.

Buser, D., Broggini, N., Wieland, M., Schenk, R.K., Denzer, A.J., Cochran, D.L., Hoffmann, B., Lussi, A., Steinemann, S.G., 2004. Enhanced bone apposition to a chemically modified SLA titanium surface. Journal of Dental Research 83, 529–533.

Campoccia, D., Montanaro, L., Arciola, C.R., 2006. The significance of infection related to orthopedic devices and issues of antibiotic resistance. Biomaterials 27, 2331–2339.

Campoccia, D., Montanaro, L., Speziale, P., Arciola, C.R., 2010. Antibiotic-loaded biomaterials and the risks for the spread of antibiotic resistance following their prophylactic and therapeutic clinical use. Biomaterials 31, 6363–6377.

Campoccia, D., Montanaro, L., Arciola, C.R., 2013. A review of the biomaterials technologies for infection-resistant surfaces. Biomaterials 34, 8533–8554.

Capriotti, L.A., Beebe Jr., T.P., Schneider, J.P., 2007. Hydroxyapatite surface-induced peptide folding. Journal of the American Chemical Society 129, 5281–5287.

Cariolou, M.A., Morse, D.E., 1988. Purification and characterization of calcium-binding conchiolin shell peptides from the mollusk, *Haliotis rufescens*, as a function of development. Journal of Comparative Physiology B: Biochemical Systemic and Environmental Physiology 157, 717–729.

Castner, D.G., Ratner, B.D., 2002. Biomedical surface science: foundations to frontiers. Surface Science 500, 28–60.

Cetinel, S., Caliskan, H.B., Yucesoy, D.T., Donatan, A.S., Yuca, E., Urgen, M., Karaguler, N.G., Tamerler, C., 2013. Addressable self-immobilization of lactate dehydrogenase across multiple length scales. Biotechnology Journal 8, 262–272.

Cha, J.N., Shimizu, K., Zhou, Y., Christiansen, S.C., Chmelka, B.F., Stucky, G.D., Morse, D.E., 1999. Silicatein filaments and subunits from a marine sponge direct the polymerization of silica and silicones in vitro. Proceedings of the National Academy of Sciences of the United States of America 96, 361–365.

Chang, C.K., Wu, J.S., Mao, D.L., Ding, C.X., 2001. Mechanical and histological evaluations of hydroxyapatite-coated and noncoated Ti6Al4V implants in tibia bone. Journal of Biomedical Materials Research 56, 17–23.

Chehroudi, B., Ratkay, J., Brunette, D.M., 1992. The role of implant surface geometry on mineralization in vivo and in vitro – a transmission and scanning electron-microscopic study. Cells and Materials 2, 89–104.

Chen, H., Su, X., Neoh, K.-G., Choe, W.-S., 2006. QCM-D analysis of binding mechanism of phage particles displaying a constrained heptapeptide with specific affinity to SiO_2 and TiO_2. Analytical Chemistry 78, 4872–4879.

Chudakov, D.M., Lukyanov, S., Lukyanov, K.A., 2005. Fluorescent proteins as a toolkit for in vivo imaging. Trends in Biotechnology 23, 605–613.

Cochran, D.L., Schenk, R.K., Lussi, A., Higginbottom, F.L., Buser, D., 1998. Bone response to unloaded and loaded titanium implants with a sandblasted and acid-etched surface: a histometric study in the canine mandible. Journal of Biomedical Materials Research 40, 1–11.

Cölfen, H., Antonietti, M., 2008. Mesocrystals and Nonclassical Crystallization. John Wiley & Sons, New York.

Cook, S.D., Thomas, K.A., Kay, J.F., 1991. Experimental coating defects in hydroxylapatite-coated implants. Clinical Orthopaedics and Related Research 280–290.

Costa, F., Carvalho, I.F., Montelaro, R.C., Gomes, P., Martins, M.C.L., 2011. Covalent immobilization of antimicrobial peptides (AMPs) onto biomaterial surfaces. Acta Biomaterialia 7, 1431–1440.

Costerton, J.W., Stewart, P.S., Greenberg, E.P., 1999. Bacterial biofilms: a common cause of persistent infections. Science 284, 1318–1322.

Cowin, S.C., 1999. Bone poroelasticity. Journal of Biomechanics 32, 217–238.

Cranford, S.W., De Boer, J., Van Blitterswijk, C., Buehler, M.J., 2013. Materiomics: an omics approach to biomaterials research. Advanced Materials 25, 802–824.

Dai, H.X., Choe, W.S., Thai, C.K., Sarikaya, M., Traxler, B.A., Baneyx, F., Schwartz, D.T., 2005. Nonequilibrium synthesis and assembly of hybrid inorganic-protein nanostructures using an engineered DNA binding protein. Journal of the American Chemical Society 127, 15637–15643.

Dalby, M.J., Gadegaard, N., Tare, R., Andar, A., Riehle, M.O., Herzyk, P., Wilkinson, C.D.W., Oreffo, R.O.C., 2007. The control of human mesenchymal cell differentiation using nanoscale symmetry and disorder. Nature Materials 6, 997–1003.

Darouiche, R.O., Mansouri, M.D., Zakarevicz, D., Alsharif, A., Landon, G.C., 2007. In vivo efficacy of antimicrobial-coated devices. Journal of Bone and Joint Surgery – American Volume 89A, 792–797.

Dash, A.K., Cudworth, G.C., 1998. Therapeutic applications of implantable drug delivery systems. Journal of Pharmacological and Toxicological Methods 40, 1–12.

De Araujo, T.S., Macedo, Z.S., De Oliveira, P.A.S.C., Valerio, M.E.G., 2007. Production and characterization of pure and Cr^{3+}-doped hydroxyapatite for biomedical applications as fluorescent probes. Journal of Materials Science 42, 2236–2243.

Delak, K., Giocondi, J., Orme, C., Evans, J.S., 2008. Modulation of crystal growth by the terminal sequences of the prismatic-associated asprich protein. Crystal Growth & Design 8, 4481–4486.
Delak, K., Harcup, C., Lakshminarayanan, R., Sun, Z., Fan, Y., Moradian-Oldak, J., Evans, J.S., 2009. The tooth enamel protein, porcine amelogenin, is an intrinsically disordered protein with an extended molecular configuration in the monomeric form. Biochemistry 48, 2272–2281.
Deporter, D., 2009. Dental implant design and optimal treatment outcomes. International Journal of Periodontics & Restorative Dentistry 29, 625–633.
Derouen, T.A., Martin, M.D., Leroux, B.G., Townes, B.D., Woods, J.S., Leitao, J., Castro-Caldas, A., Luis, H., Bernardo, M., Rosenbaum, G., Martins, I.P., 2006. Neurobehavioral effects of dental amalgam in children – a randomized clinical trial. JAMA – Journal of the American Medical Association 295, 1784–1792.
Deville, S., Saiz, E., Nalla, R.K., Tomsia, A.P., 2006a. Freezing as a path to build complex composites. Science 311, 515–518.
Deville, S., Saiz, E., Tomsia, A.P., 2006b. Freeze casting of hydroxyapatite scaffolds for bone tissue engineering. Biomaterials 27, 5480–5489.
Dickerson, M.B., Jones, S.E., Cai, Y., Ahmad, G., Naik, R.R., Kroeger, N., Sandhage, K.H., 2008. Identification and design of peptides for the rapid, high-yield formation of nanoparticulate TiO_2 from aqueous solutions at room temperature. Chemistry of Materials 20, 1578–1584.
Dietz, H., Berkemeier, F., Bertz, M., Rief, M., 2006. Anisotropic deformation response of single protein molecules. Proceedings of the National Academy of Sciences of the United States of America 103, 12724–12728.
Discher, D.E., Janmey, P., Wang, Y.L., 2005. Tissue cells feel and respond to the stiffness of their substrate. Science 310, 1139–1143.
Dsouza, R.N., Cavender, A., Sunavala, G., Alvarez, J., Ohshima, T., Kulkarni, A.B., Macdougall, M., 1997. Gene expression patterns of murine dentin matrix protein 1 (Dmp1) and dentin sialophosphoprotein (DSPP) suggest distinct developmental functions in vivo. Journal of Bone and Mineral Research 12, 2040–2049.
Du, C., Falini, G., Fermani, S., Abbott, C., Moradian-Oldak, J., 2005. Supramolecular assembly of amelogenin nanospheres into birefringent microribbons. Science 307, 1450–1454.
Elliott, J.C., 1994. Structure and Chemistry of Apatites and Other Calcium Orthophosphates. Elsevier, New York.
Etienne, O., Picart, C., Taddei, C., Haikel, Y., Dimarcq, J.L., Schaaf, P., Voegel, J.C., Ogier, J.A., Egles, C., 2004. Multilayer polyelectrolyte films functionalized by insertion of defensin: a new approach to protection of implants from bacterial colonization. Antimicrobial Agents and Chemotherapy 48, 3662–3669.
Evans, J.S., Samudrala, R., Walsh, T.R., Oren, E.E., Tamerler, C., 2008. Molecular design of inorganic-binding polypeptides. Mrs Bulletin 33, 514–518.
Evans, J.S., 2008. "Tuning in" to mollusk shell nacre- and prismatic-associated protein terminal sequences. Implications for biomineralization and the construction of high performance inorganic-organic composites. Chemical Reviews 108, 4455–4462.
Fan, D., Iijima, M., Bromley, K.M., Yang, X., Mathew, S., Moradian-Oldak, J., 2011. The cooperation of enamelin and amelogenin in controlling octacalcium phosphate crystal morphology. Cells Tissues Organs 194, 194–198.
Fang, Y., Poulsen, N., Dickerson, M.B., Cai, Y., Jones, S.E., Naik, R.R., Kroeger, N., Sandhage, K.H., 2008. Identification of peptides capable of inducing the formation of titania but not silica via a subtractive bacteriophage display approach. Journal of Materials Chemistry 18, 3871–3875.

Finney, N.S., 2006. Combinatorial discovery of fluorophores and fluorescent probes. Current Opinion in Chemical Biology 10, 238–245.

Fjell, C.D., Jenssen, H., Hilpert, K., Cheung, W.A., Pante, N., Hancock, R.E.W., Cherkasov, A., 2009. Identification of novel antibacterial peptides by chemoinformatics and machine learning. Journal of Medicinal Chemistry 52, 2006–2015.

Fong, H., White, S.N., Paine, M.L., Luo, W., Snead, M.L., Sarikaya, M., 2003. Enamel structure properties controlled by engineered proteins in transgenic mice. Journal of Bone and Mineral Research 18, 2052–2059.

Fratzl, P., Weinkamer, R., 2007. Nature's hierarchical materials. Progress in Materials Science 52, 1263–1334.

Fratzl, P., Gupta, H.S., Paschalis, E.P., Roschger, P., 2004. Structure and mechanical quality of the collagen-mineral nano-composite in bone. Journal of Materials Chemistry 14, 2115–2123.

Frenkel, S.R., Simon, J., Alexander, H., Dennis, M., Ricci, J.L., 2002. Osseointegration on metallic implant surfaces: effects of microgeometry and growth factor treatment. Journal of Biomedical Materials Research 63, 706–713.

Fukumoto, S., Tsubakino, H., Inoue, S., Liu, L., Terasawa, M., Mitamura, T., 1999. Surface modification of titanium by nitrogen ion implantation. Materials Science and Engineering A-Structural Materials Properties Microstructure and Processing 263, 205–209.

Gajjeraman, S., Narayanan, K., Hao, J., Qin, C., George, A., 2007. Matrix macromolecules in hard tissues control the nucleation and hierarchical assembly of hydroxyapatite. Journal of Biological Chemistry 282, 1193–1204.

Gaskin, D.J.H., Starck, K., Vulfson, E.N., 2000. Identification of inorganic crystal-specific sequences using phage display combinatorial library of short peptides: a feasibility study. Biotechnology Letters 22, 1211–1216.

Geetha, M., Singh, A.K., Asokamani, R., Gogia, A.K., 2009. Ti based biomaterials, the ultimate choice for orthopaedic implants – a review. Progress in Materials Science 54, 397–425.

Giepmans, B.N.G., Adams, S.R., Ellisman, M.H., Tsien, R.Y., 2006. Review – the fluorescent toolbox for assessing protein location and function. Science 312, 217–224.

Giuliani, A., Pirri, G., Nicoletto, S.F., 2007. Antimicrobial peptides: an overview of a promising class of therapeutics. Central European Journal of Biology 2, 1–33.

Glimcher, M., Nimni, M., 1992. Collagen cross-linking and biomineralization. Connective Tissue Research 27, 73–83.

Goldberg, H.A., Warner, K.J., Li, M.C., Hunter, G.K., 2001. Binding of bone sialoprotein, osteopontin and synthetic polypeptides to hydroxyapatite. Connective Tissue Research 42, 25–37.

Gordan, V.V., Garvan, C.W., Blaser, P.K., Mondragon, E., Mjoer, I.A., 2009. A long-term evaluation of alternative treatments to replacement of resin-based composite restorations Results of a seven-year study. Journal of the American Dental Association 140, 1476–1484.

Gottenbos, B., Van Der Mei, H.C., Klatter, F., Nieuwenhuis, P., Busscher, H.J., 2002. In vitro and in vivo antimicrobial activity of covalently coupled quaternary ammonium silane coatings on silicone rubber. Biomaterials 23, 1417–1423.

Gu, L.-S., Kim, Y.K., Liu, Y., Takahashi, K., Arun, S., Wimmer, C.E., Osorio, R., Ling, J.-Q., Looney, S.W., Pashley, D.H., Tay, F.R., 2011. Immobilization of a phosphonated analog of matrix phosphoproteins within cross-linked collagen as a templating mechanism for biomimetic mineralization. Acta Biomaterialia 7, 268–277.

Gungormus, M., Fong, H., Kim, I.W., Evans, J.S., Tamerler, C., Sarikaya, M., 2008. Regulation of in vitro calcium phosphate mineralization by combinatorially selected hydroxyapatite-binding peptides. Biomacromolecules 9, 966–973.

Gungormus, M., Branco, M., Fong, H., Schneider, J.P., Tamerler, C., Sarikaya, M., 2010. Self assembled bi-functional peptide hydrogels with biomineralization-directing peptides. Biomaterials 31, 7266–7274.

Gungormus, M., Oren, E.E., Horst, J.A., Fong, H., Hnilova, M., Somerman, M.J., Snead, M.L., Samudrala, R., Tamerler, C., Sarikaya, M., 2012. Cementomimetics-constructing a cementum-like biomineralized microlayer via amelogenin-derived peptides. International Journal of Oral Science 4, 69–77.

Guo, Y., Shi, D., Lian, J., Dong, Z., Wang, W., Cho, H., Liu, G., Wang, L., Ewing, R.C., 2008. Quantum dot conjugated hydroxylapatite nanoparticles for in vivo imaging. Nanotechnology 19.

Hanawa, T., Kamiura, Y., Yamamoto, S., Kohgo, T., Amemiya, A., Ukai, H., Murakami, K., Asaoka, K., 1997. Early bone formation around calcium-ion-implanted titanium inserted into rat tibia. Journal of Biomedical Materials Research 36, 131–136.

Hanawa, T., 2009. An overview of biofunctionalization of metals in Japan. Journal of the Royal Society Interface 6, S361–S369.

Harbers, G.M., Emoto, K., Greef, C., Metzger, S.W., Woodward, H.N., Mascali, J.J., Grainger, D.W., Lochhead, M.J., 2007. Functionalized poly(ethylene glycol)-based bioassay surface chemistry that facilitates bio-immobilization and inhibits nonspecific protein, bacterial, and mammalian cell adhesion. Chemistry of Materials 19, 4405–4414.

Harris, L.G., Mead, L., Muller-Oberlander, E., Richards, R.G., 2006. Bacteria and cell cytocompatibility studies on coated medical grade titanium surfaces. Journal of Biomedical Materials Research Part A 78A, 50–58.

Heimann, R.B., Kurzweg, H., Ivey, D.G., Wayman, M.L., 1998. Microstructural and in vitro chemical investigations into plasma-sprayed bioceramic coatings. Journal of Biomedical Materials Research 43, 441–450.

Hench, L.L., Wilson, J., 1993. An Introduction to Bioceramics. World Scientific Publishing Co., Singapore.

Hetrick, E.M., Schoenfisch, M.H., 2006. Reducing implant-related infections: active release strategies. Chemical Society Reviews 35, 780–789.

Hilpert, K., Elliott, M.R., Volkmer-Engert, R., Henklein, P., Donini, O., Zhou, Q., Winkler, D.F.H., Hancock, R.E.W., 2006. Sequence requirements and an optimization strategy for short antimicrobial peptides. Chemistry & Biology 13, 1101–1107.

Hnilova, M., Oren, E.E., Seker, U.O.S., Wilson, B.R., Collino, S., Evans, J.S., Tamerler, C., Sarikaya, M., 2008. Effect of molecular conformations on the adsorption behavior of gold-binding peptides. Langmuir 24, 12440–12445.

Hnilova, M., Karaca, B.T., Park, J., Jia, C., Wilson, B.R., Sarikaya, M., Tamerler, C., 2012a. Fabrication of hierarchical hybrid structures using bio-enabled layer-by-layer self-assembly. Biotechnology and Bioengineering 109, 1120–1130.

Hnilova, M., Liu, X., Yuca, E., Jia, C., Wilson, B., Karatas, A.Y., Gresswell, C., Ohuchi, F., Kitamura, K., Tamerler, C., 2012b. Multifunctional protein-enabled patterning on arrayed ferroelectric materials. ACS Applied Materials & Interfaces 4, 1865–1871.

Hoffman, R.M., 2002. Green fluorescent protein imaging of tumour growth, metastasis, and angiogenesis in mouse models. Lancet Oncology 3, 546–556.

Hsieh, M.-F., Li, J.K.-J., Lin, C.-A.J., Huang, S.-H., Sperling, R.A., Parak, W.J., Chang, W.H., 2009. Tracking of cellular uptake of hydrophilic CdSe/ZnS quantum dots/hydroxyapatite composites nanoparticles in MC3T3-E1 osteoblast cells. Journal of Nanoscience and Nanotechnology 9, 2758–2762.

Huang, Y., Chiang, C.Y., Lee, S.K., Gao, Y., Hu, E.L., De Yoreo, J., Belcher, A.M., 2005. Programmable assembly of nanoarchitectures using genetically engineered viruses. Nano Letters 5, 1429–1434.

Hulbert, S.F., Cooke, F.W., Klawitter, J.J., Leonard, R.B., Sauer, B.W., Moyle, D.D., Skinner, H.B., 1973. Attachment of prostheses to the musculo-skeletal system by tissue ingrowth and mechanical interlocking. Journal of Biomedical Materials Research 7, 1–23.

Iijima, M., Moradian-Oldak, J., 2004. Interactions of amelogenins with octacalcium phosphate crystal faces are dose dependent. Calcified Tissue International 74, 522–531.

Ingham, A.B., Moore, R.J., 2007. Recombinant production of antimicrobial peptides in heterologous microbial systems. Biotechnology and Applied Biochemistry 47, 1–9.

Jaeger, M., Zilkens, C., Zanger, K., Krauspe, R., 2007. Significance of nano- and microtopography for cell-surface interactions in orthopaedic implants. Journal of Biomedicine and Biotechnology.

Jayaraman, M., Meyer, U., Buhner, M., Joos, U., Wiesmann, H.P., 2004. Influence of titanium surfaces on attachment of osteoblast-like cells in vitro. Biomaterials 25, 625–631.

Jenssen, H., Hamill, P., Hancock, R.E.W., 2006. Peptide antimicrobial agents. Clinical Microbiology Reviews 19, 491–511.

Jiang, Z., Vasil, A.I., Hale, J.D., Hancock, R.E.W., Vasil, M.L., Hodges, R.S., 2008. Effects of net charge and the number of positively charged residues on the biological activity of amphipathic alpha-helical cationic antimicrobial peptides. Biopolymers 90, 369–383.

Jiang, P., Lin, L., Zhang, F., Dong, X., Ren, L., Lin, C., 2013. Electrochemical construction of micro–nano spongelike structure on titanium substrate for enhancing corrosion resistance and bioactivity. Electrochimica Acta 107, 16–25.

Jose, B., Antoci, V., Zeiger, A.R., Wickstrom, E., Hickok, N.J., 2005. Vancomycin covalently bonded to titanium beads kills *Staphylococcus aureus*. Chemistry & Biology 12, 1041–1048.

Junker, R., Dimakis, A., Thoneick, M., Jansen, J.A., 2009. Effects of implant surface coatings and composition on bone integration: a systematic review. Clinical Oral Implants Research 20, 185–206.

Kacar, T., Ray, J., Gungormus, M., Oren, E.E., Tamerler, C., Sarikaya, M., 2009a. Quartz binding peptides as molecular linkers towards fabricating multifunctional micropatterned substrates. Advanced Materials 21, 295–299.

Kacar, T., Zin, M.T., So, C., Wilson, B., Ma, H., Gul-Karaguler, N., Jen, A.K.Y., Sarikaya, M., Tamerler, C., 2009b. Directed self-immobilization of alkaline phosphatase on micro-patterned substrates via genetically fused metal-binding peptide. Biotechnology and Bioengineering 103, 696–705.

Kannan, S., Goetz-Neunhoeffer, F., Neubauer, J., Ferreira, J.M.F., 2008. Ionic substitutions in biphasic hydroxyapatite and β-tricalcium phosphate mixtures: structural analysis by Rietveld refinement. Journal of the American Ceramic Society 91, 1–12.

Kar, A., Raja, K.S., Misra, M., 2006. Electrodeposition of hydroxyapatite onto nanotubular TiO_2 for implant applications. Surface and Coatings Technology 201, 3723–3731.

Kasaj, A., Willershausen, B., Reichert, C., Gortan-Kasaj, A., Zafiropoulos, G.-G., Schmidt, M., 2008. Human periodontal fibroblast response to a nanostructured hydroxyapatite bone replacement graft in vitro. Archives of Oral Biology 53, 683–689.

Kashiwagi, K., Tsuji, T., Shiba, K., 2009. Directional BMP-2 for functionalization of titanium surfaces. Biomaterials 30, 1166–1175.

Kazemzadeh-Narbat, M., Kindrachuk, J., Duan, K., Jenssen, H., Hancock, R.E.W., Wang, R., 2010. Antimicrobial peptides on calcium phosphate-coated titanium for the prevention of implant-associated infections. Biomaterials 31, 9519–9526.

Kelly, M., Williams, R., Aojula, A., O'neill, J., Trzinscka, Z., Grover, L., Scott, R.A.H., Peacock, A.F.A., Logan, A., Stamboulis, A., De Cogan, F., 2015. Peptide aptamers: novel coatings for orthopaedic implants. Materials Science & Engineering C: Materials for Biological Applications 54, 84–93.

Khatayevich, D., Gungormus, M., Yazici, H., So, C., Cetinel, S., Ma, H., Jen, A., Tamerler, C., Sarikaya, M., 2010. Biofunctionalization of materials for implants using engineered peptides. Acta Biomaterialia 6, 4634–4641.

Kim, J., Arola, D.D., Gu, L., Kim, Y.K., Mai, S., Liu, Y., Pashley, D.H., Tay, F.R., 2010. Functional biomimetic analogs help remineralize apatite-depleted demineralized resin-infiltrated dentin via a bottom-up approach. Acta Biomaterialia 6, 2740–2750.

Kitaori, T., Ito, H., Schwarz, E.A., Tsutsumi, R., Yoshitomi, H., Oishi, S., Nakano, M., Fujii, N., Nagasawa, T., Nakamura, T., 2009. Stromal cell-derived factor 1/CXCR4 signaling is critical for the recruitment of mesenchymal stem cells to the fracture site during skeletal repair in a mouse model. Arthritis and Rheumatism 60, 813–823.

Klein, C.P., Patka, P., Van Der Lubbe, H.B., Wolke, J.G., De Groot, K., 1991. Plasma-sprayed coatings of tetracalcium phosphate, hydroxyl-apatite, and alpha-TCP on titanium alloy: an interface study. Journal of Biomedical Materials Research 25, 53–65.

Kokubo, T., Kim, H.M., Kawashita, M., Nakamura, T., 2004. Bioactive metals: preparation and properties. Journal of Materials Science: Materials in Medicine 15, 99–107.

Kramer, R.M., Li, C., Carter, D.C., Stone, M.O., Naik, R.R., 2004. Engineered protein cages for nanomaterial synthesis. Journal of the American Chemical Society 126, 13282–13286.

Krauland, E.M., Peelle, B.R., Wittrup, K.D., Belcher, A.M., 2007. Peptide tags for enhanced cellular and protein adhesion to single-crystal line sapphire. Biotechnology and Bioengineering 97, 1009–1020.

Kretsinger, J.K., Haines, L.A., Ozbas, B., Pochan, D.J., Schneider, J.P., 2005. Cytocompatibility of self-assembled β-hairpin peptide hydrogel surfaces. Biomaterials 26, 5177–5186.

Kriplani, U., Kay, B.K., 2005. Selecting peptides for use in nanoscale materials using phage-displayed combinatorial peptide libraries. Current Opinion in Biotechnology 16, 470–475.

Ku, Y., Chung, C.P., Jang, J.H., 2005. The effect of the surface modification of titanium using a recombinant fragment of fibronectin and vitronectin on cell behavior. Biomaterials 26, 5153–5157.

Kulkarni, M., Mazare, A., Gongadze, E., Š, P., Kralj-Iglič, V., Milošev, I., Schmuki, P., Iglič, A., Mozetič, M., 2015. Titanium nanostructures for biomedical applications. Nanotechnology 26, 062002.

Kulp, J.L., Sarikaya, M., Evans, J.S., 2004. Molecular characterization of a prokaryotic polypeptide sequence that catalyzes Au crystal formation. Journal of Materials Chemistry 14, 2325–2332.

Kunze, J., Mueller, L., Macak, J.M., Greil, P., Schmuki, P., Mueller, F.A., 2008. Time-dependent growth of biomimetic apatite on anodic TiO_2 nanotubes. Electrochimica Acta 53, 6995–7003.

Kurzweg, H., Heimann, R.B., Troczynski, T., Wayman, M.L., 1998. Development of plasma-sprayed bioceramic coatings with bond coats based on titania and zirconia. Biomaterials 19, 1507–1511.

Kwakman, P.H.S., Velde, A.A.T., Vandenbroucke-Grauls, C.M.J.E., Van Deventer, S.J.H., Zaat, S.A.J., 2006. Treatment and prevention of *Staphylococcus epidermidis* experimental biomaterial-associated infection by bactericidal peptide 2. Antimicrobial Agents and Chemotherapy 50, 3977–3983.

Le Guéhennec, L., Soueidan, A., Layrolle, P., Amouriq, Y., 2007. Surface treatments of titanium dental implants for rapid osseointegration. Dental Materials 23, 844–854.

Lee, S.W., Mao, C.B., Flynn, C.E., Belcher, A.M., 2002. Ordering of quantum dots using genetically engineered viruses. Science 296, 892–895.

Leeuwenburgh, S.C.G., Wolke, J.G.C., Siebers, T.C., Schoonman, J., Jansen, J.A., 2006. In vitro and in vivo reactivity of porous, electrosprayed calcium phosphate coatings. Biomaterials 27, 3368–3378.

Levy, Y., Onuchic, J.N., 2006. Mechanisms of protein assembly: lessons from minimalist models. Accounts of Chemical Research 39, 135–142.

Li, Q.-L., Ning, T.-Y., Cao, Y., Zhang, W.-B., Mei, M.L., Chu, C.H., 2014a. A novel self-assembled oligopeptide amphiphile for biomimetic mineralization of enamel. BMC Biotechnology 14.

Li, Y., Carrera, C., Chen, R., Li, J., Lenton, P., Rudney, J.D., Jones, R.S., Aparicio, C., Fok, A., 2014b. Degradation in the dentin-composite interface subjected to multi-species biofilm challenges. Acta Biomaterialia 10, 375–383.

Lin, S., Legeros, R.Z., Legeros, J.P., 2003. Adherent octacalciumphosphate coating on titanium alloy using modulated electrochemical deposition method. Journal of Biomedical Materials Research Part A 66, 819–828.

Liou, Y.C., Tocilj, A., Davies, P.L., Jia, Z.C., 2000. Mimicry of ice structure by surface hydroxyls and water of a beta-helix antifreeze protein. Nature 406, 322–324.

Lipman, H., 1935. Staining the skeleton of cleared embryos with Alizarin red S. Stain Technology 10, 61–63.

Liu, C., Huang, Y., Shen, W., Cui, J., 2001. Kinetics of hydroxyapatite precipitation at pH 10 to 11. Biomaterials 22, 301–306.

Liu, X.Y., Chu, P.K., Ding, C.X., 2004. Surface modification of titanium, titanium alloys, and related materials for biomedical applications. Materials Science & Engineering R: Reports 47, 49–121.

Liu, T.Y., Chen, S.Y., Liu, D.M., Liou, S.C., 2005. On the study of BSA-loaded calcium-deficient hydroxyapatite nano-carriers for controlled drug delivery. Journal of Controlled Release 107, 112–121.

Lo, C.M., Wang, H.B., Dembo, M., Wang, Y.L., 2000. Cell movement is guided by the rigidity of the substrate. Biophysical Journal 79, 144–152.

Long, M., Rack, H.J., 1998. Titanium alloys in total joint replacement – a materials science perspective. Biomaterials 19, 1621–1639.

Love, J.C., Estroff, L.A., Kriebel, J.K., Nuzzo, R.G., Whitesides, G.M., 2005. Self-assembled monolayers of thiolates on metals as a form of nanotechnology. Chemical Reviews 105, 1103–1169.

Lowenstam, H.A., Weiner, S., 1989. On Biomineralization. Oxford University Press, New York.

Lowenstam, H.A., 1981. Minerals formed by organisms. Science 211, 1126–1131.

Luo, Q., Huang, Y., Zha, G., Chen, Y., Deng, X., Zhang, K., Zhu, W., Zhao, S., Li, X., 2015. Topography-dependent antibacterial, osteogenic and anti-aging properties of pure titanium. Journal of Materials Chemistry B 3, 784–795.

Ma, H., Zin, M.T., Zareie, M.H., Kang, M.-S., Kang, S.-H., Kim, K.-S., Reed, B.W., Behar, C.T., Sarikaya, M., Jen, A.K.Y., 2007. Assembly of nanomaterials through highly ordered self-assembled monolayers and peptide-organic hybrid conjugates as templates. Journal of Nanoscience and Nanotechnology 7, 2549–2566.

Ma, M.-Y., Zhu, Y.-J., Li, L., Cao, S.-W., 2008. Nanostructured porous hollow ellipsoidal capsules of hydroxyapatite and calcium silicate: preparation and application in drug delivery. Journal of Materials Chemistry 18, 2722–2727.

MacDonald, D.E., Rapuano, B.E., Deo, N., Stranick, M., Somasundaran, P., Boskey, A.L., 2004. Thermal and chemical modification of titanium-aluminum-vanadium implant materials: effects on surface properties, glycoprotein adsorption, and MG63 cell attachment. Biomaterials 25, 3135–3146.

Maia, F.R., Bidarra, S.J., Granja, P.L., Barrias, C.C., 2013. Functionalization of biomaterials with small osteoinductive moieties. Acta Biomaterialia 9, 8773–8789.

Mann, S., 1993. Molecular tectonics in biomineralization and biomimetic materials chemistry. Nature 365, 499–505.

Mann, S., 1996. Biomimetic Materials Chemistry. Wiley-VCH, New York.
Mann, S., 2001. Biomineralization: Principles and Concepts in Bioinorganic Materials Chemistry. Oxford University, New York.
Martin, H.J., Schulz, K.H., Bumgardner, J.D., Walters, K.B., 2007. XPS study on the use of 3-aminopropyltriethoxysilane to bond chitosan to a titanium surface. Langmuir 23, 6645–6651.
Mayer, G., Sarikaya, M., 2002. Rigid biological composite materials: structural examples for biomimetic design. Experimental Mechanics 42, 395–403.
Meloan, S., Puchtler, H., 1985. Chemical mechanisms of staining methods: von Kossa's technique. What von Kossa really wrote and a modified reaction for selective demonstration of inorganic phosphate. Journal of Histotechnology 8, 11–13.
Meyers, S.R., Khoo, X., Huang, X., Walsh, E.B., Grinstaff, M.W., Kenan, D.J., 2009. The development of peptide-based interfacial biomaterials for generating biological functionality on the surface of bioinert materials. Biomaterials 30, 277–286.
Mohorcic, M., Jerman, I., Zorko, M., Butinar, L., Orel, B., Jerala, R., Friedrich, J., 2010. Surface with antimicrobial activity obtained through silane coating with covalently bound polymyxin B. Journal of Materials Science: Materials in Medicine 21, 2775–2782.
Morra, M., 2006. Biochemical modification of titanium surfaces: peptides and ECM proteins. European Cells & Materials 12, 1–15.
Mrksich, M., Whitesides, G.M., 1996. Using self-assembled monolayers to understand the interactions of man-made surfaces with proteins and cells. Annual Review of Biophysics and Biomolecular Structure 25, 55–78.
Munch, E., Launey, M.E., Alsem, D.H., Saiz, E., Tomsia, A.P., Ritchie, R.O., 2008. Tough, bio-inspired hybrid materials. Science 322, 1516–1520.
Naik, R.R., Brott, L.L., Clarson, S.J., Stone, M.O., 2002a. Silica-precipitating peptides isolated from a combinatorial phage display peptide library. Journal of Nanoscience and Nanotechnology 2, 95–100.
Naik, R.R., Stringer, S.J., Agarwal, G., Jones, S.E., Stone, M.O., 2002b. Biomimetic synthesis and patterning of silver nanoparticles. Nature Materials 1, 169–172.
Nam, K.T., Lee, Y.J., Krauland, E.M., Kottmann, S.T., Belcher, A.M., 2008. Peptide-mediated reduction of silver ions on engineered biological scaffolds. ACS Nano 2, 1480–1486.
Nancollas, G.H., Wu, W., 2000. Biomineralization mechanisms: a kinetics and interfacial energy approach. Journal of Crystal Growth 211, 137–142.
Narayanan, R., Seshadri, S.K., Kwon, T.Y., Kim, K.H., 2007. Electrochemical nano-grained calcium phosphate coatings on Ti-6Al-4V for biomaterial applications. Scripta Materialia 56, 229–232.
Narayanan, R., Seshadri, S.K., Kwon, T.Y., Kim, K.H., 2008. Calcium phosphate-based coatings on titanium and its alloys. Journal of Biomedical Materials Research Part B: Applied Biomaterials 85B, 279–299.
Niemeyer, C.M., 2001. Nanoparticles, proteins, and nucleic acids: biotechnology meets materials science. Angewandte Chemie: International Edition 40, 4128–4158.
Nomura, S., Hiltner, A., Lando, J.B., Baer, E., 1977. Interaction of water with native collagen. Biopolymers 16, 231–246.
Ogawa, T., Saruwatari, L., Takeuchi, K., Aita, H., Ohno, N., 2008. Ti nano-nodular structuring for bone integration and regeneration. Journal of Dental Research 87, 751–756.
Oh, S.H., Finones, R.R., Daraio, C., Chen, L.H., Jin, S.H., 2005. Growth of nano-scale hydroxyapatite using chemically treated titanium oxide nanotubes. Biomaterials 26, 4938–4943.

Omar, O., Lenneras, M., Svensson, S., Suska, F., Emanuelsson, L., Hall, J., Nannmark, U., Thomsen, P., 2010. Integrin and chemokine receptor gene expression in implant-adherent cells during early osseointegration. Journal of Materials Science: Materials in Medicine 21, 969–980.

Opdam, N.J.M., Bronkhorst, E.M., Loomans, B.A.C., Huysmans, M.C.D.N.J.M., 2010. 12-Year survival of composite vs. amalgam restorations. Journal of Dental Research 89, 1063–1067.

Oren, E.E., Tamerler, C., Sahin, D., Hnilova, M., Seker, U.O.S., Sarikaya, M., Samudrala, R., 2007. A novel knowledge-based approach to design inorganic-binding peptides. Bioinformatics 23, 2816–2822.

Orsini, G., Assenza, B., Scarano, A., Piattelli, M., Piattelli, A., 2000. Surface analysis of machined versus sandblasted and acid-etched titanium implants. International Journal of Oral & Maxillofacial Implants 15, 779–784.

Padovano, J.D., Ravindran, S., Snee, P.T., Ramachandran, A., Bedran-Russo, A.K., George, A., 2015. DMP1-derived peptides promote remineralization of human dentin. Journal of Dental Research 94, 608–614.

Paine, M.L., Snead, M.L., 1997. Protein interactions during assembly of the enamel organic extracellular matrix. Journal of Bone and Mineral Research 12, 221–227.

Paine, M.L., Luo, W., Zhu, D.H., Bringas, P., Snead, M.L., 2003. Functional domains for amelogenin revealed by compound genetic defects. Journal of Bone and Mineral Research 18, 466–472.

Palmquist, A., Lindberg, F., Emanuelsson, L., Branemark, R., Engqvist, H., Thomsen, P., 2010. Biomechanical, histological, and ultrastructural analyses of laser micro- and nano-structured titanium alloy implants: a study in rabbit. Journal of Biomedical Materials Research Part A 92A, 1476–1486.

Pampena, D.A., Robertson, K.A., Litvinova, O., Lajoie, G., Goldberg, H.A., Hunter, G.K., 2004. Inhibition of hydroxyapatite formation by osteopontin phosphopeptides. Biochemical Journal 378, 1083–1087.

Park, J., Bauer, S., Von Der Mark, K., Schmuki, P., 2007. Nanosize and vitality: TiO_2 nanotube diameter directs cell fate. Nano Letters 7, 1686–1691.

Pasupuleti, M., Schmidtchen, A., Malmsten, M., 2012. Antimicrobial peptides: key components of the innate immune system. Critical Reviews in Biotechnology 32, 143–171.

Pender, M.J., Sowards, L.A., Hartgerink, J.D., Stone, M.O., Naik, R.R., 2006. Peptide-mediated formation of single-wall carbon nanotube composites. Nano Letters 6, 40–44.

Pokroy, B., Quintana, J.P., Caspi, E.A.N., Berner, A., Zolotoyabko, E., 2004. Anisotropic lattice distortions in biogenic aragonite. Nature Materials 3, 900–902.

Pokroy, B., Fitch, A.N., Lee, P.L., Quintana, J.P., Caspi, E.A.N., Zolotoyabko, E., 2006. Anisotropic lattice distortions in the mollusk-made aragonite: a widespread phenomenon. Journal of Structural Biology 153, 145–150.

Pokroy, B., Demensky, V., Zolotoyabko, E., 2009. Nacre in mollusk shells as a multilayered structure with strain gradient. Advanced Functional Materials 19, 1054–1059.

Price, J.S., Tencer, A.F., Arm, D.M., Bohach, G.A., 1996. Controlled release of antibiotics from coated orthopedic implants. Journal of Biomedical Materials Research 30, 281–286.

Raja, K.S., Misra, M., Paramguru, K., 2005. Deposition of calcium phosphate coating on nanotubular anodized titanium. Materials Letters 59, 2137–2141.

Rakngarm, A., Mutoh, Y., 2009. Characterization and fatigue damage of plasma sprayed HAp top coat with Ti and HAp/Ti bond coat layers on commercially pure titanium substrate. Journal of the Mechanical Behavior of Biomedical Materials 2, 444–453.

Rathbone, C.R., Cross, J.D., Brown, K.V., Murray, C.K., Wenke, J.C., 2011. Effect of various concentrations of antibiotics on osteogenic cell viability and activity. Journal of Orthopaedic Research 29, 1070–1074.

Rautray, T.R., Narayanan, R., Kwon, T.-Y., Kim, K.-H., 2010. Surface modification of titanium and titanium alloys by ion implantation. Journal of Biomedical Materials Research Part B: Applied Biomaterials 93B, 581–591.

Reddy, K.V.R., Yedery, R.D., Aranha, C., 2004. Antimicrobial peptides: premises and promises. International Journal of Antimicrobial Agents 24, 536–547.

Redepenning, J., Schlessinger, T., Burnham, S., Lippiello, L., Miyano, J., 1996. Characterization of electrolytically prepared brushite and hydroxyapatite coatings on orthopedic alloys. Journal of Biomedical Materials Research 30, 287–294.

Rehman, I., Bonfield, W., 1997. Characterization of hydroxyapatite and carbonated apatite by photo acoustic FTIR spectroscopy. Journal of Materials Science: Materials in Medicine 8, 1–4.

Reznikov, N., Shahar, R., Weiner, S., 2014. Bone hierarchical structure in three dimensions. Acta Biomaterialia 10, 3815–3826.

Robinson, R.A., 1952. An electron-microscopic study of the crystalline inorganic component of bone and its relationship to the organic matrix. Journal of Bone & Joint Surgery.

Rossler, S., Sewing, A., Stolzel, M., Born, R., Scharnweber, D., Dard, M., Worch, H., 2003. Electrochemically assisted deposition of thin calcium phosphate coatings at near-physiological pH and temperature. Journal of Biomedical Materials Research Part A 64A, 655–663.

Roy, M.D., Stanley, S.K., Amis, E.J., Becker, M.L., 2008. Identification of a highly specific hydroxyapatite-binding peptide using phage display. Advanced Materials 20, 1830–1836.

Ruoslahti, E., 1996. RGD and other recognition sequences for integrins. Annual Review of Cell and Developmental Biology 12, 697–715.

Russell, A.D., Tattawasart, U., Maillard, J.Y., Furr, J.R., 1998. Possible link between bacterial resistance and use of antibiotics and biocides. Antimicrobial Agents and Chemotherapy 42, 2151.

Ryu, D.D.Y., Nam, D.H., 2000. Recent progress in biomolecular engineering. Biotechnology Progress 16, 2–16.

Saiz, E., Zimmermann, E.A., Lee, J.S., Wegst, U.G.K., Tomsia, A.P., 2013. Perspectives on the role of nanotechnology in bone tissue engineering. Dental Materials 29, 103–115.

Sanghvi, A.B., Miller, K.P.H., Belcher, A.M., Schmidt, C.E., 2005. Biomaterials functionalization using a novel peptide that selectively binds to a conducting polymer. Nature Materials 4, 496–502.

Sano, K.I., Shiba, K., 2003. A hexapeptide motif that electrostatically binds to the surface of titanium. Journal of the American Chemical Society 125, 14234–14235.

Sano, K.I., Sasaki, H., Shiba, K., 2005. Specificity and biomineralization activities of Ti-binding peptide-1 (TBP-1). Langmuir 21, 3090–3095.

Sano, K., Sasaki, H., Shiba, K., 2006. Utilization of the pleiotropy of a peptidic aptamer to fabricate heterogeneous nanodot-containing multilayer nanostructures. Journal of the American Chemical Society 128, 1717–1722.

Sarikaya, M., Tamerler, C., 2009. Peptide-based functional nanostructures. Abstracts of Papers of the American Chemical Society 238.

Sarikaya, M., Tamerler, C., Jen, A.K.Y., Schulten, K., Baneyx, F., 2003. Molecular biomimetics: nanotechnology through biology. Nature Materials 2, 577–585.

Sarikaya, M., Tamerler, C., Schwartz, D.T., Baneyx, F.O., 2004. Materials assembly and formation using engineered polypeptides. Annual Review of Materials Research 34, 373–408.

Sarikaya, M., 1999. Biomimetics: materials fabrication through biology. Proceedings of the National Academy of Sciences of the United States of America 96, 14183–14185.
Sauro, S., Osorio, R., Watson, T.F., Toledano, M., 2015. Influence of phosphoproteins' biomimetic analogs on remineralization of mineral-depleted resin-dentin interfaces created with ion-releasing resin-based systems. Dental Materials 31, 759–777.
Schliephake, H., Aref, A., Scharnweber, D., Roessler, S., Sewing, A., 2009. Effect of modifications of dual acid-etched implant surfaces on periimplant bone formation. Part II: calcium phosphate coatings. Clinical Oral Implants Research 20, 38–44.
Seeman, N.C., Belcher, A.M., 2002. Emulating biology: building nanostructures from the bottom up. Proceedings of the National Academy of Sciences of the United States of America 99, 6451–6455.
Seker, U.O.S., Wilson, B., Dincer, S., Kim, I.W., Oren, E.E., Evans, J.S., Tamerler, C., Sarikaya, M., 2007a. Adsorption behavior of linear and cyclic genetically engineered platinum binding peptides. Langmuir 23, 7895–7900.
Seker, U.O.S., Wilson, B.R., Tamerler, C., Sarikaya, M., 2007b. Thermodynamical analysis of the gold surface recognition by a gold binding peptide. Abstracts of Papers of the American Chemical Society 233.
Seker, U.O.S., Wilson, B., Sahin, D., Tamerler, C., Sarikaya, M., 2009. Quantitative affinity of genetically engineered repeating polypeptides to inorganic surfaces. Biomacromolecules 10, 250–257.
Shiba, K., 2010. Exploitation of peptide motif sequences and their use in nanobiotechnology. Current Opinion in Biotechnology 21, 412–425.
Shimotoyodome, A., Koudate, T., Kobayashi, H., Nakamura, J., Tokimitsu, I., Hase, T., Inoue, T., Matsukubo, T., Takaesu, Y., 2007. Reduction of *Streptococcus mutans* adherence and dental biofilm formation by surface treatment with phosphorylated polyethylene glycol. Antimicrobial Agents and Chemotherapy 51, 3634–3641.
Shirkhanzadeh, M., 1998. Direct formation of nanophase hydroxyapatite on cathodically polarized electrodes. Journal of Materials Science: Materials in Medicine 9, 67–72.
Slocik, J.M., Naik, R.R., 2006. Biologically programmed synthesis of bimetallic nanostructures. Advanced Materials 18, 1988–1992.
Ślósarczyk, A., Paszkiewicz, Z., Paluszkiewicz, C., 2005. FTIR and XRD evaluation of carbonated hydroxyapatite powders synthesized by wet methods. Journal of Molecular Structure 744–747, 657–661.
Smith, D.C., 1993. Dental implants: materials and design considerations. International Journal of Prosthodontics 6, 106–117.
Snead, M.L., Zhu, D., Lei, Y., White, S.N., Snead, C.M., Luo, W., Paine, M.L., 2006. Protein self-assembly creates a nanoscale device for biomineralization. Materials Science & Engineering C: Biomimetic and Supramolecular Systems 26, 1296–1300.
Socransky, S.S., Haffajee, A.D., 2002. Dental biofilms: difficult therapeutic targets. Periodontology 2000 28, 12–55.
Spencer, P., Ye, Q., Park, J., Topp, E.M., Misra, A., Marangos, O., Wang, Y., Bohaty, B.S., Singh, V., Sene, F., Eslick, J., Camarda, K., Katz, J.L., 2010. Adhesive/dentin interface: the weak link in the composite restoration. Annals of Biomedical Engineering 38, 1989–2003.
Stojanovic, D., Jokic, B., Veljovic, D., Petrovic, R., Uskokovic, P.S., Janackovic, D., 2007. Bioactive glass-apatite composite coating for titanium implant synthesized by electrophoretic deposition. Journal of the European Ceramic Society 27, 1595–1599.
Taller, A., Grohe, B., Rogers, K.A., Goldberg, H.A., Hunter, G.K., 2007. Specific adsorption of osteopontin and synthetic polypeptides to calcium oxalate monohydrate crystals. Biophysical Journal 93, 1768–1777.

Tamerler, C., Sarikaya, M., 2007. Molecular biomimetics: utilizing naturels molecular ways in practical engineering. Acta Biomaterialia 3, 289–299.

Tamerler, C., Sarikaya, M., 2008. Molecular biomimetics: genetic synthesis, assembly, and formation of materials using peptides. Mrs Bulletin 33, 504–510.

Tamerler, C., Sarikaya, M., 2009a. Genetically designed peptide-based molecular materials. ACS Nano 3, 1606–1615.

Tamerler, C., Sarikaya, M., 2009b. Molecular biomimetics: nanotechnology and bionanotechnology using genetically engineered peptides. Philosophical Transactions of the Royal Society A: Mathematical Physical and Engineering Sciences 367, 1705–1726.

Tamerler, C., Dincer, S., Heidel, D., Zareie, M.H., Sarikaya, M., 2003. Biomimetic multifunctional molecular coatings using engineered proteins. Progress in Organic Coatings 47, 267–274.

Tamerler, C., Oren, E.E., Duman, M., Venkatasubramanian, E., Sarikaya, M., 2006. Adsorption kinetics of an engineered gold binding peptide by surface plasmon resonance spectroscopy and a quartz crystal microbalance. Langmuir 22, 7712–7718.

Tamerler, C., Kacar, T., Sahin, D., Fong, H., Sarikaya, M., 2007. Genetically engineered polypeptides for inorganics: a utility in biological materials science and engineering. Materials Science & Engineering C: Biomimetic and Supramolecular Systems 27, 558–564.

Tamerler, C., Khatayevich, D., Gungormus, M., Kacar, T., Oren, E.E., Hnilova, M., Sarikaya, M., 2010. Molecular biomimetics: GEPI-based biological routes to technology. Biopolymers 94, 78–94.

Tamerler, C., 2011. Biology enabled nanotechnology: biomolecular approaches in materials assembly and synthesis. Current Opinion in Biotechnology 22, S30.

Tan, K., Cheang, P., Ho, I.A.W., Lam, P.Y.P., Hui, K.M., 2007. Nanosized bioceramic particles could function as efficient gene delivery vehicles with target specificity for the spleen. Gene Therapy 14, 828–835.

Taubman, M.A., Valverde, P., Han, X.Z., Kawai, T., 2005. Immune response: the key to bone resorption in periodontal disease. Journal of Periodontology 76, 2033–2041.

Thai, C.K., Dai, H.X., Sastry, M.S.R., Sarikaya, M., Schwartz, D.T., Baneyx, F., 2004. Identification and characterization of Cu_2O- and ZnO-binding polypeptides by *Escherichia coli* cell surface display: toward an understanding of metal oxide binding. Biotechnology and Bioengineering 87, 129–137.

Tomasio, S.D.M., Walsh, T.R., 2007. Atomistic modelling of the interaction between peptides and carbon nanotubes. Molecular Physics 105, 221–229.

Tomsia, A.P., Launey, M.E., Lee, J.S., Mankani, M.H., Wegst, U.G.K., Saiz, E., 2011. Nanotechnology approaches to improve dental implants. International Journal of Oral & Maxillofacial Implants 26, 25–44.

Trisi, P., Lazzara, R., Rao, W., Rebaudi, A., 2002. Bone-implant contact and bone quality: evaluation of expected and actual bone contact on machined and Osseotite implant surfaces. International Journal of Periodontics & Restorative Dentistry 22, 535–545.

Tye, C.E., Rattray, K.R., Warner, K.J., Gordon, J.A.R., Sodek, J., Hunter, G.K., Goldberg, H.A., 2003. Delineation of the hydroxyapatite-nucleating domains of bone sialoprotein. Journal of Biological Chemistry 278, 7949–7955.

Uckay, I., Hoffmeyer, P., Lew, D., Pittet, D., 2013. Prevention of surgical site infections in orthopaedic surgery and bone trauma: state-of-the-art update. Journal of Hospital Infection 84, 5–12.

Utku, F.S., Klein, E., Saybasili, H., Yucesoy, C.A., Weiner, S., 2008. Probing the role of water in lamellar bone by dehydration in the environmental scanning electron microscope. Journal of Structural Biology 162, 361–367.

Utku, F.S., Seckin, E., Goller, G., Tamerler, C., Urgen, M., 2014. Carbonated hydroxyapatite deposition at physiological temperature on ordered titanium oxide nanotubes using pulsed electrochemistry. Ceramics International 40, 15479–15487.

Utku, F.S., Seckin, E., Goller, G., Tamerler, C., Urgen, M., 2015a. Electrochemically designed interfaces: hydroxyapatite coated macro-mesoporous titania surfaces. Applied Surface Science 350, 62–68.

Utku, F.S., Yuca, E., Seckin, E., Goller, G., Karatas, A.Y., Urgen, M., Tamerler, C., 2015b. Protein-mediated hydroxyapatite composite layer formation on nanotubular titania. Bioinspired, Biomimetic and Nanobiomaterials 4, 155–165.

Van de Sande, F.H., Opdam, N.J., Da Rosa Rodolpho, P.A., Correa, M.B., Demarco, F.F., Cenci, M.S., 2013. Patient risk factors' influence on survival of posterior composites. Journal of Dental Research 92, S78–S83.

Variola, F., Brunski, J.B., Orsini, G., De Oliveira, P.T., Wazen, R., Nanci, A., 2011. Nanoscale surface modifications of medically relevant metals: state-of-the art and perspectives. Nanoscale 3, 335–353.

Vreuls, C., Zocchi, G., Genin, A., Archambeau, C., Martial, J., Van De Weerdt, C., 2010. Inorganic-binding peptides as tools for surface quality control. Journal of Inorganic Biochemistry 104, 1013–1021.

Wang, L., Nancollas, G.H., 2009. Pathways to biomineralization and biodemineralization of calcium phosphates: the thermodynamic and kinetic controls. Dalton Transactions 2665–2672.

Wang, H., Lin, C., Hu, R., 2009. Effects of structure and composition of the CaP composite coatings on apatite formation and bioactivity in simulated body fluid. Applied Surface Science 255, 4074–4081.

Wazen, R.M., Tye, C.E., Goldberg, H.A., Hunter, G.K., Smith, C.E., Nanci, A., 2007. In vivo functional analysis of polyglutamic acid domains in recombinant bone sialoprotein. Journal of Histochemistry & Cytochemistry 55, 35–42.

Wegst, U.G.K., Bai, H., Saiz, E., Tomsia, A.P., Ritchie, R.O., 2014. Bioinspired structural materials. Nature Materials (advance online publication).

Wei, J.H., Kacar, T., Tamerler, C., Sarikaya, M., Ginger, D.S., 2009. Nanopatterning peptides as bifunctional inks for templated assembly. Small 5, 689–693.

Weiner, S., Traub, W., 1986. Organization of hydroxyapatite crystals within collagen fibrils. FEBS Letters 206, 262–266.

Weiner, S., Wagner, H.D., 1998. The material bone: structure mechanical function relations. Annual Review of Materials Science 28, 271–298.

Wen, X., Cawthorn, W.P., Macdougald, O.A., Stupp, S.I., Snead, M.L., Zhou, Y., 2011. The influence of Leucine-rich amelogenin peptide on MSC fate by inducing Wnt10b expression. Biomaterials 32, 6478–6486.

Whaley, S.R., English, D.S., Hu, E.L., Barbara, P.F., Belcher, A.M., 2000. Selection of peptides with semiconductor binding specificity for directed nanocrystal assembly. Nature 405, 665–668.

Wiedenmann, J., Oswald, F., Nienhaus, G.U., 2009. Fluorescent proteins for live cell imaging: opportunities, limitations, and challenges. IUBMB Life 61, 1029–1042.

Wininger, D.A., Fass, R.J., 1996. Antibiotic-impregnated cement and beads for orthopedic infections. Antimicrobial Agents and Chemotherapy 40, 2675–2679.

Woesz, A., Weaver, J.C., Kazanci, M., Dauphin, Y., Aizenberg, J., Morse, D.E., Fratzl, P., 2006. Micromechanical properties of biological silica in skeletons of deep-sea sponges. Journal of Materials Research 21, 2068–2078.

Woodbury, R.G., Wendin, C., Clendenning, J., Melendez, J., Elkind, J., Bartholomew, D., Brown, S., Furlong, C.E., 1998. Construction of biosensors using a gold-binding polypeptide and a miniature integrated surface plasmon resonance sensor. Biosensors & Bioelectronics 13, 1117–1126.

Xiao, S.J., Textor, M., Spencer, N.D., Wieland, M., Keller, B., Sigrist, H., 1997. Immobilization of the cell-adhesive peptide Arg–Gly–Asp–Cys (RGDC) on titanium surfaces by covalent chemical attachment. Journal of Materials Science: Materials in Medicine 8, 867–872.

Yang, P., Quan, Z., Li, C., Kang, X., Lian, H., Lin, J., 2008. Bioactive, luminescent and mesoporous europium-doped hydroxyapatite as a drug carrier. Biomaterials 29, 4341–4347.

Yazici, H., Fong, H., Wilson, B., Oren, E.E., Amos, F.A., Zhang, H., Evans, J.S., Snead, M.L., Sarikaya, M., Tamerler, C., 2013. Biological response on a titanium implant-grade surface functionalized with modular peptides. Acta Biomaterialia 9, 5341–5352.

Yeung, T., Georges, P.C., Flanagan, L.A., Marg, B., Ortiz, M., Funaki, M., Zahir, N., Ming, W.Y., Weaver, V., Janmey, P.A., 2005. Effects of substrate stiffness on cell morphology, cytoskeletal structure, and adhesion. Cell Motility and the Cytoskeleton 60, 24–34.

Yokoo, N., Togashi, T., Umetsu, M., Tsumoto, K., Hattori, T., Nakanishi, T., Ohara, S., Takami, S., Naka, T., Abe, H., Kumagai, I., Adschiri, T., 2010. Direct and selective immobilization of proteins by means of an inorganic material-binding peptide: discussion on functionalization in the elongation to material-binding peptide. Journal of Physical Chemistry B 114, 480–486.

Yoshinari, M., Kato, T., Matsuzaka, K., Hayakawa, T., Shiba, K., 2010. Prevention of biofilm formation on titanium surfaces modified with conjugated molecules comprised of antimicrobial and titanium-binding peptides. Biofouling 26, 103–110.

Yuca, E., Karatas, A.Y., Seker, U.O.S., Gungormus, M., Dinler-Doganay, G., Sarikaya, M., Tamerler, C., 2011. In vitro labeling of hydroxyapatite minerals by an engineered protein. Biotechnology and Bioengineering 108, 1021–1030.

Yucesoy, D.T., Hnilova, M., Boone, K., Arnold, P.M., Snead, M.L., Tamerler, C., 2015a. Chimeric peptides as implant functionalization agents for titanium alloy implants with antimicrobial properties. JOM 67, 754–766.

Yucesoy, D.T., Karaca, B.T., Cetinel, S., Caliskan, H.B., Adali, E., Gul-Karaguler, N., Tamerler, C., 2015b. Direct bioelectrocatalysis at the interfaces by genetically engineered dehydrogenase. Bioinspired Biomimetic and Nanobiomaterials 4, 79–89.

Zaheer, A., Lenkinski, R.E., Mahmood, A., Jones, A.G., Cantley, L.C., Frangioni, J.V., 2001. In vivo near-infrared fluorescence imaging of osteoblastic activity. Nature Biotechnology 19, 1148–1154.

Zaslansky, P., Friesem, A.A., Weiner, S., 2006. Structure and mechanical properties of the soft zone separating bulk dentin and enamel in crowns of human teeth: insight into tooth function. Journal of Structural Biology 153, 188–199.

Zasloff, M., 2002. Antimicrobial peptides of multicellular organisms. Nature 415, 389–395.

Zhang, S., Gangal, G., Uludag, H., 2007. 'Magic bullets' for bone diseases: progress in rational design of bone-seeking medicinal agents. Chemical Society Reviews 36, 507–531.

Zhang, Y., Yuan, Y., Liu, C., 2008. Fluorescent labeling of nanometer hydroxyapatite. Journal of Materials Science & Technology 24, 187–191.

Zhang, Q., Leng, Y., Lu, X., Xin, R., Yang, X., Chen, J., 2009. Bioactive films on metallic surfaces for osteoconduction. Journal of Biomedical Materials Research Part A 88A, 481–490.

Zhang, S., Karaca, B.T., Vanoosten, S.K., Yuca, E., Mahalingam, S., Edirisinghe, M., Tamerler, C., 2015. Coupling infusion and gyration for the nanoscale assembly of functional polymer nanofibers integrated with genetically engineered proteins. Macromolecular Rapid Communications 36, 1322–1328.

Zhao, L., Chu, P.K., Zhang, Y., Wu, Z., 2009. Antibacterial coatings on titanium implants. Journal of Biomedical Materials Research Part B: Applied Biomaterials 91B, 470–480.

Zhou, Y., Snead, M.L., Tamerler, C., 2015. Bio-inspired hard-to-soft interface for implant integration to bone. Nanomedicine: Nanotechnology Biology and Medicine 11, 431–434.

Zimmer, M., 2002. Green fluorescent protein (GFP): applications, structure, and related photophysical behavior. Chemical Reviews 102, 759–781.

Zin, M.T., Ma, H., Sarikaya, M., Jen, A.K.Y., 2005. Assembly of gold nanoparticles using genetically engineered polypeptides. Small 1, 698–702.

Zin, M.T., Munro, A.M., Gungormus, M., Wong, N.Y., Ma, H., Tamerler, C., Ginger, D.S., Sarikaya, M., Jen, A.K.Y., 2007. Peptide-mediated surface-immobilized quantum dot hybrid nanoassemblies with controlled photoluminescence. Journal of Materials Chemistry 17, 866–872.

Stem cells and dental tissue reconstruction

13

G.T.-J. Huang, F. Garcia-Godoy
University of Tennessee Health Science Center, Memphis, TN, United States

13.1 Introduction

Cell-based tissue engineering and regeneration is a very important approach to repair relatively large tissue or organ defects that have gone beyond what cell-free approach can accomplish. It involves the delivery of exogenous cells obtained from either autologous or allogenic source. The advantage of using stem/progenitor cells instead of differentiated cells for such purposes is that these cells can proliferate to the needed amount before or after transplantation. Before stem cells were discovered in dental tissues, research on dental tissue regeneration was limited. In 2000, dental pulp stem cells (DPSCs) harbored in the pulp of permanent teeth were discovered and reported (Gronthos et al., 2000). DPSCs are mesenchymal/stromal stem cell (MSC)-like populations with more specific properties for differentiating into dental cell lineages. Since then, there has been vigorous research effort to characterize dental stem cells (DSCs) and to test various tissue engineering approaches to regenerate dental tissues using these stem cells. DSCs have also shown potential for regeneration of non-dental tissues. On the other hand, nonoral source MSCs such as bone marrow-derived MSCs (BMMSCs) and adipose tissue MSCs (AdMSCs) have been explored for their use for dental tissue regeneration. This chapter presents the general characteristics of stem cells with a focus on DSCs and reviews the use of these stem cells for dental tissue regeneration, particularly regarding pulp–dentin, periodontal ligament (PDL), and whole tooth regeneration.

13.2 Dental stem cells

Stem cell biology examines the dynamics of cell physiology as to how stem cells maintain their stemness and give rise to specialized cells. This field has become a fundamental underpinning for understanding developmental biology and establishing cell-based regenerative therapies. DSCs exist in different parts or developmental stages of dental tissues, as illustrated in Fig. 13.1. These DSCs will be reviewed in the following discussion. The basic stem cell concepts and properties will first be briefly introduced.

Material-Tissue Interfacial Phenomena. http://dx.doi.org/10.1016/B978-0-08-100330-5.00013-3

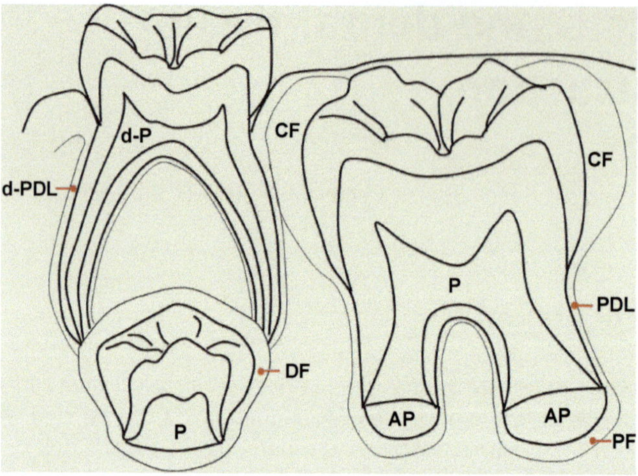

Figure 13.1 Dental tissues that give rise to dental stem cells. *P*, pulp of permanent teeth—it gives rise to dental pulp stem cells; *d-P*, pulp of shedding deciduous teeth—gives rise to stem cells from exfoliated deciduous teeth; *PDL*, periodontal ligament—gives rise to periodontal ligament stem cells (PDLSCs); *d-PDL*, PDL of deciduous teeth—gives rise to deciduous PDLSCs; *DF*, dental follicle—gives dental follicle stem cells (DFSCs); *CF*, coronal follicle—gives DFSCs; *PF*, periapical follicle—gives periapical follicle stem cells; *AP*, apical papilla—gives stem cells from apical papilla.

13.2.1 Key properties of stem cells

The two most important characteristics of stem cells are that they can self-renew and differentiate into different lineages of specialized cells. Commonly discussed stem cells for therapeutic use are pluripotent stem cells and multipotent stem cells. The former are capable of differentiating into all types, and the latter are capable of giving rise to multiple lineages of cells (Robey and Bianco, 2006). In terms of maturity, pluripotent stem cells are less mature than multipotent stem cells and it is determined at the epigenetic level. Pluripotent genes such as NANOG, OCT4, and SOX2 are highly expressed in pluripotent stem cells, less expressed in multipotent stem cells, and are normally not expressed in differentiated cells. The promoter regions of these genes are least methylated at the pluripotent state, whereas heavily methylated when the cells are differentiated.

13.2.2 Embryonic, induced pluripotent, and multipotent stem cells

13.2.2.1 Human embryonic stem cells

The human embryonic stem cell (hESC) line was established in 1998 (Thomson et al., 1998). These cells are maintained in undifferentiated state and expanded on feeder cells or in a feeder-free culture system. Because hESCs can continuously expand in culture and can differentiate into any cell type, they have been considered as a good cell source for stem cell–based regenerative therapies. The drawback for their clinical use is their allogeneic source, which may be rejected by the recipients. Also, hESCs may form teratoma in vivo if any cell failed to differentiate. Currently, there are a number of clinical trials treating retinal degenerative diseases using hESC-derived retina pigmented epithelial cells, and so far none have shown the development of tumors (Peterson and Loring, 2014). One report using hESCs for retina regeneration to restore the eyesight of patients showed no adverse effects after 4 months of cell transplantation (Schwartz et al., 2012).

13.2.2.2 Induced pluripotent stem cells

The establishment of induced pluripotent stem cells (iPSCs) has been considered a groundbreaking discovery in stem cell biology and medicine (Huang, 2010). With this approach, almost any cell type can be reprogrammed into pluripotent stem cells by delivering four factors, *c-MYC*, *KLF4*, *OCT4*, and *SOX2* (Takahashi and Yamanaka, 2006; Takahashi et al., 2007). Therefore, patient-specific iPSCs can be established for various medical purposes. Although there is a concern regarding the clinical use of iPSCs because mutations may occur during the reprogramming (Gore et al., 2011; Lister et al., 2011), iPSCs may replace the need of embryonic stem cells as a cell source for clinical medicine in the future if these cells are proven to be clinically safe. The ongoing clinical trials with iPSCs will address these issues (Cyranoski, 2013). It has been shown that transplantation of human iPSC-derived neural stem cells (NSCs) enhanced axonal sparing, regrowth without tumor formation; prevented the demyelination after spinal cord injury; and promoted functional recovery in an animal study model (Kobayashi et al., 2012).

iPSCs were first established by delivering the four factors into dermal fibroblasts (DFs). Subsequently, other sources of cells such as oral stem cells have been shown to be more feasible and accessible for reprogramming into iPSCs (Fig. 13.2) (Miyoshi et al., 2010; Tamaoki et al., 2010; Wada et al., 2011; Yan et al., 2010).

13.2.2.3 Multipotent stem cells

Stem cells that are not as potent as pluripotent stem cells are multipotent stem cells, and they include stem cells from fetal tissues. Adult stem cells (also known as postnatal stem cells) are multipotent stem cells that are not capable of giving rise to all cell types. Some reports showed that certain adult stem cells can become cells of all germ layers and form teratomalike tissues in vivo demonstrating their near-pluripotent capacity (Marynka-Kalmani et al., 2010; Pelaez et al., 2013). There are two main types of adult stem cells in the bone marrow, hematopoietic stem cells and MSCs. Bone marrow–derived MSCs (BMMSCs) are the best characterized MSCs, and they were described as colony-forming unit-fibroblasts (CFU-Fs) in vitro (Caplan, 1991; Cohnheim, 1867; Friedenstein et al., 1976; Pittenger et al., 1999). DSCs are MSC-like stem cells with trilineage differentiation potential, ie, osteo-, adipo-, and chondrogenic differentiation (Huang et al., 2009b; Morsczeck et al., 2013). Compared with BMMSCs, DSCs are in general less adipogenic and chondrogenic.

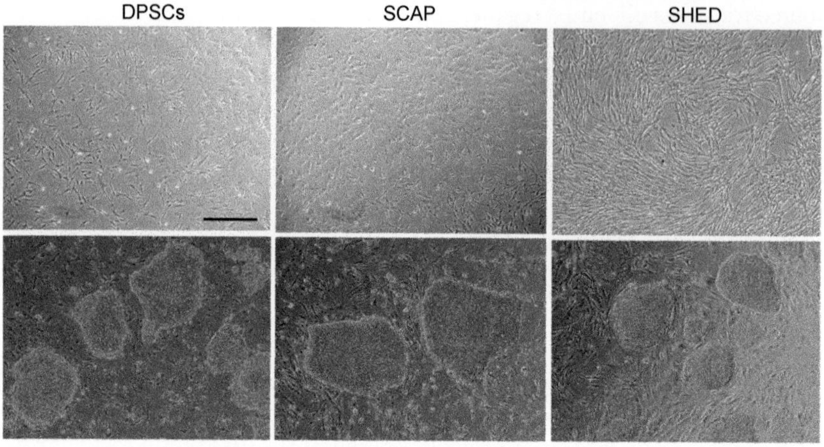

Figure 13.2 Induced pluripotent stem cells reprogrammed from human dental stem cells: dental pulp stem cells (DPSCs), stem cells from apical papilla (SCAP), and stem cells from exfoliated deciduous teeth (SHED). Top panel: DSCs before reprogramming. Lower panel: established iPSC colonies grown on mouse embryonic fibroblasts feeder cells after successful reprogramming and passaging in cultures. Scale bars: 500 μm.
Adapted from Yan X, Qin H, Qu C, Tuan RS, Shi S, Huang GT. iPS cells reprogrammed from human mesenchymal-like stem/progenitor cells of dental tissue origin. Stem Cells Dev 2010;19(4):469–80, with permission.

13.2.3 Stem cells in pulp and apical papilla

13.2.3.1 Dental pulp stem cells

DPSCs were isolated from postnatal teeth and compared with BMMSCs (Gronthos et al., 2000). Although DPSCs display features similar to BMMSCs including certain cell surface markers such as STRO-1, CD90, and CD146, DPSCs have two key different properties from BMMSCs. One is their greater population doubling (PD) in culture. BMMSCs have relatively limited growth potential, having only 30–50 PDs following ex vivo expansion (Bianco et al., 2001; Bruder et al., 1997), whereas DPSCs can reach >100 PDs (Huang et al., 2009b). In fact, DSCs tend to have greater growth potential than BMMSCs in vitro (Huang et al., 2009b).

The other key difference is the type of tissue regenerated in vivo. Although DPSCs share a similar pattern of gene expression with BMMSCs in vitro during induced odontogenic and/or osteogenic differentiation, DPSCs form ectopic pulp–dentin complex, whereas BMMSCs form bone and marrow when mixed with osteoinductive materials such as hydroxyapatite/tricalcium phosphate (HA/TCP) and transplanted into an in vivo study model (Gronthos et al., 2000; Shi and Gronthos, 2003).

While examining the gene profiles, there is preferential gene expression between DPSCs and BMMSCs (Shi et al., 2001). Higher expression levels of alkaline phosphomonoesterase (ALP), dentin sialophosphoprotein (DSPP), and dentin matrix acidic phosphoprotein 1 (DMP-1) were found in DPSCs after osteoinduction compared with BMMSCs (Yamada et al., 2006a). In terms of other differentiation capacities, DPSCs are weaker in chondrogenic and adipogenic potential compared with BMMSCs (Sonoyama et al., 2008; Zhang et al., 2006). Conversely, the neurogenicity of DPSCs is more potent than that of BMMSCs, most probably due to their neural crest (NC) origin.

Although DPSCs are a good cell source for dental tissue regeneration (Huang, 2009b), two features also make them a good source for nondental tissue regeneration. The first is their angiogenic and angioinductive property. A highly angiogenic subfraction of side population (SP) cells, $CD31^-/CD146^-$, was identified from the porcine DPSCs expressing CD34 and vascular endothelial growth factor receptor-2 (VEGFR2)/Flk1, which are similar to endothelial progenitor cells (Iohara et al., 2008). Porcine $CD31^-/CD146^-$ SP cell fractions transplanted into the striatum of adult rats induced neovascularization of the ischemic zone and enhanced subsequent neuronal regeneration (Sugiyama et al., 2011). Such an angioinductive capacity was tested for therapeutic potential in the repair of myocardial infarction (MI). Rats with induced MI showed an improvement in cardiac function 4 weeks after being injected with human DPSCs intramyocardially. Although no DPSCs were observed within the infarct, angiogenesis was increased relative to control treated animals (Gandia et al., 2008). The other feature is their neurogenic and neuroinductive capacity. As mentioned earlier, $CD31^-/CD146^-$ SP cell fractions have such a capacity that can enhance neuronal regeneration (Sugiyama et al., 2011). Although DPSCs can only be guided to neural-like cells with limited neuronal activities (Aanismaa et al., 2012; Arthur et al., 2008), they are capable of expressing a plethora of neurotrophic factors that induce endogenous axon guidance (Arthur et al., 2009), promoting proliferation and differentiation of endogenous neural cells in the hippocampus of mice (Huang et al., 2008a), and facilitating locomotor recovery after complete transection of the rat spinal cord (Sakai et al., 2012).

DPSCs treated with small molecules pluripotin (SC1), 6-bromoindirubin-3'-oxime (BIO), or rapamycin showed increased expression of STRO-1 and pluripotent genes NANOG, OCT4, and SOX2, indicating that their stemness may be extended in cultures by such a treatment (Al-Habib et al., 2013). Culturing DPSCs in the presence of platelet-derived growth factor (PDGF), (epidermal growth factor (EGF), and Leukemia inhibitory factor (LIF) also increases the expression of the pluripotent genes NANOG and OCT4 (Atari et al., 2012). DPSCs have been reprogrammed to iPSCs showing hESC characteristics, which may potentially be utilized for various medical applications (Tamaoki et al., 2010; Yan et al., 2010).

13.2.3.2 Stem cells from apical papilla

At the final stage of tooth development, most developing tissues have lost or disappeared, such as dental epithelium and dental papilla that make up the crown. After tooth eruption, the root continues to develop, and therefore a developing tissue still exists at this stage until the root apex is mature. This tissue is termed the apical papilla (Fig. 13.3), and MSC-like populations were isolated in the tissue termed stem cells from apical papilla (SCAP) (Abe et al., 2007; Degistirici et al., 2008; Huang et al., 2008b; Sonoyama et al., 2006, 2008). SCAP are similar to DPSCs in many aspects except the following two key features: (1) SCAP express CD24, and its expression is downregulated upon osteoinduction and (2) SCAP express survivin (Sonoyama et al., 2006).

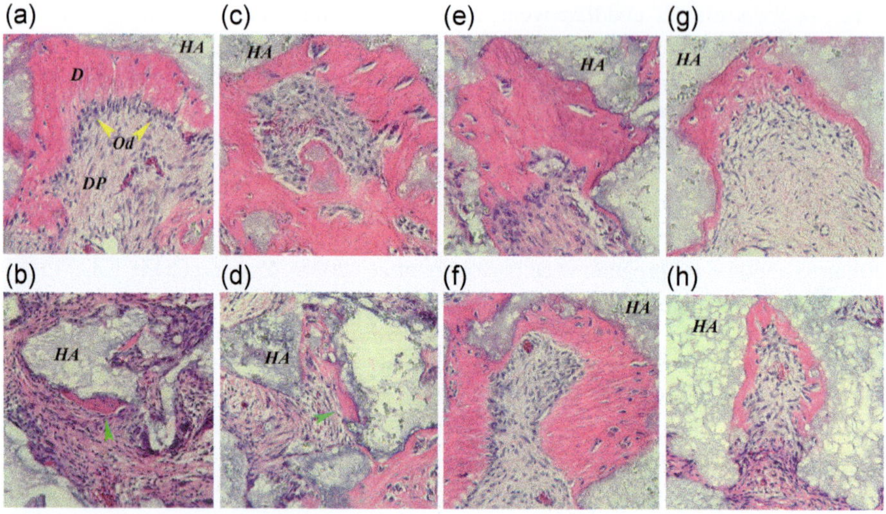

Figure 13.3 In vivo formation of pulp–dentin complexes by dental pulp stem cells (DPSCs)-inflamed pulp (DPSCs-IP). Cells mixed with hydroxyapatite (HA)/tricalcium phosphate were subcutaneously transplanted into Begie XIDIII nu/nu mice. After 8 weeks, the resected tissues were processed for hematoxylin & eosin staining. (a) DPSCs from normal pulps as the control. (b) DPSCs-IP multiple colony (MC), sample #1, 17-year-old male tooth #19. (c–f) DPSCs-IP, sample #2, 19-year-old male tooth #30. [(c) MC, (d) SC-4a, (e) SC-5a, and (f) SC-6b)]. (g, h) DPSCs-IP sample #3, 15-year-old male tooth #30. [(g) MC and (h) SC-6a]. SC: single colony. *Green arrows*, mineralized tissue; *yellow arrows*, odontoblastlike cells. Adapted from Alongi DJ, Yamaza T, Song Y, Fouad AF, Romberg EE, Shi S, et al. Stem/progenitor cells from inflamed human dental pulp retain tissue regeneration potential. Regen Med 2010;5(4):617–31, with permission.

SCAP have been shown to regenerate new vascularized pulplike tissue with the deposition of a new layer of dentinlike tissue in the root canal space of a tooth fragment model, which utilizes the in vivo environment of immunocompromised mice (Huang et al., 2009c). The discovery of SCAP has allowed a paradigm shift in the treatment of permanent immature teeth with endodontic infection (Huang, 2009a; Huang et al., 2008b). It has been considered that SCAP residing in the apical papilla that survives the endodontic infection may be chemoattracted into the canal space to regenerate the lost pulp tissue, although certain hurdles remain to be overcome (Huang and Garcia-Godoy, 2014).

SCAP express neuronal markers such as neuron-specific enolase (NSE), neurofilament M (NFM), and neuronal nuclear antigen (NeuN) after neurogenic induction. In fact, SCAP already express βIII-tubulin, NFM, NSE, and very low levels of 2',3'-Cyclic-nucleotide 3'-phosphodiesterase (CNPase) in culture without specific differentiation induction (Zou et al., 2012). Treatment with basic fibroblast growth factor (bFGF) can further enhance the stemness of SCAP with increased expression of STRO-1, NANOG, OCT4, SOX2, and REX1 as well as the ability to form colony-forming unit (Wu et al., 2012). SCAP have also been reprogrammed into iPSCs as a cell source for neuronogenesis (Zou et al., 2012).

The apical papilla is a padlike tissue at the apex of immature root (Degistirici et al., 2008; Sonoyama et al., 2008). Further apical to the apical papilla, there is a layer of soft tissue termed periapical follicle, which is the developing tissue that will mature into PDL and cementum.

13.2.3.3 Stem cells from human exfoliated deciduous teeth

Stem cells also exist in the dental pulp of exfoliated primary teeth (Miura et al., 2003) (Fig. 13.1). Since these cells are normally from children shedding teeth around ages 6–12, they are relatively more immature stem cells than DPSCs or SCAP, which are usually obtained from the third molars of older individuals at ages 16–22. Stem cells from human exfoliated deciduous teeth (SHED) are also MSC-like with multi-differentiation potential and express embryonic stem cell markers OCT4, NANOG, stage-specific embryonic antigens (SSEA-3, SSEA-4), and tumor recognition antigens (TRA-1-60 and TRA-1-81) (Kerkis et al., 2006). They have a relatively high PD (>140) and can form sphere culture and expand in a manner similar to neurospheres formed by NSCs (Miura et al., 2003). Although they are from pulp tissue, their ability to form ectopic pulp-dentin complex in vivo is lacking or much weaker than that of DPSCs and SCAP (Miura et al., 2003). As a result, using SHED as a cell source to regenerate pulp tissue, the newly generated dentin on dentinal wall is minimal (Sakai et al., 2010).

Two important features of SHED that can be used for nondental tissue regeneration are their osteoinductive capacity and neurogenic potential. It was shown that SHED could not differentiate directly into osteoblasts, whereas they appeared to induce new bone formation by forming an osteoinductive template to recruit host osteogenic cells (Miura et al., 2003; Seo et al., 2008). Nonetheless, compared with BMMSCs, SHED-induced bone formation lacks the bona fide feature of bone/marrow structures.

SHED have strong neurogenic potential, and they readily express a variety of neural cell markers. SHED form neurospherelike aggregates similar to NSCs when cultured in neurogenic medium, and the expression of βIII-tubulin, GAD, and NeuN is increased (Miura et al., 2003). When injected into the dentate gyrus of the hippocampus of immunocompromised mice, SHED can survive in the mouse brain and express neural markers such as NFM. SHED can also be converted to dopaminergic neuron-like cells in vitro and appear to help in recovery from behavioral disorders associated with Parkinson disease after transplantation into the brain of parkinsonian rats (Wang et al., 2010). Similar to DPSCs, SHED also can differentiate to endothelium. Sakai et al. (2010) showed in the capillary sprouting assay in 3D collagen matrices that SHED treated with vascular endothelial growth factor increased sprouting and that VEGFR1 signaling is required for endothelial differentiation.

13.2.4 Stem cells in periodontal ligament

The PDL is a unique tissue that connects alveolar bone to tooth via a layer of mineralized tissue—cementum, which is very similar to bone. There are several cell types in PDL including fibroblasts, cementoblasts, and osteoblasts. Cementoblasts have been speculated to originate from Hertwig epithelial root sheath (HERS) via epithelial–mesenchymal transition (Thomas, 1995) and migrate from the paravascular cells in endosteal spaces of the alveolar bone (McCulloch et al., 1987), or the paravascularly located stem cells in the PDL (Seo et al., 2004).

13.2.4.1 Periodontal ligament stem cells

Periodontal ligament stem cells (PDLSCs) have been isolated from the PDL of third molars (Fig. 13.1). They are also MSC-like populations expressing STRO-1 and CD146 as well as scleraxis—a tendon cell–specific transcription factor (Seo et al., 2004). They also demonstrate trilineage differentiation potential (Gay et al., 2007; Seo et al., 2004). PDLSCs generate a periodontiumlike tissue when mixed with HA/TCP and transplanted into immunocompromised mice. The regenerated tissues showed cementum-like and PDL-like structures with dense collagenous fibers resembling Sharpey fibers (Seo et al., 2004). The isolation of PDLSCs allowed the study of cementogenesis of PDLSCs promoted by the HERS cells (Sonoyama et al., 2007), indicating that cementoblasts may be derived from PDLSCs. Additionally, STRO-1 and CD146 are detected in the paravascular niche of the PDL, and when the PDL is inflamed, STRO-1- and CD146-expressing cells are observed on the cementum surface (Chen et al., 2006), suggesting that paravascular PDLSCs may migrate to the cementum side becoming cementoblasts.

Similar to other DSCs mentioned, PDLSCs were also found to express pluripotent genes NANOG, OCT4, SOX2 ,and KLF4 as well as NC markers nestin, Slug, p75, and SOX10 (Huang et al., 2009a). Subpopulations of PDLSCs such as connexin 43 $(Cx43)^+$ and frizzled-9 $(CD349)^+$ cells express pluripotency-associated genes OCT4, NANOG, and SOX2, as well as NC-specific markers (Pelaez et al., 2013; Trubiani et al., 2010). Furthermore, these cells form teratomalike tissues encompassing the three embryological germ layers: endoderm, mesoderm, and ectoderm (Pelaez et al., 2013).

PDLSCs appear to participate in the regeneration of alveolar bone in addition to their cementogenic potential when transplanted into the periodontal defect (Seo et al., 2004), suggesting that they may also be osteogenic. In vitro studies also indicated the highly osteogenic potential of PDLSCs (Kato et al., 2011; Singhatanadgit et al., 2009); however, either ectopic or orthotopic in vivo bone regeneration showed that the newly formed bone is similar but not identical to the real bone, ie, lacking ability to form bone marrow despite mineralized tissues being present that express bone matrix proteins such as osteopontin, bone sialoprotein (BSP), and osteoclacin (Hiraga et al., 2009; Moshaverinia et al., 2014; Tour et al., 2012). The chondrogenic potential of PDLSCs was examined by stimulation of cells with transforming growth factor (TGF)-β3, bone morphogenetic protein (BMP)-6, or combination of both using standard pellet cultures (Choi et al., 2013). Although PDLSC pellets were able to express chondrogenic genes including aggrecan, collagen type II, and SOX9, and the pellets stained positive with alcian blue and safranin O, they lacked the typical chondrocyte and cartilage morphology (Choi et al., 2013). The STRO-1^+/CD146^+ subpopulation of PDLSCs appear to form more mature cartilage pellets after chondrogenic induction (Xu et al., 2009).

13.2.5 Stem cells in dental follicle

Dental follicle surrounds the entire developing tooth prior to eruption (Fig. 13.1). The coronal part of the follicle will eventually merge into gingival tissues as the tooth erupts. Little is known about the merging process. As soon as the root begins to form, the radicular part of the follicle gives rise to the periodontium, ie, the cementum, PDL, and alveolar bone. As the root continues to develop, the radicular follicle is located at the apex and is considered as the periapical follicle (Han et al., 2010). Precursor cells have been isolated from human dental follicle of impacted third molars termed dental follicle precursor cells (DFPCs) (Morsczeck et al., 2005).

13.2.5.1 Dental follicle stem/precursor cells

Based on the properties of DFSCs reported in the studies, stem cells exist in dental follicles, although they were first named DFPCs (Kémoun et al., 2007; Morsczeck et al., 2005). STRO-1 and BMP receptors are expressed in dental follicles in vivo (Kémoun et al., 2007). In cultures, they are MSC-like expressing STRO-1, NOTCH-1, Nestin, CD44, and fibroblast growth factor receptor1-IIIC (Kémoun et al., 2007; Morsczeck et al., 2005). Expression of cementum attachment protein and cementum protein-23, two putative cementoblast markers, has been detected in EMD-stimulated whole dental follicle and in cultured DFSCs stimulated with EMD or BMP2 and BMP7 (Kémoun et al., 2007). DFSCs demonstrate osteogenic differentiation capacity in vitro after induction and form tissues expressing BSP, osteocalcin (OCN), and collagen type I in vivo (Morsczeck et al., 2005; Morsczeck et al., 2008).

Like other DSCs, DFSCs also possess the trilineage differentiation potential (Kémoun et al., 2007). The neurogenic potential of DFSCs was tested and found to be similar to that of SHED inasmuch as they form neurospherelike cultures and differentiate into neural-like cells expressing βIII-tubulin and NSE (Völlner et al., 2009). The bone regeneration potential of human DFSCs was also studied using a rat calvarial defect model (Honda et al., 2011). Although DFSCs appear to promote bone formation, it is unclear whether the transplanted DFSCs become osteoblasts and form new bone in vivo.

13.2.5.2 Periapical follicle stem cells

As mentioned earlier, dental follicle becomes separated into coronal and radicular parts as the root develops (Fig. 13.1). The continued existence of the radicular dental follicle was not discussed until the identification of apical papilla in human immature permanent teeth (Sonoyama et al., 2006, 2008). However, the terminology of apical papilla varies. Abe et al. (2007) named it the "apical pulp" and the isolated cells were called the "apical pulp-derived cells; Degistirici et al. (2008) named it padlike and the outgrown explant cells were called dental NC-derived progenitor cells. The reason why Sonoyama et al. named it apical papilla is because it is considered as the dental papilla. Once the crown dentin is laid down and the root formation begins at the cervical loop, the dental papilla becomes the young pulp and the apical portion of the papilla continues to form root dentin in concert with the HERS (Huang et al., 2008b; Sonoyama et al., 2008).

Jo et al. (2007) reported the identification of periapical follicle stem cells (PAFSCs) isolated from what they considered as periapical follicle. However, their data did not clearly specify the exact location of the periapical follicle and its relationship to the apical papilla. Subsequently, Han et al. (2010) defined periapical follicle to be located outside the apical papilla. The authors reported that PAFSCs are MSC-like expressing STRO-1 and CD146 and have osteogenic and adipogenic potential. They proliferate faster than PDLSCs in vitro and form typical cementum-/PDL-like tissue in vivo (Han et al., 2010). PAFSCs appear to enhance the dentinogenesis of SCAP as the conditioned medium from PAFSCs appears to induce the ALP activity and osteo- and/or dentinogenic differentiation of SCAP in cultures (Wu et al., 2013).

13.2.6 Stem cells in inflamed dental tissues

13.2.6.1 Dental pulp stem cells from inflamed pulp

DPSCs have been isolated from inflamed pulp termed DPSCs-IP (Alongi et al., 2010). Overall, these DPSCs-IP appear to have lower PDs and less osteo- and/or odontogenic capacities in cultures compared with DPSCs from normal pulps. Some of these DPSCs-IP are capable of forming pulp–dentin complex in immunocompromised mice (Fig. 13.3). Other features such as levels of STRO-1 expression, morphology, proliferation rate, and colony forming in cultures do not differ from those of DPSCs from normal pulp (Pereira et al., 2012). These data suggest that DPSCs-IP may be used for various clinical application such as dental pulp regeneration.

13.2.6.2 Periodontal ligament stem cells from inflamed periodontal ligament

PDLSCs could be isolated from inflamed PDL tissues human periodontal ligament stem cells from inflamed PDL (ihPDLSCs) (Park et al., 2011). PDLSCs and ihPDLSCs expressed the same stem cell markers such as CD146 and STRO-1, and they had the same multipotent cell differentiation potential. From a clinical perspective, one may remove the inflamed PDL to isolate ihPDLSCs and replant the autologous cells for periodontal regeneration.

13.2.6.3 Inflamed periapical progenitor cells

The inflamed periapical tissues also contain progenitor cells. Osteogenic cells were first found in periapical lesions that have the potential to differentiate into mature osteoblastic cells (Maeda et al., 2004). Subsequently, Liao et al. detected STRO-1, CD146, and CD90 paravascularly in periapical lesions and cells isolated from the lesions formed CFU-Fs (Fig. 13.4(a)). These cultured cells expressed STRO-1, CD73, CD90, CD105, and CD146 (Fig. 13.4(b)) and are highly osteogenic and also showed adipogenic potential. When cells are mixed with HA/TCP and implanted into the immunocompromised mice, mineral tissue is formed but the amount is less when compared with DPSCs (Fig. 13.4(c)). It is to be noted that these cells divide slower than DPSCs, do not form high-density CFU-Fs after passaging, and only reach a PD of 23–26. Therefore, the authors considered that these cells are progenitors, not stem cells, and named

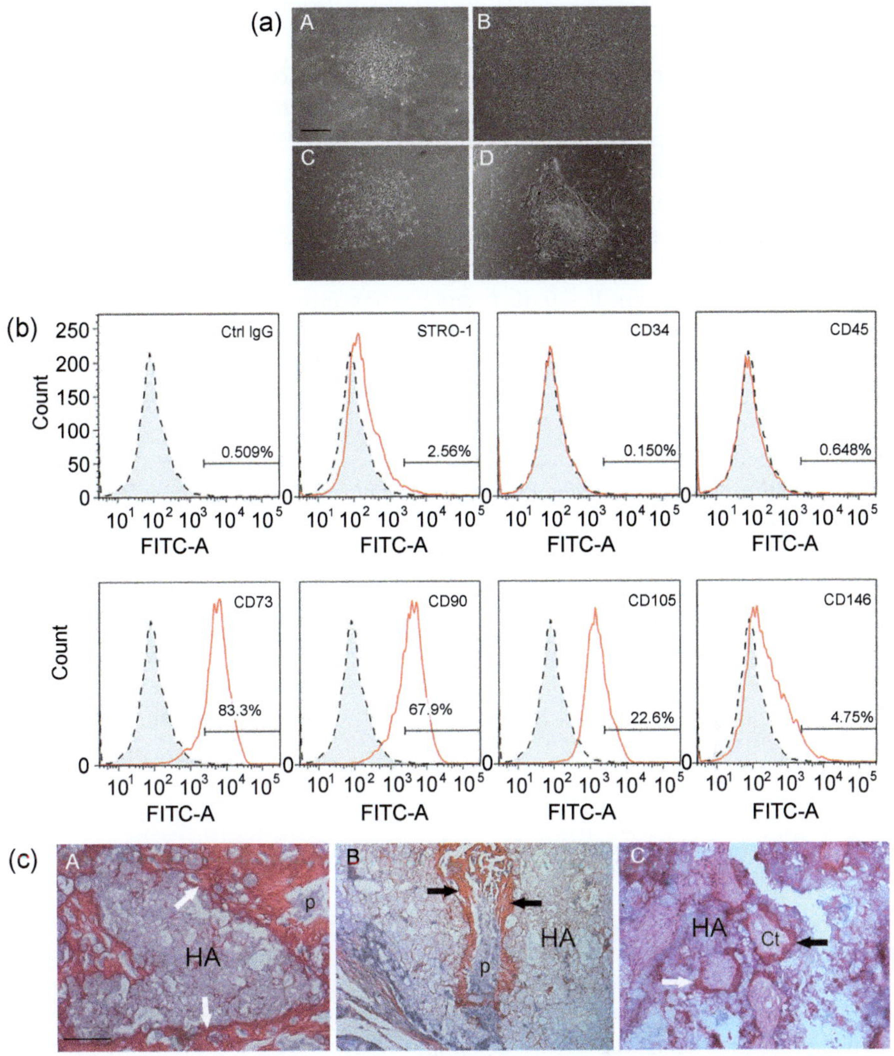

Figure 13.4 Isolation and characterization of inflamed periapical progenitor cells (iPAPCs). (a) Growth of cells isolated from inflamed periapical tissues at passage 0. (A–C) Colony-forming unit-fibroblasts of loose or denser colonies are shown. (D) Formation of an epithelial cell island, likely derived from epithelial cell rest of Malassez. Scale bar: 500 μm.
(b) Immunophenotyping of cells from inflamed periapical tissues. Heterogeneous pooled population of cells at passages two were analyzed with flow cytometry to detect cell surface marker expression. Dashed peaks are the controls, and solid peaks are the specific antibody staining. (c) In vivo formation of mineralized tissues. Cells mixed with hydroxyapatite (HA)/tricalcium phosphate were subcutaneously transplanted into severe combined immunodeficiency mice. After 8 weeks, the resected tissues were processed for hematoxylin & eosin staining. (A) DPSCs as positive controls. (B, C) iPAPCs. *p*, Dental pulplike; *Ct*, soft connective tissue. Arrows indicate mineralized tissue. Scale bar: 200 μm.
Adapted from Liao J, Al Shahrani M, Al-Habib M, Tanaka T, Huang GT. Cells isolated from inflamed periapical tissue express mesenchymal stem cell markers and are highly osteogenic. J Endod 2011;37(9):1217–24, with permission.

them "inflamed periapical progenitor cells (iPAPCs)'' (Liao et al., 2011). Dokic et al isolated these cells from periapical lesion (PL) and named them PL-MSCs, which also formed lose CFU-Fs expressing STRO-1, CD146, CD90, CD44, CD29, CD166, CD46, and CD105, and have trilineage differentiation potential. They further demonstrated that these PL-MSCs have immunosuppressive properties capable of inhibiting phytohemagglutinin-induced proliferation of peripheral blood mononuclear cells (PB-MNCs) and production of interleukin (IL)-2, interferon γ, and IL-5 in the coculture. These cells also suppressed the production of IL-1β, IL-6, and tumor necrosis factor-α by the inflammatory cells isolated from the periapical lesions via soluble mediators, whereas the suppression of IL-8 production required a direct cell-to-cell contact (Dokic et al., 2012). This immunosuppressive property was not strong enough to prevent xenographic rejection, as the transplantation of PL-MSCs into 1-day-old BALB/c mice did not lead to the formation of detectable tissues (Dokic et al., 2012).

The isolation of these cells may have significant indications if considering using periapical stem/progenitor cells for pulp regeneration. Current endodontic revitalization/revascularization protocols intend to bring stem/progenitor cells in the periapical tissues into the pulp space via creating a hemorrhage in the periapical area allowing blood clot formation in the canal. The blood clot may carry stem/progenitor cells for tissue regeneration (Lovelace et al., 2011). However, animal studies and human cases have indicated that the generated tissues in the canal via the revitalization technique may not lead to pulp–dentin regeneration (Lin et al., 2014; Wang et al., 2010b).

13.3 Dental tissue regeneration

In the field of tissue engineering and regeneration, approaches to regenerate tissues involve the use or nonuse of exogenous cell transplantation, meaning either cell-based or cell-free respectively. The tissue regeneration potential of the aforementioned stem cells is summarized in Table 13.1. The following sections will focus on the stem cell–based approach for dental tissue regeneration.

13.3.1 Dentin-pulp regeneration

While regenerating pulp–dentin was considered an almost impossible task, attempts to regenerate pulplike tissue in the canal space was made in the early 1960s. Inducing hemorrhage to form blood clots in the canal as mentioned earlier was tested 40–50 years ago in the hope to regenerate pulp tissue (Myers and Fountain, 1974; Ostby, 1961). No pulp or dentin except minimal amounts of fibrous tissues were grown into the canal. The emergence of tissue engineering sciences in the late 1990s drew researchers to test the newly developed synthetic material polyglycolic acid seeded with pulp fibroblasts for pulp regeneration, and pulplike tissue was formed in both in vitro and in vivo study models (Buurma et al., 1999; Gu et al., 1996; Mooney et al., 1996). Subsequently, DSCs were discovered as described earlier allowing researchers to further investigate pulp–dentin regeneration using these stem cells.

Table 13.1 Dental stem cells for tissue regeneration

Cell type	Dental tissue regeneration	Nondental tissue regeneration
DPSCs	• Dentin-pulp-like tissues • Bioroot	• Bonelike tissues • Neurogenic • Angiogenic
Stem cells from exfoliated deciduous teeth	• Pulplike	• Bonelike tissues • Neurogenic • Angiogenic
Stem cells from apical papilla	• Dentin-pulp-like tissues • Bioroot	—
PDLSCs	• Periodontal tissues	• Bonelike • Cartilagelike
Dental follicle stem/progenitor cells	• Periodontal tissues • Tooth root • Pulp–dentin tissues	—
Periapical follicle stem cells	• Peridontal tissues • Tooth root	—
DPSCs from inflamed pulp	• Dentin-pulp-like tissues	—
PDLSCs from inflamed PDL	—	—
Inflamed periapical progenitor cells	• Mineral tissues	—

DPSC, dental pulp stem cells; *PDL*, periodontal ligament; *PDLSC*, periodontal ligament stem cells.

Regenerative endodontics have also emerged as a new discipline in the field of endodontics (Murray et al., 2007). The cell-free approach for revitalization/revascularization has not shown pulp–dentin regeneration, whereas researchers focusing on stem cell-based approach in animal models have demonstrated the possibility of pulp and dentin regeneration in the root canal space (Fig. 13.5) (Huang et al., 2010; Iohara et al., 2011; Nakashima and Huang, 2013). Using an immunocompromised mouse model, Huang et al. (2010) demonstrated that human pulplike and/or dentinlike tissues can be de novo regenerated in emptied root canal space with blood supply from one end of the canal. Heterogeneous population of human DPSCs or SCAP were used in their study. In a dog model to test orthotopic pulp/dentin regeneration, Iohara et al. (2011) demonstrated the complete regeneration of pulp in mature teeth using $CD105^+$ subpopulation of DPSCs.

There has long been speculation that the undifferentiated mesenchymal cells residing in the periapical tissue or in the alveolar bone can be brought into the root canal space via induction of hemorrhage leading to blood clot formation, which may allow pulplike tissue regeneration with newly differentiated odontoblasts (Myers & Fountain, 1974). This idea continues to be the key concept of the recent revitalization protocol in regenerative endodontics as mentioned earlier; however, it has been questioned and discussed from several perspectives (Huang and Garcia-Godoy, 2014). One important point to note is whether nonodontoblastic lineages can differentiate into odontoblasts. Based on the studies, it is unlikely that odontoblasts can derive

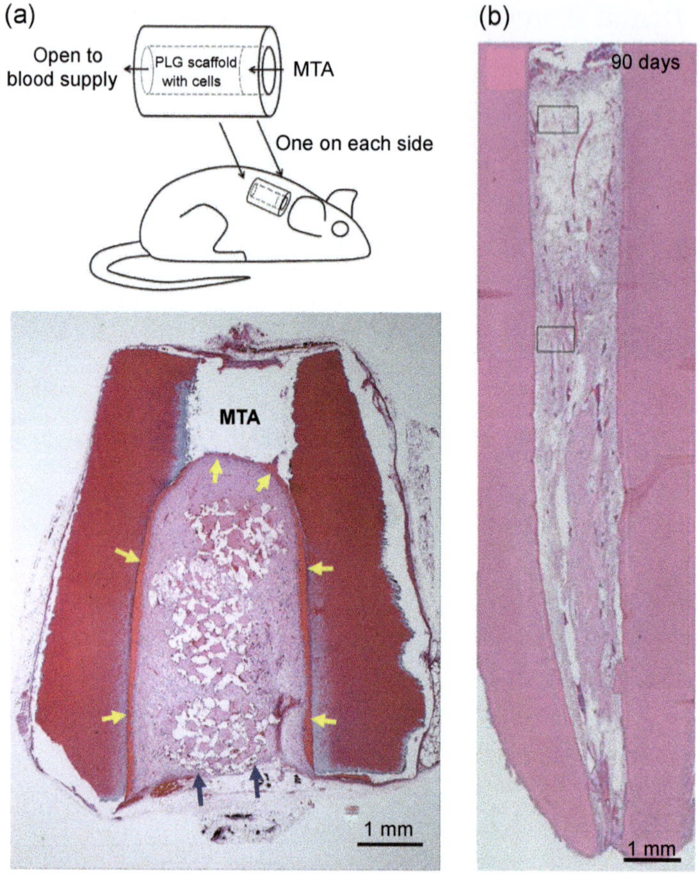

Figure 13.5 Complete pulp regeneration in animal models. (a) Top: Schematics of SCID mouse subcutaneous study model for human pulp–dentin regeneration. The canal space of human tooth root fragments (~6–7 mm long) was enlarged to ~1–2.5 mm in diameter. One end of the canal opening was sealed with MTA cement. SCID, severe combined immunodeficient; MTA, mineral trioxide aggregate. Bottom: Pulp–dentin regeneration using human stem cells from apical papilla (SCAP) seeded in polylactide glycolide (PLG) synthetic scaffolds The implanted tooth fragment containing SCAP/PLG was removed after 3 months in the subcutaneous space of SCID mice and processed for histological analysis. Blue *arrows* indicate the apex of the canal where the blood supply can enter; *yellow arrows* indicate the newly deposited dentinlike mineral tissue onto the canal dentinal wall and the MTA surface. *(Adapted from Huang GT. Pulp and dentin tissue engineering and regeneration: current progress. Regen Med 2009b;4(5):697–707, with permission.)* (b) Complete orthotopic regeneration of pulp tissue after autologous transplantation of $CD105^+$ cells with SDF-1 in the emptied root canal after pulpectomy in dogs showing histological image at 90 days after transplantation of pulp $CD105^+$ cells with SDF-1 (Stromal cell-derived factor 1). The regenerated pulp is vascularized and innervated and forms a layer of new dentinlike mineral onto the canal dentinal wall. *(Adapted from Iohara K, Imabayashi K, Ishizaka R, Watanabe A, Nabekura J, Ito M, et al. Complete pulp regeneration after pulpectomy by transplantation of CD105+ stem cells with stromal cell-derived factor-1. Tissue Eng Part A 2011;17(15–16):1911–20, with permission.)*

from PDL or periapical bone. When BMMSCs, PDLSCs, or DPSCs are transplanted into the subcutaneous space of immunocompromised mice, they form bone with marrowlike, cementum-/PDL-like, or dentin-pulp-like complexes, respectively (Gronthos et al., 2000; Seo et al., 2004). Besides DPSCs, SCAP can also form dentin-pulp-like complex (Sonoyama et al., 2006).

Local MSCs are normally committed to differentiate into tissue cells where they reside. PDLSCs in PDL differentiate into cementogenic or osteogenic cells, and MSCs in the periapical alveolar bone differentiate into osteoblasts (Chadipiralla et al., 2010). This commitment appears to be determined by the local microenvironment where specific signals are to guide such differentiation. When undifferentiated cells are displaced in a different microenvironment, they might be converted into other cell lineages. Huo et al. cultured dermal MSCs with conditioned medium of embryonic tooth germ cells and determined if these cells would differentiate into odontogenic lineage. They found that the capacity of dermal MSCs to form ectopic dentinlike mineral tissue in vivo is much weaker compared with DPSCs (Huo et al., 2010). Furthermore, no odontoblast marker DSP can be detected, suggesting that to guide nonodontogenic type of stem cells into odontogenic cells is difficult.

It is possible that such conversion from cementum- or bone-committed PDLSCs into odontoblastic cells may be difficult under natural condition. Perhaps, by artificially loading PDLSCs onto the decellularized pulp extracellular matrix, these cells may be converted into odontoblast markers (Ravindran et al., 2014). Similarly, transplanting $CD31^-$ SP from BMMSCs or AdMSCs into root canal space can regenerated pulplike tissues, similar to using $CD31^-$ SP from DPSCs (Ishizaka et al., 2012). The environment in the root canal space may provide signals to guide these cells toward generating pulplike tissues.

The treatment of root canal dentin wall may affect odontoblast differentiation from stem cells. Factors imbedded in dentin may play an important role in guiding the odontoblast differentiation, for example, TGF-β family and DMP-1 (Jussila et al., 2013; Qin et al., 2007). Using a tooth slice/SHED model for pulp regeneration, Casagrande et al. demonstrated that when the dentin wall surface was treated with 5.25% NaOCl for 5 days, which damaged the dentin proteins, no recognizable odontoblasts were observed along the dentin wall. In contrast, if the dentin wall was treated with 10% ethylenediaminetetraacetic acid (EDTA) for 1 min, which mobilizes dentin proteins, the regenerated pulp resembled natural pulp with well-aligned odontoblastlike cells along the dentin wall (Casagrande et al., 2010). Furthermore, they found that BMP2, and not BMP7, plays the key role in guiding SHED to become odontoblastlike cells expressing DSPP, DMP-1, and Matrix extracellular phosphoglycoprotein (MEPE) (Casagrande et al., 2010). In the pulp regeneration model, if the root canal space is treated with a combination of 17% EDTA for 10 min, 19% citric acid for 1 min (both for removing smear layers), and 5.25% NaOCl for 10–15 min, which resembles the clinical disinfection protocols, the odontoblast layer was able to form but was disorganized and inconsistent (Huang et al., 2010). Studies have shown reduced SCAP viability after seeding onto the 6% NaOCl-treated dentin (Trevino et al., 2011). To minimize the adverse effect, 5.25% NaOCl treatment followed by 17% EDTA rinse appears to salvage the condition (Galler et al., 2011). The use of 1.5% NaOCl followed by 17% EDTA treatment of dentin is more optimal in the case of regenerative approach (Martin et al., 2014).

13.3.2 Periodontal tissue regeneration

Non–cell-based periodontal regeneration therapy has been tested for many decades including the use of growth factors. However, the outcomes have been inconsistent leading to the popularity of extracting periodontally involved teeth, which are replaced with dental implants. Cell-based regenerative periodontal therapy has gained attention and has been investigated in animal models as well as in humans in attempts to regenerate complete periodontium, including PDL with well-oriented collagen fibers, alveolar bone, and cementum. In a dog model, autologous PDL cell sheets were fabricated using a temperature-responsive cell culture dish. The cell sheet with reinforced hyaluronic acid carrier was applied to the artificially created defect. Eight weeks after surgery, periodontal tissue healing with bone, PDL, and cementum formation was observed histologically (Akizuki et al., 2005). In a similar study using a dog model, three-layered sheets of PDL-derived cells supported with woven polyglycolic acid were transplanted autonomously to dental root surfaces with three-wall periodontal defects. Both new bone and cementum connected with well-oriented collagen fibers were observed 6 weeks after transplantation (Iwata et al., 2009). A minipig model was also used to demonstrate that periodontal defects may be repaired by applying autologous PDLSCs leading to regeneration of PDL, regaining the alveolar bone to a normal level (Fig. 13.6 top panel) (Liu et al., 2008).

Despite the promising results from large animal studies using cell-based periodontal therapies, minimal information is available regarding such therapies for humans. A human clinical case report has demonstrated that using ex vivo expanded autologous BMMSCs facilitated the repair of periodontal defects with reduction of pocket depths at 1-year recall (Yamada et al., 2006b). Three clinical cases of patients with periodontal bone loss were treated with PDL progenitors (PDLPs). Sixteen teeth with at least one deep intrabony defect of probing depth ≥6 mm received PDLP transplantation and the clinical outcomes were monitored for a duration of 32–72 months. There were no adverse effects, and significant pocket reduction and attachment gain were observed. This study demonstrated clinical potential efficacy and safety in utilizing autologous PDL cells for treatment of human periodontitis (Fig. 13.6 bottom panel) (Feng et al., 2010).

Another cell source for periodontal regeneration is DFSCs. Because DF is the precursor of PDL, the stem cells in the DF could potentially be a good source for periodontal regeneration. As mentioned, periodontal regeneration includes regeneration of cementum, PDL, and bone. Among the three types of tissues, PDL appears to be the most important tissue to regenerate because without regeneration of PDL, the adjacent cementum and bone are unlikely to establish a normal architecture with the root. In fact, without PDL, the root will become ankylose and may be replaced by bone. Studies of DFSC osteogenic differentiation (Honda et al., 2011; Mori et al., 2012; Viale-Bouroncle et al., 2011), however, are more reported than those of periodontal regeneration. Guo et al. reported the regeneration of complex periodontal tissues using heterogeneous dental follicle cells from human impacted molars. These cells express NOTCH-1, STRO-1, ALP, type I collagen, type III collagen, and osteocalcin even at passage 30. Cells at this passage were mixed with ceramic bovine bone and implanted into the dorsum of immunodeficient mice and the formation of a cementum–PDL complex was observed 6 weeks after implantation (Guo et al., 2012a).

Of note, PDL regeneration for avulsed teeth using cell sheet of PDLSCs plus platelet-rich fibrin granules was demonstrated in a dog model (Zhao et al., 2013), indicating that utilization of PDL regeneration technologies can improve the survival of teeth that normally have poor treatment outcome using currently existing clinical protocols.

13.3.3 Whole tooth regeneration

Although dental implants have become a practical and reliable solution to restore lost teeth, the lack of morphological and biological similarity of and integration into the natural dentition in the jaws calls for search for more advanced technology. Regeneration of teeth that are similar to natural ones in the edentulous regions appears to be the ultimate quest to restore the dentition. Several approaches either to regenerate a complete tooth or just a root have been tested and are summarized in the following sections.

13.3.3.1 Tooth regeneration using tooth germ cells

Forming a whole tooth requires the cells of both ectodermal and mesodermal origin, therefore obtaining cells from a tooth germ, which is made of two germ layers, to regenerate a whole tooth by re-creating organogenesis is certainly a logical approach. Earlier studies using cells isolated from tooth buds and seeded onto scaffolds followed by transplantation into an ectopic in vivo environment have shown the regeneration of toothlike structures (Duailibi et al., 2004; Nakao et al., 2007; Young et al., 2002). Orthotopic regeneration of engineered teeth have been shown in larger animal studies but lack functional restoration. In a dog model, bell-stage tooth bud cells seeded onto scaffolds and transplanted back to the original tooth sockets formed dentin structure, but there was no enamel or root formation (Honda et al., 2006). In a miniswine model, ex vivo expanded bell-stage tooth bud cells cultured onto cylinder-shaped scaffolds were autografted back to the original alveolar sockets. Tooth formation with root structures along with periodontium was observed (Kuo et al., 2008). However, there was no evidence of complete eruption into functional occlusion.

In a mouse model, a system was established to demonstrate fully functional bioengineered tooth replacement (Ikeda et al., 2009; Nakao et al., 2007; Oshima et al., 2011). The initial phase is a standard in vitro process that begins with separating cells from the ectodermal epithelial layer and mesodermal layer of the tooth germ and culturing them separately. They are then seeded onto a scaffold to allow reestablishing a bioengineered tooth germ, which is subsequently either implanted into an edentulous region in the jaw allowing natural development and eruption or implanted into the subrenal capsular space of the mice. The latter approach will form an ectopic "tooth unit" encompassing a whole tooth, PDL, and bone. This

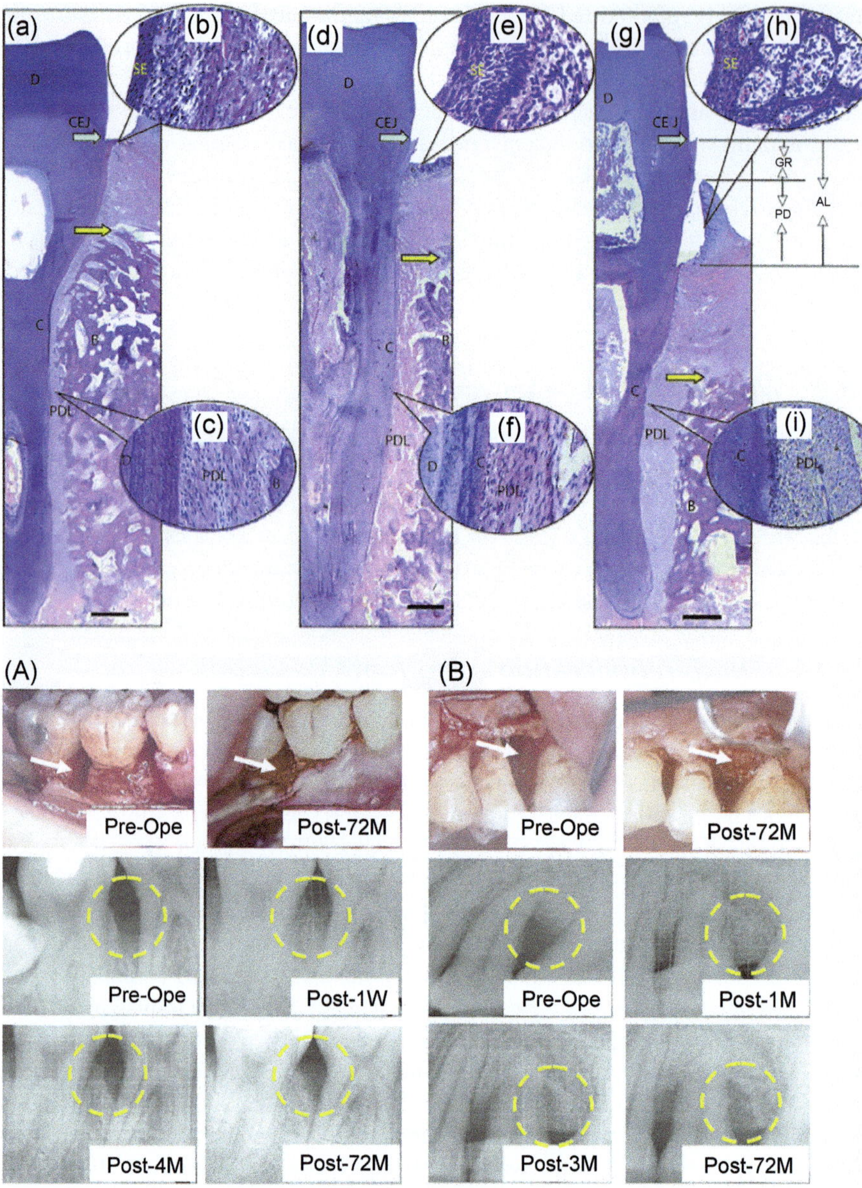

Figure 13.6 Periodontal tissue regeneration using periodontal ligament stem cells (PDLSCs) in a miniswine model and in humans. Top panel (miniswine): A buccal–lingual direction histopathological section showed junctional epithelia attached on the cementoenamel junction in normal periodontal tissues (a). The sulcular epithelium was thin and flat, and less infiltration of inflammatory cells could be observed in the connective tissues of the normal periodontal tissues (b). Sharpey fibers were a typical characteristic in the structure of normal periodontal tissues (c). Although the position of junctional epithelium was below the cementoenamel junction, the periodontal tissue regeneration in PDLSC-mediated group (d) was much better

tooth unit is then implanted into the alveolar bone; this process is similar to placing a dental implant (Fig. 13.7). Through either approaches, functional tooth can be regenerated with normal occlusion.

The aforementioned approaches require the presence of existing tooth germ. Another concept for tooth regeneration is to identify a way to reignite the early tooth forming signals in the gingival tissues to develop a whole teeth. Angelova Volponi et al. (2013) showed that epithelial cells derived from adult human gingival tissue are capable of responding to tooth-inducing signals from mouse embryonic tooth mesenchyme cells and form teeth. This finding suggests that the adult gingival epithelium

than that in the HA/TCP group. The sulcular epithelium in the PDLSC-mediated group was thicker, and the epithelial pegs and dermal papillae were short and blunt with less inflammatory cells in the PDLSC-mediated group (e), New bone, cememtum, and periodontal ligament were regenerated in the periodontal defect area in the PDLSC-mediated group (f), and the height of the new alveolar bone was much higher than that in the HA/TCP group (g), but still lower than the normal level (a). Histopathological photomicrography showed that plenty of new bone and periodontal tissues including cememtum and periodontal ligament were regenerated in the periodontal defective area, and the newly formed Sharpey fibers plugged into the newly regenerated cementum in the PDLSC-mediated group (f). Typical periodontitis including marked periodontal tissue reduction (GR, AL) and infiltration of inflammatory cells were still found in the HA/TCP group (g). The epithelial pegs and dermal papillae were long and slender with infiltration of inflammatory cells underlying connective tissue (h). Fibers lacking the typical structure of Sharpey fibers filled in the periodontal defect in the HA/TCP group (i). Scale bar: 1 mm. B, bone (*yellow arrow* showed the top of the new bone); *D*, dentin; *C*, cementum; *PDL*, periodontal ligament; *CEJ*, cemetoenamel junction (*blue arrows*; CEJ is covered by junctional epithelium in normal periodontal tissue); *SE*, sulcular epithelium; *GR*, gingival recession (the height from CEJ to the margin of gingival); *PD*, probing depth (the depth of periodontal pocket); *AL*, attachment loss (the length from CEJ to the bottom of the pocket; in this study, the bottom of the pocket was below the CEJ, so AL is equal to the GR plus PD). *(Adapted from Liu Y, Zheng Y, Ding G, Fang D, Zhang C, Bartold PM, et al. Periodontal ligament stem cell-mediated treatment for periodontitis in miniature swine. Stem Cells 2008:2007–0734, with permission.).* Bottom panel: Clinical evaluation of autologous PDLP-mediated treatment for periodontitis in humans. (A) Patient no. 1 showed periodontal tissue destruction at preoperation caused by periodontitis in tooth no. 30 (*arrow* in Pre-Ope). After 72 months of autologous PDLP implantation, surgical reentry to the implanted area showed periodontal tissue regeneration (*arrow* in Post-72M). X-ray analysis showed bone resorption at preoperation (*yellow circle* in Pre-Ope) and PDLP/carrier material implantation at 1 week postoperation (*yellow circle* in Post-1W), 4 months postoperation (*yellow circle* in Post-4M), and 72 months postoperation (*yellow circle* in Post-72M). (B) Patient no. 2 showed periodontal tissue destruction at preoperation caused by periodontitis in tooth no. 13 (*arrow* in Pre-Ope). After 72 months of autologous PDLP implantation, surgical reentry to the implanted area showed periodontal tissue regeneration (*arrow* in Post-72M). X-ray analysis showed bone resorption at preoperation (*yellow circle* in Pre-Ope) and PDLP/carrier material implantation at 1 month postoperation (*yellow circle* in Post-1M), 3 months postoperation (*yellow circle* in Post-3M), and 72 months postoperation (*yellow circle* in Post-72M). *M*, months; W, week. *(Adapted from Feng F, Akiyama K, Liu Y, Yamaza T, Wang TM, Chen JH, et al. Utility of PDL progenitors for in vivo tissue regeneration: a report of 3 cases. Oral Dis 2010;16(1):20–8, with permission.)*

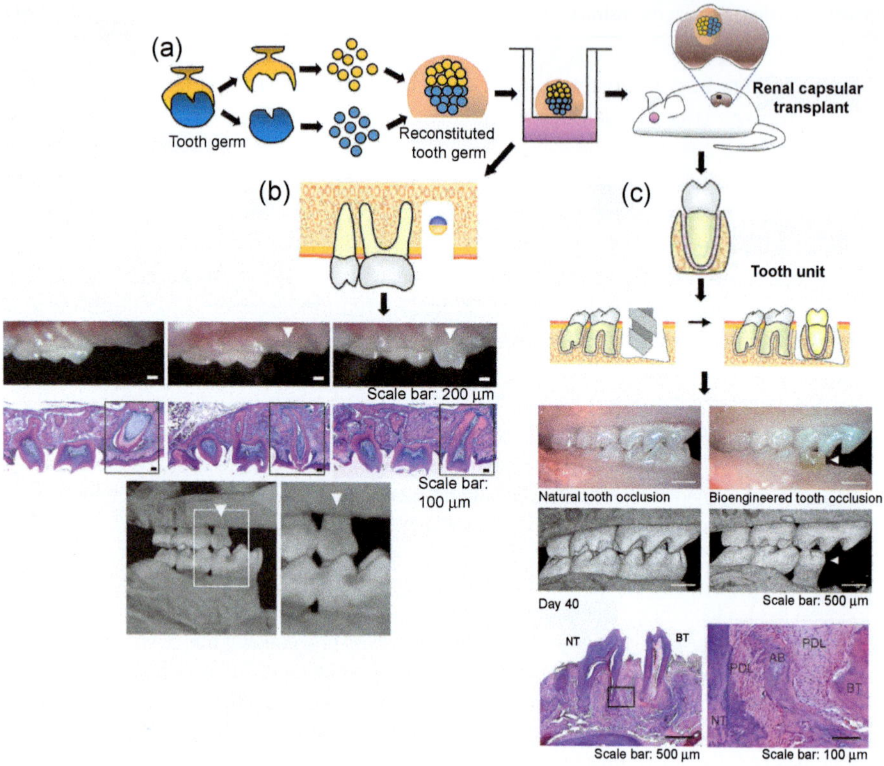

Figure 13.7 Bioengineering and regeneration of whole tooth in mouse model. (a) Schematic representation of the tooth bioengineering technology beginning with a tooth germ (cap stage) separated into epithelial and mesenchymal layers. Cells from the two layers are isolated, cultured, and reconstituted into tooth germ in collagen gel and maintained as organ culture for 5–7 days. Subsequently, the reconstituted tooth germ may undergo two different approaches to regenerated functional tooth. (b) Direct transplantation of the engineered tooth germ into a created socket of the edentulous region allowing the tooth to develop, erupt, and reach the occlusion. Oral photographs of a bioengineered tooth during eruption and occlusion processes, including before eruption (left), immediately after eruption (center), and full occlusion (right). Histological images showing the corresponding steps during the tooth eruption to full occlusion with normal tooth morphology and tissues including enamel, dentin, pulp and PDL. Micro–computed tomographic (CT) images (black and white) images of the occlusion of the bioengineered tooth. The bioengineered tooth is indicated by the *arrowhead*. (c) The engineered tooth germ is transplanted into the subrenal capsular space to allow the formation of a tooth unit encompassing the entire mature tooth plus surrounding bone. The tooth socket is created and the tooth unit is inserted. Oral photographs (upper) and micro-CT (lower) images showing occlusion of natural (left) and bioengineered teeth (right). Bottom images showing histological analysis of the engrafted bioengineered tooth unit at 40 days post transplantation was also performed. NT, natural tooth; BT, bioengineered tooth; AB, alveolar bone; PDL, periodontal ligament. Adapted from Ikeda E, Morita R, Nakao K, Ishida K, Nakamura T, Takano-Yamamoto T, et al. Fully functional bioengineered tooth replacement as an organ replacement therapy. Proc Natl Acad Sci USA 2009;106(32):13475–80; Oshima M, Mizuno M, Imamura A, Ogawa M, Yasukawa M, Yamazaki H, et al. Functional tooth regeneration using a bioengineered tooth unit as a mature organ replacement regenerative therapy. PLoS One 2011;6(7):e21531, with permission.

can be induced to regain the ability to interact with the underlying mesenchyme, leading to the formation of a regenerated tooth.

13.3.3.2 Bioroot engineering

Sonoyama et al. first demonstrated the generation of a bioroot in a miniswine model in which SCAP were loaded onto an HA/TCP scaffold made into a root form and PDLSCs were loaded onto gelfoam that encircled the HA/TCP root before being implanted into the socket of the lower jaw. A bioroot with PDL tissues was regenerated and restored to function by placing an artificial crown onto the bioroot (Sonoyama et al., 2006). The bioroot structure was composed of randomly deposited dentin by the SCAP with a layer of PDL. The research team subsequently utilized allogeneic DPSCs and PDLSCs to repeat the study, and they were able to obtain similar results with dentinlike structures and functional PDL-like tissues. There was mature alignment of the PDL fibers after the bioroot was restored into function (Wei et al., 2013).

13.3.3.3 Regeneration of root by dental follicle stem cells

Honda et al. isolated enamel organ epithelium, dental pulp, and dental follicle from the third molar of 6-month-old pigs. DFSCs were expanded from the DF in cultures. Then they loaded DFSCs into the bottom of an eppendorf tube, followed by successively loading dental pulp cells, enamel epithelial cells, and again DFSCs into the tube. This combination mimics the tooth primordia, which was then inserted into a cavity of the shaft of the bone, followed by transplanting into the omentum of immunodeficient rats. A tooth root–like structure containing dentin, pulp, cementum, and PDL-like tissue was observed (Honda et al., 2011).

In a rat model, DFCs seeded onto EDTA treated dentin matrix (TDM) and transplanted in alveolar fossa microenvironment can regenerate a bioroot containing pulp- and PDL-like tissues with odontoblast layer, new dentin, and cementum (Guo et al., 2009, 2012b; Yang et al., 2012). This root formation appears to require specific environment, because after transplantation in skull and omental pockets, it did not regenerate the rootlike structures (Guo et al., 2012b). These studies suggest that although DFSCs do not express odontoblast markers before and after cultivation in a standard medium for osteogenic differentiation, TDM can induce the differentiation of DFSCs into odontoblastlike cells (Guo et al., 2009).

13.4 Conclusions and prospects

Major advancement has taken place since the first DSCs, DPSCs, were isolated and reported in 2000 (Gronthos et al., 2000). These DSCs have been extensively studied to explore their potential for regeneration of dental or nondental tissues. For their natural capabilities to differentiate into odontogenic cell types, they have been tested to regenerate tooth and its adjacent structures— pulp, dentin, cementum, PDL, and bone. Such potential has promoted the clinical direction toward regeneration rather than artificial restoration. For example, regenerative endodontics aims to regenerate partial or complete pulp tissue in the canal space as well as form new dentin on the existing canal walls (Huang, 2011). Cell-based regenerative endodontics has reached the first phase of clinical trial (Nakashima and Iohara, 2014). Similarly, in regenerative periodontics, cell-based therapy has shown promising results in the large animal studies and a clinical trial was mounted (https://clinicaltrials.gov/ct2/show/NCT00221130); however, we are yet to see the published report. On the other hand, a cell therapy trial to enhance tooth socket bone healing to receive dental implants was reported, and it has been proved to be safe and effective (Kaigler et al., 2013). Whole tooth regeneration has yet to reach clinical trials. As for nondental tissue regeneration including neurogenesis and osteogenesis using DSCs, more research in the animal models is needed before they are ready for clinical trials. For neurogenesis, the problems lie in the complexity of neurogenesis and regeneration per se. As for bone regeneration, adipose tissue–derived MSCs and BMMSCs are been tested in clinical trials (Grayson et al., 2015). Clinical trials using DSCs for bone regeneration are yet to be performed.

Acknowledgments

The work was supported in part by grants from the National Institute of Dental and Craniofacial Research (NIH/NIDCR) R01DE019156 (GT.-J.H.).

References

Aanismaa R, Hautala J, Vuorinen A, Miettinen S, Narkilahti S. Human dental pulp stem cells differentiate into neural precursors but not into mature functional neurons. Stem Cell Discov 2012;2:85–91.

Abe S, Yamaguchi S, Amagasa T. Multilineage cells from apical pulp of human tooth with immature apex. Oral Sci Int 2007;4(1):45–58.

Akizuki T, Oda S, Komaki M, Tsuchioka H, Kawakatsu N, Kikuchi A, et al. Application of periodontal ligament cell sheet for periodontal regeneration: a pilot study in beagle dogs. J Periodontal Res 2005;40(3):245–51.

Al-Habib M, Yu Z, Huang GTJ. Small molecules affect human dental pulp stem cell properties via multiple signaling pathways. Stem Cells Dev 2013;22(17):2402–13.

Alongi DJ, Yamaza T, Song Y, Fouad AF, Romberg EE, Shi S, et al. Stem/progenitor cells from inflamed human dental pulp retain tissue regeneration potential. Regen Med 2010;5(4):617–31.

Angelova Volponi A, Kawasaki M, Sharpe PT. Adult human gingival epithelial cells as a source for whole-tooth bioengineering. J Dent Res 2013;92(4):329–34.

Arthur A, Rychkov G, Shi S, Koblar SA, Gronthos S. Adult human dental pulp stem cells differentiate toward functionally active neurons under appropriate environmental cues. Stem Cells 2008;26(7):1787–95.

Arthur A, Shi S, Zannettino AC, Fujii N, Gronthos S, Koblar SA. Implanted adult human dental pulp stem cells induce endogenous axon guidance. Stem Cells 2009;27(9):2229–37.

Atari M, Gil-Recio C, Fabregat M, García-Fernández D, Barajas M, Carrasco MA, et al. Dental pulp of the third molar: a new source of pluripotent-like stem cells. J Cell Sci 2012;125(14):3343–56.
Bianco P, Riminucci M, Gronthos S, Robey PG. Bone marrow stromal stem cells: nature, biology, and potential applications. Stem Cells 2001;19(3):180–92.
Bruder SP, Jaiswal N, Haynesworth SE. Growth kinetics, self-renewal, and the osteogenic potential of purified human mesenchymal stem cells during extensive subcultivation and following cryopreservation. J Cell Biochem 1997;64(2):278–94.
Buurma B, Gu K, Rutherford RB. Transplantation of human pulpal and gingival fibroblasts attached to synthetic scaffolds. Eur J Oral Sci 1999;107(4):282–9.
Caplan AI. Mesenchymal stem cells. J Orthop Res 1991;9(5):641–50.
Casagrande L, Demarco FF, Zhang Z, Araujo FB, Shi S, Nor JE. Dentin-derived BMP-2 and odontoblast differentiation. J Dent Res 2010;89(6):603–8.
Chadipiralla K, Yochim JM, Bahuleyan B, Huang CY, Garcia-Godoy F, Murray PE, et al. Osteogenic differentiation of stem cells derived from human periodontal ligaments and pulp of human exfoliated deciduous teeth. Cell Tissue Res 2010;340(2):323–33.
Chen SC, Marino V, Gronthos S, Bartold PM. Location of putative stem cells in human periodontal ligament. J Periodontal Res 2006;41(6):547–53.
Choi S, Cho TJ, Kwon SK, Lee G, Cho J. Chondrogenesis of periodontal ligament stem cells by transforming growth factor-beta3 and bone morphogenetic protein-6 in a normal healthy impacted third molar. Int J Oral Sci 2013;5(1):7–13.
Cohnheim J. Ueber entzündung und eiterung. Arch Path Anat Physiol Klin Med 1867;40(1).
Cyranoski D. Stem cells cruise to clinic. Nature 2013;494:413.
Degistirici O, Jaquiery C, Schonebeck B, Siemonsmeier J, Gotz W, Martin I, et al. Defining properties of neural crest-derived progenitor cells from the apex of human developing tooth. Tissue Eng Part A 2008;14(2):317–30.
Dokic J, Tomic S, Cerovic S, Todorovic V, Rudolf R, Colic M. Characterization and immunosuppressive properties of mesenchymal stem cells from periapical lesions. J Clin Periodontol 2012;39(9):807–16.
Duailibi MT, Duailibi SE, Young CS, Bartlett JD, Vacanti JP, Yelick PC. Bioengineered teeth from cultured rat tooth bud cells. J Dent Res 2004;83(7):523–8.
Feng F, Akiyama K, Liu Y, Yamaza T, Wang TM, Chen JH, et al. Utility of PDL progenitors for in vivo tissue regeneration: a report of 3 cases. Oral Dis 2010;16(1):20–8.
Friedenstein AJ, Gorskaja JF, Kulagina NN. Fibroblast precursors in normal and irradiated mouse hematopoietic organs. Exp Hematol 1976;4(5):267–74.
Galler KM, D'Souza RN, Federlin M, Cavender AC, Hartgerink JD, Hecker S, et al. Dentin conditioning codetermines cell fate in regenerative endodontics. J Endod 2011;37(11):1536–41.
Gandia C, Arminan A, Garcia-Verdugo JM, Lledo E, Ruiz A, Minana MD, et al. Human dental pulp stem cells improve left ventricular function, induce angiogenesis, and reduce infarct size in rats with acute myocardial infarction. Stem Cells 2008;26(3):638–45.
Gay I, Chen S, MacDougall M. Isolation and characterization of multipotent human periodontal ligament stem cells. Orthod Craniofacial Res 2007;10(3):149–60.
Gore A, Li Z, Fung HL, Young JE, Agarwal S, Antosiewicz-Bourget J, et al. Somatic coding mutations in human induced pluripotent stem cells. Nature 2011;471(7336):63–7.
Grayson WL, Bunnell BA, Martin E, Frazier T, Hung BP, Gimble JM. Stromal cells and stem cells in clinical bone regeneration. Nat Rev Endocrinol March 2015;11(3):140–50, http://dx.doi.org/10.1038/nrendo.2014.234. Epub 2015 January 6.
Gronthos S, Mankani M, Brahim J, Robey PG, Shi S. Postnatal human dental pulp stem cells (DPSCs) in vitro and in vivo. Proc Natl Acad Sci USA 2000;97(25):13625–30.

Gu K, Smoke RH, Rutherford RB. Expression of genes for bone morphogenetic proteins and receptors in human dental pulp. Arch Oral Biol 1996;41(10):919–23.
Guo W, He Y, Zhang X, Lu W, Wang C, Yu H, et al. The use of dentin matrix scaffold and dental follicle cells for dentin regeneration. Biomaterials 2009;30(35):6708–23.
Guo W, Chen L, Gong K, Ding B, Duan Y, Jin Y. Heterogeneous dental follicle cells and the regeneration of complex periodontal tissues. Tissue Eng Part A 2012a;18(5–6):459–70.
Guo W, Gong K, Shi H, Zhu G, He Y, Ding B, et al. Dental follicle cells and treated dentin matrix scaffold for tissue engineering the tooth root. Biomaterials 2012b;33(5):1291–302.
Han C, Yang Z, Zhou W, Jin F, Song Y, Wang Y, et al. Periapical follicle stem cell: a promising candidate for cementum/periodontal ligament regeneration and bio-root engineering. Stem Cells Dev 2010;19(9):1405–15.
Hiraga T, Ninomiya T, Hosoya A, Takahashi M, Nakamura H. Formation of bone-like mineralized matrix by periodontal ligament cells in vivo: a morphological study in rats. J Bone Min Metab 2009;27(2):149–57.
Honda MJ, Ohara T, Sumita Y, Ogaeri T, Kagami H, Ueda M. Preliminary study of tissue-engineered odontogenesis in the canine jaw. J Oral Maxillofac Surg 2006;64(2):283–9.
Honda MJ, Imaizumi M, Suzuki H, Ohshima S, Tsuchiya S, Satomura K. Stem cells isolated from human dental follicles have osteogenic potential. Oral Surg Oral Med Oral Pathol Oral Radiol Endod 2011;111(6):700–8.
Huang GT, Garcia-Godoy F. Missing concepts in de novo pulp regeneration. J Dent Res 2014;93(8):717–24.
Huang AHC, Snyder BR, Cheng PH, Chan AW. Putative dental pulp-derived stem/stromal cells promote proliferation and differentiation of endogenous neural cells in the Hippocampus of mice. Stem Cells 2008a;26(10):2654–63.
Huang GTJ, Sonoyama W, Liu Y, Liu H, Wang S, Shi S. The hidden treasure in apical papilla: the potential role in pulp/dentin regeneration and BioRoot engineering. J Endod 2008b;34(6):645–51.
Huang CY, Pelaez D, Dominguez-Bendala J, Garcia-Godoy F, Cheung HS. Plasticity of stem cells derived from adult periodontal ligament. Regen Med 2009a;4(6):809–21.
Huang GT, Gronthos S, Shi S. Mesenchymal stem cells derived from dental tissues vs. those from other sources: their biology and role in regenerative medicine. J Dent Res 2009b;88(9):792–806.
Huang GTJ, Yamaza T, Shea LD, Djouad F, Kuhn NZ, Tuan RS, et al. Stem/progenitor cell–mediated de novo regeneration of dental pulp with newly deposited continuous layer of dentin in an in vivo model. Tissue Eng Part A 2009c;16(2):605–15.
Huang GT-J, Yamaza T, Shea LD, Djouad F, Kuhn NZ, Tuan RS, et al. Stem/progenitor cell–mediated de novo regeneration of dental pulp with newly deposited continuous layer of dentin in an in vivo model. Tissue Eng Part A 2010;16(2):605–15.
Huang GT-J. Apexification: the beginning of its end. J Int Endo 2009a;42(10):855–66.
Huang GT. Pulp and dentin tissue engineering and regeneration: current progress. Regen Med 2009b;4(5):697–707.
Huang GT-J. Induced pluripotent stem cells—a new foundation in medicine. J Exp Clin Med 2010;2(5):202–17.
Huang GT. Dental pulp and dentin tissue engineering and regeneration: advancement and challenge. Front Biosci 2011;3:788–800.
Huo N, Tang L, Yang Z, Qian H, Wang Y, Han C, et al. Differentiation of dermal multipotent cells into odontogenic lineage induced by embryonic and neonatal tooth germ cell-conditioned medium. Stem Cells Dev 2010;19(1):93–104.
Ikeda E, Morita R, Nakao K, Ishida K, Nakamura T, Takano-Yamamoto T, et al. Fully functional bioengineered tooth replacement as an organ replacement therapy. Proc Natl Acad Sci USA 2009;106(32):13475–80.

Iohara K, Zheng L, Wake H, Ito M, Nabekura J, Wakita H, et al. A novel stem cell source for vasculogenesis in ischemia: subfraction of side population cells from dental pulp. Stem Cells 2008;26(9):2408–18.

Iohara K, Imabayashi K, Ishizaka R, Watanabe A, Nabekura J, Ito M, et al. Complete pulp regeneration after pulpectomy by transplantation of CD105+ stem cells with stromal cell-derived factor-1. Tissue Eng Part A 2011;17(15–16):1911–20.

Ishizaka R, Iohara K, Murakami M, Fukuta O, Nakashima M. Regeneration of dental pulp following pulpectomy by fractionated stem/progenitor cells from bone marrow and adipose tissue. Biomaterials 2012;33(7):2109–18.

Iwata T, Yamato M, Tsuchioka H, Takagi R, Mukobata S, Washio K, et al. Periodontal regeneration with multi-layered periodontal ligament-derived cell sheets in a canine model. Biomaterials 2009;30(14):2716–23.

Jo YY, Lee HJ, Kook SY, Choung HW, Park JY, Chung JH, et al. Isolation and characterization of postnatal stem cells from human dental tissues. Tissue Eng 2007;13(4):767–73.

Jussila M, Juuri E, Thesleff I. Tooth morphogenesis and renewal. 1st ed. Hoboken, New Jersey: Wiley-Blackwell; 2013.

Kaigler D, Pagni G, Park CH, Braun TM, Holman LA, Yi E, et al. Stem cell therapy for craniofacial bone regeneration: a randomized, controlled feasibility trial. Cell Transpl 2013;22(5):767–77.

Kato T, Hattori K, Deguchi T, Katsube Y, Matsumoto T, Ohgushi H, et al. Osteogenic potential of rat stromal cells derived from periodontal ligament. J Tissue Eng Regen Med 2011;5(10):798–805.

Kémoun P, Laurencin-Dalicieux S, Rue J, Farges J-C, Gennero I, Conte-Auriol F, et al. Human dental follicle cells acquire cementoblast features under stimulation by BMP-2/-7 and enamel matrix derivatives (EMD) in vitro. Cell Tissue Res 2007;329(2):283–94.

Kerkis I, Kerkis A, Dozortsev D, Stukart-Parsons GC, Gomes Massironi SM, Pereira LV, et al. Isolation and characterization of a population of immature dental pulp stem cells expressing OCT-4 and other embryonic stem cell markers. Cells Tissues Organs 2006;184(3–4):105–16.

Kobayashi Y, Okada Y, Itakura G, Iwai H, Nishimura S, Yasuda A, et al. Pre-evaluated safe human iPSC-derived neural stem cells promote functional recovery after spinal cord injury in common marmoset without tumorigenicity. PLoS One 2012;7(12):e52787.

Kuo T-F, Huang A-T, Chang H-H, Lin F-H, Chen S-T, Chen R-S, et al. Regeneration of dentin-pulp complex with cementum and periodontal ligament formation using dental bud cells in gelatin-chondroitin-hyaluronan tri-copolymer scaffold in swine. J Biomed Mater Res Part A September 2008 15;86(4):1062–8.

Liao J, Al Shahrani M, Al-Habib M, Tanaka T, Huang GT. Cells isolated from inflamed periapical tissue express mesenchymal stem cell markers and are highly osteogenic. J Endod 2011;37(9):1217–24.

Lin LM, Ricucci D, Huang GTJ. Regeneration of the dentine–pulp complex with revitalization/revascularization therapy: challenges and hopes. Int Endod J August 2014;47(8):713–24. http://dx.doi.org/10.1111/iej.12210. Epub 2013 December 11.

Lister R, Pelizzola M, Kida YS, Hawkins RD, Nery JR, Hon G, et al. Hotspots of aberrant epigenomic reprogramming in human induced pluripotent stem cells. Nature 2011;471(7336):68–73.

Liu Y, Zheng Y, Ding G, Fang D, Zhang C, Bartold PM, et al. Periodontal ligament stem cell-mediated treatment for periodontitis in miniature swine. Stem Cells 2008. pp. 2007–0734.

Lovelace TW, Henry MA, Hargreaves KM, Diogenes A. Evaluation of the delivery of mesenchymal stem cells into the root canal space of necrotic immature teeth after clinical regenerative endodontic procedure. J Endod 2011;37(2):133–8.

Maeda H, Wada N, Nakamuta H, Akamine A. Human periapical granulation tissue contains osteogenic cells. Cell Tissue Res 2004;315(2):203–8.

Martin DE, De Almeida JF, Henry MA, Khaing ZZ, Schmidt CE, Teixeira FB, et al. Concentration-dependent effect of sodium hypochlorite on stem cells of apical papilla survival and differentiation. J Endod 2014;40(1):51–5.

Marynka-Kalmani K, Treves S, Yafee M, Rachima H, Gafni Y, Cohen MA, et al. The lamina propria of adult human oral mucosa harbors a novel stem cell population. Stem Cells 2010;28(5):984–95.

McCulloch CA, Nemeth E, Lowenberg B, Melcher AH. Paravascular cells in endosteal spaces of alveolar bone contribute to periodontal ligament cell populations. Anat Rec 1987;219(3):233–42.

Miura M, Gronthos S, Zhao M, Lu B, Fisher LW, Robey PG, et al. SHED: stem cells from human exfoliated deciduous teeth. Proc Natl Acad Sci USA 2003;100(10):5807–12.

Miyoshi K, Tsuji D, Kudoh K, Satomura K, Muto T, Itoh K, et al. Generation of human induced pluripotent stem cells from oral mucosa. J Biosci Bioeng September 2010;110(3):345–50. http://dx.doi.org/10.1016/j.jbiosc.2010.03.004. Epub 2010 April 8.

Mooney DJ, Powell C, Piana J, Rutherford B. Engineering dental pulp-like tissue in vitro. Biotechnol Prog 1996;12(6):865–8.

Mori G, Ballini A, Carbone C, Oranger A, Brunetti G, Di Benedetto A, et al. Osteogenic differentiation of dental follicle stem cells. Int J Med Sci 2012;9(6):480–7.

Morsczeck C, Gotz W, Schierholz J, Zeilhofer F, Kuhn U, Mohl C, et al. Isolation of precursor cells (PCs) from human dental follicle of wisdom teeth. Matrix Biol 2005;24(2):155–65.

Morsczeck C, Schmalz G, Reichert T, Völlner F, Galler K, Driemel O. Somatic stem cells for regenerative dentistry. Clin Oral Investig 2008. [Epub ahead of print].

Morsczeck C, Huang GT-J, Shi S. Stem and progenitor cells of dental and gingival tissue origin. Stem Cells Craniofacial Dev Regen 2013;285.

Moshaverinia A, Chen C, Xu X, Akiyama K, Ansari S, Zadeh HH, et al. Bone regeneration potential of stem cells derived from periodontal ligament or gingival tissue sources encapsulated in RGD-modified alginate scaffold. Tissue Eng Part A February 2014;20(3-4):611–21. http://dx.doi.org/10.1089/ten.TEA.2013.0229. Epub 2013 November 6.

Murray PE, Garcia-Godoy F, Hargreaves KM. Regenerative endodontics: a review of current status and a call for action. J Endod 2007;33(4):377–90.

Myers WC, Fountain SB. Dental pulp regeneration aided by blood and blood substitutes after experimentally induced periapical infection. Oral Surg Oral Med Oral Pathol 1974;37(3):441–50.

Nakao K, Morita R, Saji Y, Ishida K, Tomita Y, Ogawa M, et al. The development of a bioengineered organ germ method. Nat Methods 2007;4(3):227–30.

Nakashima M, Huang GT-J. Pulp and dentin regeneration. In: Huang GT-J, Thesleff I, editors. Stem cells in craniofacial development and regeneration. Hoboken, New Jersey: Wiley-Blackwell; 2013. p. 461–84.

Nakashima M, Iohara K. Mobilized dental pulp stem cells for pulp regeneration: initiation of clinical trial. J Endod 2014;40(Suppl. 4):S26–32.

Oshima M, Mizuno M, Imamura A, Ogawa M, Yasukawa M, Yamazaki H, et al. Functional tooth regeneration using a bioengineered tooth unit as a mature organ replacement regenerative therapy. PLoS One 2011;6(7):e21531.

Ostby BN. The role of the blood clot in endodontic therapy. An experimental histologic study. Acta Odontol Scand 1961;19:324–53.

Park JC, Kim JM, Jung IH, Kim JC, Choi SH, Cho KS, Kim CS. Isolation and characterization of human periodontal ligament (pdl) stem cells (pdlscs) from the inflamed pdl tissue: In vitro and in vivo evaluations. J Clin Periodontol 2011;38(8):721–31.

Pelaez D, Huang CY, Cheung HS. Isolation of pluripotent neural crest-derived stem cells from adult human tissues by connexin-43 enrichment. Stem Cells Dev 2013;22(21):2906–14.
Pereira LO, Rubini MR, Silva JR, Oliveira DM, Silva ICR, Poças-Fonseca MJ, et al. Comparison of stem cell properties of cells isolated from normal and inflamed dental pulps. Int Endod J 2012;45(12):1080–90.
Peterson SE, Loring JF. Genomic instability in pluripotent stem cells: implications for clinical applications. J Biol Chem 2014;289(8):4578–84.
Pittenger MF, Mackay AM, Beck SC, Jaiswal RK, Douglas R, Mosca JD, et al. Multilineage potential of adult human mesenchymal stem cells. Science 1999;284(5411):143–7.
Qin C, D'Souza R, Feng JQ. Dentin matrix protein 1 (DMP1): new and important roles for biomineralization and phosphate homeostasis. J Dent Res 2007;86(12):1134–41.
Ravindran S, Zhang Y, Huang CC, George A. Odontogenic induction of dental stem cells by extracellular matrix-inspired three-dimensional scaffold. Tissue Eng Part A 2014;20(1–2):92–102.
Robey PG, Bianco P. The use of adult stem cells in rebuilding the human face. J Am Dent Assoc 2006;137(7):961–72.
Sakai VT, Zhang Z, Dong Z, Neiva KG, Machado MAAM, Shi S, et al. Shed differentiate into functional odontoblasts and endothelium. J Dent Res 2010;89(8):791–6.
Sakai K, Yamamoto A, Matsubara K, Nakamura S, Naruse M, Yamagata M, et al. Human dental pulp-derived stem cells promote locomotor recovery after complete transection of the rat spinal cord by multiple neuro-regenerative mechanisms. J Clin Invest 2012;122(1):80–90.
Schwartz SD, Hubschman JP, Heilwell G, Franco-Cardenas V, Pan CK, Ostrick RM, et al. Embryonic stem cell trials for macular degeneration: a preliminary report. Lancet 2012;379(9817):713–20.
Seo BM, Miura M, Gronthos S, Bartold PM, Batouli S, Brahim J, et al. Investigation of multipotent postnatal stem cells from human periodontal ligament. Lancet 2004;364(9429):149–55.
Seo BM, Sonoyama W, Yamaza T, Coppe C, Kikuiri T, Akiyama K, et al. SHED repair critical-size calvarial defects in mice. Oral Dis 2008;14:428–34.
Shi S, Gronthos S. Perivascular niche of postnatal mesenchymal stem cells in human bone marrow and dental pulp. J Bone Min Res 2003;18(4):696–704.
Shi S, Robey PG, Gronthos S. Comparison of human dental pulp and bone marrow stromal stem cells by cDNA microarray analysis. Bone 2001;29(6):532–9.
Singhatanadgit W, Donos N, Olsen I. Isolation and characterization of stem cell clones from adult human ligament. Tissue Eng Part A 2009;15(9):2625–36.
Sonoyama W, Liu Y, Fang D, Yamaza T, Seo B-M, Zhang C, et al. Mesenchymal stem cell-mediated functional tooth regeneration in swine. PLoS One 2006;1(1):e79.
Sonoyama W, Seo B-M, Yamaza T, Shi S. Human Hertwig's epithelial root sheath cells play crucial roles in cementum formation. J Dent Res 2007;86(7):594–9.
Sonoyama W, Liu Y, Yamaza T, Tuan RS, Wang S, Shi S, et al. Characterization of the apical papilla and its residing stem cells from human immature permanent teeth: a pilot study. J Endod 2008;34(2):166–71.
Sugiyama M, Iohara K, Wakita H, Hattori H, Ueda M, Matsushita K, et al. Dental pulp-derived $CD31^{-}/CD146^{-}$ side population stem/progenitor cells enhance recovery of focal cerebral ischemia in rats. Tissue Eng Part A 2011;17(9–10):1303–11.
Takahashi K, Yamanaka S. Induction of pluripotent stem cells from mouse embryonic and adult fibroblast cultures by defined factors. Cell 2006;126(4):663–76.
Takahashi K, Tanabe K, Ohnuki M, Narita M, Ichisaka T, Tomoda K, et al. Induction of pluripotent stem cells from adult human fibroblasts by defined factors. Cell 2007;131(5):861–72.

Tamaoki N, Takahashi K, Tanaka T, Ichisaka T, Aoki H, Takeda-Kawaguchi T, et al. Dental pulp cells for induced pluripotent stem cell banking. J Dent Res 2010;89(8):773–8.

Thomas HF. Root formation. Int J Dev Biol 1995;39(1):231–7.

Thomson JA, Itskovitz-Eldor J, Shapiro SS, Waknitz MA, Swiergiel JJ, Marshall VS, et al. Embryonic stem cell lines derived from human blastocysts. Science 1998;282(5391):1145–7.

Tour G, Wendel M, Moll G, Tcacencu I. Bone repair using periodontal ligament progenitor cell-seeded constructs. J Dent Res 2012;91(8):789–94.

Trevino EG, Patwardhan AN, Henry MA, Perry G, Dybdal-Hargreaves N, Hargreaves KM, et al. Effect of irrigants on the survival of human stem cells of the apical papilla in a platelet-rich plasma scaffold in human root tips. J Endod 2011;37(8):1109–15.

Trubiani O, Zalzal SF, Paganelli R, Marchisio M, Giancola R, Pizzicannella J, et al. Expression profile of the embryonic markers NANOG, OCT-4, SSEA-1, SSEA-4, and frizzled-9 receptor in human periodontal ligament mesenchymal stem cells. J Cell Physiol 2010;225(1):123–31.

Viale-Bouroncle S, Vollner F, Mohl C, Kupper K, Brockhoff G, Reichert TE, et al. Soft matrix supports osteogenic differentiation of human dental follicle cells. Biochem Biophys Res Commun 2011;410(3):587–92.

Völlner F, Ernst W, Driemel O, Morsczeck C. A two-step strategy for neuronal differentiation in vitro of human dental follicle cells. Differentiation 2009;77(5):433–41.

Wada N, Wang B, Lin NH, Laslett AL, Gronthos S, Bartold PM. Induced pluripotent stem cell lines derived from human gingival fibroblasts and periodontal ligament fibroblasts. J Periodontal Res 2011;46(4):438–47.

Wang J, Wang X, Sun Z, Yang H, Shi S, Wang S. Stem cells from human-exfoliated deciduous teeth can differentiate into dopaminergic neuron-like cells. Stem Cells Dev September 2010;19(9):1375–83. http://dx.doi.org/110.1089/scd.2009.0258.

Wang X, Thibodeau B, Trope M, Lin LM, Huang GT. Histologic characterization of regenerated tissues in canal space after the revitalization/revascularization procedure of immature dog teeth with apical periodontitis. J Endod 2010b;36(1):56–63.

Wei F, Song T, Ding G, Xu J, Liu Y, Liu D, et al. Functional tooth restoration by allogeneic mesenchymal stem cell-based bio-root regeneration in swine. Stem Cells Dev 2013;22(12):1752–62.

Wu J, Huang GT, He W, Wang P, Tong Z, Jia Q, et al. Basic fibroblast growth factor enhances stemness of human stem cells from the apical papilla. J Endod 2012;38(5):614–22.

Wu J, Jia Q, He W, Liu J, Hou L, Zhang J, et al. Conditioned medium from periapical follicle cells induces the odontogenic differentiation of stem cells from the apical papilla in vitro. J Endod 2013;39(8):1015–22.

Xu J, Wang W, Kapila Y, Lotz J, Kapila S. Multiple differentiation capacity of STRO-1+/CD146+ PDL mesenchymal progenitor cells. Stem Cells Dev 2009;18(3):487–96.

Yamada Y, Fujimoto A, Ito A, Yoshimi R, Ueda M. Cluster analysis and gene expression profiles: a cDNA microarray system-based comparison between human dental pulp stem cells (hDPSCs) and human mesenchymal stem cells (hMSCs) for tissue engineering cell therapy. Biomaterials 2006a;27(20):3766–81.

Yamada Y, Ueda M, Hibi H, Baba S. A novel approach to periodontal tissue regeneration with mesenchymal stem cells and platelet-rich plasma using tissue engineering technology: a clinical case report. Int J Periodontics Restorative Dent 2006b;26(4):363–9.

Yan X, Qin H, Qu C, Tuan RS, Shi S, Huang GT. iPS cells reprogrammed from human mesenchymal-like stem/progenitor cells of dental tissue origin. Stem Cells Dev 2010;19(4):469–80.

Yang B, Chen G, Li J, Zou Q, Xie D, Chen Y, et al. Tooth root regeneration using dental follicle cell sheets in combination with a dentin matrix - based scaffold. Biomaterials 2012;33(8):2449–61.

Young CS, Terada S, Vacanti JP, Honda M, Bartlett JD, Yelick PC. Tissue engineering of complex tooth structures on biodegradable polymer scaffolds. J Dent Res 2002;81(10):695–700.

Zhang W, Walboomers XF, Shi S, Fan M, Jansen JA. Multilineage differentiation potential of stem cells derived from human dental pulp after cryopreservation. Tissue Eng 2006;12(10):2813–23.

Zhao YH, Zhang M, Liu NX, Lv X, Zhang J, Chen FM, et al. The combined use of cell sheet fragments of periodontal ligament stem cells and platelet-rich fibrin granules for avulsed tooth reimplantation. Biomaterials 2013;34(22):5506–20.

Zou XY, Yang HY, Yu Z, Tan XB, Yan X, Huang GT. Establishment of transgene-free induced pluripotent stem cells reprogrammed from human stem cells of apical papilla for neural differentiation. Stem Cell Res Ther 2012;3(5):43.

Index

'*Note*: Page numbers followed by "f" indicate figures and "t" indicate tables.'

D

M

S